THE WOMAN'S BOOK OF YOGA AND HEALTH

THE WOMAN'S BOOK OF

Yoga and Health

A Lifelong Guide to Wellness

Linda Sparrowe

WITH YOGA SEQUENCES BY
Patricia Walden

FOREWORD BY
Judith Hanson Lasater, Ph.D., P.T.

PHOTOGRAPHY BY
David Martinez

Shambhala Boston & London 2002

Contents

Foreword by Judith Hanson Lasater   vii

Introduction   ix

How to Use This Book   xiii

PART ONE *Essential Yoga Sequences*   1

CHAPTER 1 The Woman's Essential Sequence   3

CHAPTER 2 The Woman's Energizing Sequence   25

CHAPTER 3 The Woman's Restorative Sequence   43

PART TWO *The Time of Awakening*   55

CHAPTER 4 Befriending Your Body   59

CHAPTER 5 Honoring Your Menstrual Cycle   88

CHAPTER 6 Supporting Your Immune System   118

PART THREE *Coming into Fullness*   133

CHAPTER 7 Preparing for Labor, Birth, and Postpartum   137

CHAPTER 8 Caring for Your Back   168

CHAPTER 9 Relieving Headaches   190

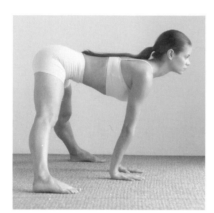

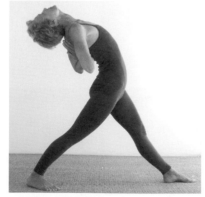

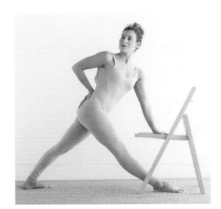

PART FOUR *Speaking the Truth*   207

CHAPTER 10 Working with Depression   211

CHAPTER 11 Easing into Menopause   233

CHAPTER 12 Improving Digestion   273

PART FIVE *Wisdom from the Heart*   295

CHAPTER 13 Minimizing Postmenopausal Symptoms   299

CHAPTER 14 Relieving Osteoporosis   322

CHAPTER 15 Strengthening Your Heart   340

Resources   353

Acknowledgments   358

Index   361

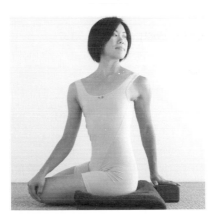

Shambhala Publications, Inc.
Horticultural Hall
300 Massachusetts Avenue
Boston, Massachusetts 02115
www.shambhala.com

9 8 7 6 5 4 3 2 1
Printed in Canada
∞ This edition is printed on acid-free paper that meets the
American National Standards Institute Z39.48 Standard.
Distributed in the United States by Random House, Inc.,
and in Canada by Random House of Canada Ltd

Interior design and composition: Greta D. Sibley & Associates

Library of Congress Cataloging-in-Publication Data
Sparrowe, Linda.
The woman's book of yoga and health : a lifelong guide to wellness /
Linda Sparrowe ; with yoga sequences by Patricia Walden ; foreword by
Judith Hanson Lasater ; photography by David Martinez.
p. cm.
Includes index.
ISBN 1-57062-470-4 (alk. paper)
1. Yoga. 2. Women—Health and hygiene. I. Walden, Patricia. II. Title.
RA781.7 .S645 2002
613.7'046'082—dc21
2002005561

Today more than ever, it's crucial that we include practices in our daily lives that promote health and spiritual growth. The state of the environment, the stresses created by the world's ever-increasing population's demand on dwindling resources, and political unrest are signposts of the critical state we face. If we want a world worth living in, and worth leaving to future generations, we need to take responsibility by creating well-being in our lives and by supporting others as they choose healthier lives. In other words, to transform the world, we first have to transform ourselves.

My personal journey with yoga began with a health challenge: when I was in my early twenties I suffered from arthritis. I was loath to take the daily barrage of pills prescribed to me and opted instead to try a yoga class offered where I worked. The results were transformative. Through careful experimentation with diet and daily yoga practice, my symptoms subsided within a couple of months. Needless to say, my dedication to practicing yoga was cemented by no longer being in pain. But I also found that I felt more alive, more open on all levels. Simply put, I was become healthier spiritually as well as physically. I feel very strongly that, while yoga may not cure all our symptoms, the regular practice of yoga can lead us home to ourselves, to our power and compassion, and therefore to greater mental and emotional health.

In fact, increasing research in the fields of health and well-being indicates that the stress-reducing effects of yoga practice, breathing techniques, and meditation are significant and powerful. But while many books have been written about the physical, emotional, and spiritual benefits of yoga, very few have focused on the special needs of women. This omission has been corrected by the publication of *The Woman's Book of Yoga and Health: A Lifelong Guide to Wellness*.

As modern women, we face the increasing stresses of work and family responsibilities, while living in a society of quick fixes, quick meals, and quick moments of family intimacy caught on the fly. We run faster and word harder, nurturing those around us and checking things off our "to do" list. But there remains in many of us a deep longing. We crave solace and comfort. We long for freedom—not the freedom *from* our lives, but the freedom we can find *within* our lives.

Yoga can help us to find this freedom, not only freedom from our aches and pains, but also from our fears, our agitation, and our sense of separateness. Yoga brings a feeling of connection—to ourselves and to the larger community of women. As we step onto our mat every day, we can be assured that other women are doing the same thing. Practicing then becomes both a personal and a universal exercise. By remembering our deep selves in the poses, we reaffirm our connection with the souls of women everywhere who are struggling to survive, to flourish, to give birth, and to raise their daughters to live with open hearts and clear minds.

As we bend and stretch in yoga class, we are training our bodies to be flexible and we learn to be adaptable as well. Adaptability is the greatest strength women carry through life—as we are suddenly thrust from childhood to womanhood through the mystery of menstruation, as we experience the miracle of pregnancy and birth, and when we inevitably transform again in the next stage of life as menses cease. Along the way we need to be flexible and adaptable as we embrace our new roles and watch our bodies change. The yoga practices in *The Woman's Book of Yoga and Health* celebrate these changes and offer us specific practices to understand and make peace with any difficulties we experience as we pass through the stages of life.

I urge you to pick up this book and commit to practicing. Do not let your doubts derail you. If nothing else, pick just one of the poses suggested by the authors and practice it every day. If you only have time for one pose, I suggest that be the Corpse Pose (Savasana), the pose of deep relaxation. Americans are sleep deprived and women suffer more than men. We are up early with the babies, car pools, meals to prepare, and jobs to get to. We are up late paying bills, folding laundry, and vegging out in front of the TV, seeking a few minutes of escape and respite from the unrelenting demands of our own standard of perfection. So practice the Corpse Pose instead; replenish your body by doing absolutely nothing for fifteen minutes every day. Even if you cannot take the time right now to practice other poses, this one is key.

It won't be long before you open the book again and add other practices. You will find that the authors, Linda Sparrowe and Patricia Walden, offer you a complete feast of yoga including, for example, poses for pregnancy and for menopause, as well as poses to bolster your immune system, to alleviate your headaches, to lighten your depression, and to ease your lower back. The pictures are artfully done and the text is instructive. But the key is you. Without your full participation, this remains a book on the shelf. You can bring these practices to life; they will help you from the first moment you try them.

So I challenge you to ask yourself, "What do I want in my life right now?" You may not have the power to change your life circumstances: an ailing parent, not as much money as you would like, a cranky teenager. But you do possess the power necessary to transform how you feel about these challenges. You can access this power and choose these feelings by using the techniques in this book.

Linda, Patricia, and I are just like you. We are women who struggle with our bodies and with our lives. We face the difficulties of relationships that do not work out and the challenges of those that do. In the midst of it all, we have found that the regular practice of yoga poses and breathing, with moments of quiet reflection, have become the foundation for our lives. We wish for you that your practice nurtures you as we have felt nurtured, and that as often as possible, you will join us on the mat for a practice that will liberate you into good health, strong energy, and a wholesome and deep connection with yourself and all other beings.

May we live like the lotus, at home in the muddy water.

—Judith Hanson Lasater, Ph.D., P.T.

Introduction

Yoga is everywhere these days, in health clubs, recreation centers, and specialized studios all over the country. Doctors recommend it for bad backs, prenatal exercise, and stress relief—and it works wonders. But yoga is much more than a prescription for what ails you; it's a lifelong companion. It originated in an age-old tradition from deep in the heart of ancient India, and it has only recently become popular as a means to support the Western way of life. The yoga we know—the postures we learn to alleviate PMS, calm jittery nerves, or bring more flexibility to aging joints—began as a way of teaching men to sit properly during meditation and developed into a way of purifying and strengthening their bodies for the rigors of such practice.

As yoga developed into a highly evolved combination of meditation practices and physical postures (some schools believe only eighty-four poses exist, others teach more than 200, and still others tout 900-plus), more and more women felt drawn to it. Unfortunately, the masculine emphasis on physical prowess and rigorous discipline continued to predominate and, as many of us in the 1970s and 1980s could attest, yoga became the vehicle by which we could attain enlightenment—or even a tight, buff body—but it was not seen as a means to heal ourselves.

So, how did yoga become a healing companion for women? Luckily women have a way of bringing out the feminine aspects of any recipient of their passions, and yoga proved no exception. Patricia explained it beautifully in a talk we gave together at the Women and Yoga conference (Kripalu, May 2000): "As more and more women became practitioners, they saw the need to make yoga uniquely their own. They midwifed a discipline that encouraged women to find their own truth, to discover the needs of their own bodies and their own minds. These yoginis worked toward creating a discipline that would help women shed society's destructive and inappropriate messages of the perfect body and the ideal woman (buxom, flat-bellied, submissive), and that allowed them to become strong and powerful, secure in their femininity, grace, and individuality."

These Western women—Angela Farmer, Felicity Green, Dona Holleman, Judith Hanson Lasater, Patricia Walden—received guidance from an Indian master, Dr. Geeta Iyengar, who also felt very strongly that women needed their own particular brand of yoga. Geeta, daughter of B. K. S. Iyengar, one of the fathers of American yoga, revolutionized the way many women practice yoga by emphasizing two things. First, she introduced restorative poses, modified versions of classic poses that often include some form of support, to bring a sense of calm and clarity to otherwise hectic lives. Second, she devised new ways of doing poses and put them in sequences that would enable women to honor their cycles, to practice according to what their bodies and minds needed at any given moment, and to reap the health benefits associated with becoming more integrated and balanced. Her sequences helped women go through the various stages of life gracefully and mindfully.

ix

This feminization of yoga has allowed both women and men a chance to get in touch with themselves on very deep levels. But Patricia and I believe that it has created something extra special for women. It gives us the vehicle to move through and honor each stage of life—from the early years of adolescence and young adulthood to the hectic times of childbearing and career development; from the midlife changes of perimenopause to the wisdom of our elder years. It shows us the deep, abiding connection between our cycles and the cycle of the universe; it allows us to silence the outside chatter, the shoulds and shouldn'ts of life, and to hear and respond to the sound of our own voices.

I wrote this book to show women how yoga can become this life-long companion that supports them at whatever stage they find themselves; to prove to them that it's never too late to start practicing. I asked Patricia to help me. Patricia's name is synonymous with American yoga, a discipline she has passionately embraced for more than twenty-five years. Her beautiful countenance graces many of the world's leading yoga videos, the most memorable being the *Yoga Journal* series of instructional tapes. She trains yoga teachers, leads workshops, teaches classes all over the world, and oversees the day-to-day operation of her own yoga studio outside of Boston, while still maintaining her own dedicated physical and spiritual practice. She's truly devoted to her teachers—B. K. S. Iyengar, his daughter Geeta, and his son Prashant—and counts both Geeta and fellow teacher Dona Holleman as two important female influences in her life.

The sequences Patricia has put together in these pages come from the Iyengar method of yoga. Even if you've just begun practicing, you have probably heard of this method, the most popular type of yoga in the West. Its teachers stress precise alignment and use myriad props to help those who are less flexible or less adept get the most advantage from the poses. Thousands of women have benefited from Patricia's yoga workshops on menstruation, depression, menopause, and post-menopause. Besides creating most of the sequences found in these pages, Patricia has shared her wisdom, gentle humor, and practical tips in every chapter.

Although I came to yoga in the early seventies, like Patricia did, in search of enlightenment, my path took a somewhat different turn. In graduate school, I devoted my time to studying the Vedas, the ancient scriptures of India; yoga philosophy; and the Sanskrit language. I had developed a strong meditation practice and a weekly yoga practice by the time I joined *Yoga Journal* as its managing editor in 1992. Besides my continuing affiliation with *Yoga Journal* as a contributing editor and writer, I also owned and served as the editorial director of *The Herb Quarterly*, the oldest publication dedicated to the healing power of plants. Along the way, I have been fortunate to learn from many wise and wonderful Western and Eastern herbal practitioners, which has allowed me to treat my family and myself with natural medicines for more than twenty years.

Patricia and I created this book to teach women of all ages to care for themselves physically, emotionally, and spiritually. We've organized the information loosely around four stages of a woman's life: the time of awakening (adolescence through the twenties); coming into fullness (the thirties and forties); speaking the truth (midlife from fifty through sixty-five); and wisdom from the heart (postmenopause and beyond). Within each stage, we begin by pointing out what there is to celebrate and then look at ways to deal with the more difficult realities we all face.

For example, even though adolescence is a difficult time for a young woman as she navigates the rough waters of puberty, filled with societal imperatives and peer pressures while she struggles to find her own voice, it is also a wondrous time of self-discovery, experimentation, and building relationships. In her thirties and forties, a woman fights to define her place in the world, establish long-term relationships, and give birth to children or new ideas; she also feels alive, in motion, full to the brim with possibilities as she builds a life for herself. The midlife years may be a confusing time of raging hormones, depleted sexual energies, and precarious body image, but these years also bring a woman more time to discover what she truly wants, more energy to speak out against injustice, more opportunities to speak her own truth. The wise older woman may fear the ravaging effects of osteoporosis and heart disease, but she is ready and willing to celebrate life in much the same way she did as a child; she combines the spirituality and intuitive nature of her preadolescent self with the wisdom and power that come from a lifetime of experience.

An ongoing yoga practice has a lot to offer no matter what stage of life you're in. Physically, it can help to improve your strength, flexibility, and balance, and to address specific problems such as PMS, back pain, hot flashes, or poor digestion. Yoga can also bring a spiritual and emotional element to your life. It requires that you focus exclusively on the present moment, which can help clear your mind and bring you a sense of peace. Patricia tells her students that daily practice can lift their spirits; give them a valuable energy boost; and provide the time they need for contemplation so they can make thoughtful, careful choices.

No matter how often you do yoga, you can't hope to prevent or heal your health problems without making other lifestyle changes. If you practice yoga, but continue to eat poorly, get very little sleep, or stay in abusive or stressful relationships (in either your personal or work life), chances are you'll continue to get sick. So, we've liberally sprinkled the book with advice about diet, simple herbal remedies, meditation techniques, and other methods of self-care. Remember, however, to talk with your doctor or holistic health care professional (preferably one who is familiar with yoga) before embarking on any new health and exercise program.

It probably won't take you long to discover several common threads among the conditions we all face as women. For example, poor posture causes far more problems than just lower back pain. And you'll be amazed by how just about everything you do affects your reproductive health.

Patricia and I truly believe women benefit as much from hearing each other's stories as they do from research, textbooks, and expert advice.

Thus, we've included anecdotes gathered from our own experiences and from the countless women we've met in classes, workshops, and conferences. We even put together a questionnaire asking women to describe how yoga has helped them physically, emotionally, or spiritually (or all three). Many women wrote back to share some amazingly personal tales and offer words of encouragement. In deference to those who asked that we not use their names, we've given pseudonyms to almost everyone. To further protect their anonymity, many of the examples are actually compilations of several women's stories.

Although much of the information you'll find in these pages is therapeutic in nature, Patricia and I urge you to resist the temptation to use this book merely as a prescription for what ails you. We obviously want you to reap the physical benefits yoga has to offer—from stretching and toning your muscles to helping you balance your immune system. We even encourage you to share what you've learned with the men in your life. After all, they could certainly benefit from the attention yoga poses bring to their sore backs, their low spirits, or their immune systems. But most important, we want yoga to become your companion for life—something that can sustain you when you're well, shore you up when you're depressed, and support you when you're sick. Yoga can teach you to love yourself from the inside out; that reminds you each time you step onto the yoga mat that you are already perfect exactly the way you are. We want you to take the lessons you learn on the mat and use them in other aspects of your life. Think of your yoga practice as a mirror to your soul, as a barometer by which to gauge your feelings, and as a prescription for healthy action. We can't promise that yoga will fix all your physical, mental, and spiritual ills, but if you make the commitment to a regular practice, we can promise that yoga will change your life.

How to Use This Book

USING THE SEQUENCES

To ensure that you remain balanced through the joys and challenges of each stage of life, Patricia has put together what we call The Woman's Essential Sequence. These twenty-six poses will take your body through its complete range of motion. They can help balance your endocrine and nervous systems; squeeze stale blood from your organs and flush them with fresh, oxygenated blood; and bring a renewed sense of calm, strength, and focus. They will also remind you to soften and relax your belly as you tone it, because—no matter what the fashion magazines preach—a tight, constricted belly serves no purpose other than to impede circulation.

If you feel healthy and generally fit, you can use The Woman's Essential Sequence as your daily yoga routine or alternate it with The Woman's Energizing Sequence and The Woman's Restorative Sequence. But if your energy feels depleted or if you are menstruating, pregnant, or suffering from any of the health problems we discuss in specific chapters, modify your practice with the appropriate poses and sequences provided in those chapters.

Although the book is divided into life stages, don't limit yourself to the chapters within your stage. Many women in their thirties and forties go through PMS and cramps every month and struggle with eating disorders. Teens and young women may suffer from headaches and backaches. And women of every age need help supporting their immune system from time to time. Browse through all the chapters and find what is applicable and useful for you.

Throughout the chapters, you'll see that we've not only given poses and sequences for each condition, we've listed their anticipated effects. Knowing why we chose a pose will help you create your own routine if you find some of our choices too difficult or too time-consuming. For example, knowing that opening your chest can help relieve deep-seated depression and that forward bends may exacerbate it, you may decide to do a series of gentle backbends and skip poses that involve bending over. When you're pregnant, if you know the focus of your practice should be making space for your baby, you'll choose poses with that principle in mind.

GETTING STARTED

The best way to approach your yoga practice is "open, empty, and bare." That means, come with an open mind, an empty stomach, and bare feet. An open mind allows you to hear what your body has to teach you—clearly and without judging. Yoga challenges you to accept what is, at this moment, while delighting in the changes that inevitably occur over time. Wait at least two to three hours after a large meal and one to two hours after a lighter one before you practice. An empty stomach ensures that you don't overtax your internal organs. Taking off your shoes and socks lets you feel the mat or floor beneath you and keeps you from slipping during standing poses. Your feet will love being active participants in your practice. You can, of course, have a pair of socks handy to wear during Corpse Pose (Savasana) to keep your feet warm.

FINDING TIME

If you can, make a commitment to practice at least a little bit every day. Some women find it easiest to choose a particular hour and stick to that; others must find time whenever they can. It's better to practice even a few minutes a day than to save up and have a two-hour routine only once a week. If you have difficulty finding enough time, begin by committing to three full practices a week, with minisessions in between.

CREATING SPACE

Choose a room where no one will interrupt you and nothing can distract you. You should have enough space around you to stretch out in all directions and an unencumbered wall for support. If you don't have adequate wall space, you can use the back of a closed door. Some women like to practice with instrumental music playing softly in the background, others need the comfort of silence. It's often easier to listen to your body and the rhythm of your breathing if you forgo distractions. Wear comfortable clothing that doesn't bind, ride up, or annoy you. Leotards or yoga clothes are nice, but shorts and a tank top or light sweats work just as well.

WHAT YOU'LL NEED

You'll notice in the photographs and pose descriptions that we use props to modify some of the postures. Although you can substitute items around the house for some of these aids (for example, a firm sofa cushion can work as a bolster), it's much better to make a commitment to have the real thing.

Have everything you need on hand before you begin. Unroll your sticky mat and place your props nearby but off your mat.

Sticky Mat

Invest in a good-quality sticky mat; I like the thicker ones the best. Although you can do yoga on your living room carpet, a sticky mat ensures that your feet won't slip out from under you when you're in a wide-angle stance such as Extended Triangle Pose. It also provides extra cushioning for seated and reclining poses.

Blankets

You will need blankets to support your back and neck in supine poses and your head and neck in inversions, as well as to raise your buttocks in seated poses to help keep your spine straight. Yoga blankets are finely woven wool or cotton, but any flat-weave, slightly stiff blanket will do. Two or three folded blankets can take the place of a bolster.

Bolsters

Yoga bolsters come in various shapes and sizes. They offer the support you need to stretch and relax in restorative poses. You'll want two firm, oblong bolsters, preferably with removable cotton coverings.

Straps

You use straps in seated or reclining poses to stretch your hamstrings and in restorative poses to avoid straining your muscles. You'll need one or two straps. Although you can use a bathrobe belt or a man's necktie for some poses, a real yoga belt with a buckle is better.

Blocks

You can use blocks in myriad ways: to help you balance, to support your hands or head if you can't reach the floor, or to provide a sitting base so you can elongate your spine. Wooden or lighter-weight Styrofoam blocks are available in yoga stores.

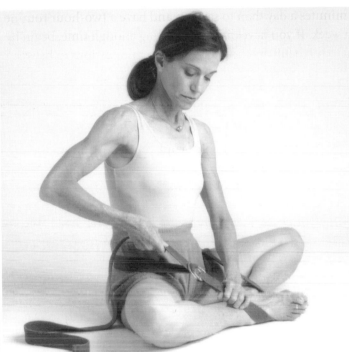

Slide the belt's end through the buckle, and keeping the strap a loose loop, slip it over your head and bring it around your back at the sacrum (below the waist). Loop it under feet so that it stretches over your ankles and rests on the tops of your thighs. Then cinch the belt securely.

Chair

Certain twisting poses, backbends, and modified inversions—such as Shoulderstand (Sarvangasana) and Half-Plough Pose (Ardha Halasana)—call for a chair. This should preferably be a metal folding chair with an open back rest so you can slide your legs through it comfortably and still have something to hold on to. A wooden kitchen chair works, too. Just make sure it is sturdy enough to hold you and can't slip out from under you. When you use a chair, be sure to place it on your sticky mat.

Eye Pillows and Weighted Sandbags

Eye pillows, or eyebags, block out external distractions and help you relax more fully. They are available in a variety of colors and come scented or unscented. Weighted sandbags (generally 10 pounds) apply pressure to specific areas of the body.

GETTING INTO AND OUT OF POSTURES

How you move into and out of a yoga pose is as important as being in the pose itself. Your first concern is your safety and comfort. Move slowly, keeping your eyes open, as you go into and release from the pose. Do standing poses—most of which begin with Mountain Pose (Tadasana) on one side first, press through your legs to come up, and then slowly reverse sides, before returning to your starting position. From standing or seated forward bends, come up slowly. Once you're fully upright, lift your head. To get out of reclining poses, always roll to one side, take a breath or two on your side, and then carefully push yourself up with your hands. After Headstand (Sirsasana), you should rest in Child's Pose (Adho Mukha Virasana) with your forehead touching the mat for a few breaths. This helps you to adjust after being upside down. Sit up slowly, stacking each vertebra on top of the next and lifting your head up last.

Many of the poses give instructions about inhaling and exhaling; most often, you rise up on the inhalation and bend or move on the exhalation. Don't worry too much about whether you're breathing properly. When in doubt, just breathe through your nose (with your mouth closed) as naturally and smoothly as you can.

BODY LANGUAGE AND WARNING SIGNS

Because we created this book to be for every woman, we may have included poses you've never done before or some you think may be much too hard for you. Before you dismiss them, however, try the modifications and variations we've provided. You'll notice we've indicated poses that should be skipped or modified due to health reasons or ability by placing a dagger next to the pose name and an explanatory footnote beneath its description.

Don't do more than your body can handle. You'll learn to distinguish between pain and intensity, but the cardinal rule is: If it hurts, stop! If you feel exhausted, rest for a few moments or modify the pose. Your breath serves as a reliable barometer. If you're working beyond your comfort zone, your breathing will become labored, erratic, or shallow. Ease up a little, modify the pose or substitute another one, or just skip the pose entirely.

Remember, don't get discouraged. Just because you can't do a specific pose one day doesn't mean it's out of reach forever. Even if you exercise regularly, your body may not be used to moving in certain ways. Be patient and listen to what your body and your breath are telling you. You don't practice to be perfect; you practice to feel better.

ROUND BODY TIPS

No one body type is necessary to practice yoga and benefit from it. If you are heavyset, follow Genia Pauli Haddon's tips for round-bodied practitioners:

- Seated forward bends. Keep your knees spread a little wider than instructed so you can accommodate your breasts and your belly comfortably when you bend. Rest your forehead on a folded blanket if you have trouble reaching the floor.

- Seated twisting poses. If necessary, widen your knees to accommodate your belly comfortably.

- Inversions. You should avoid poses such as Headstand (Sirsasana), Shoulderstand (Sarvangasana), and Plough Pose (Halasana), because there is a high risk of spinal injury if you lose your balance. Cultivate balance first through Mountain Pose (Tadasana) and other standing poses, which you can do with your back against a wall until you become proficient. Use props whenever appropriate to compensate for tight joints or an expansive belly. You can also substitute Downward-Facing Dog Pose (Adho Mukha Svanasana) for Headstand (Sirsasana) and Legs-Up-the-Wall Pose (Viparita Karani) for Shoulderstand (Sarvangasana) to get many of the same benefits.

A BASIC ANATOMY LESSON

As you read through the chapters and follow the instructions for the poses, you will run across various terms for bones, muscles, and other parts of the body that may be unfamiliar. The figures provided illustrate the terms we discuss often throughout the book. Detailed illustrations for specific areas, such as the endocrine and reproductive systems and the spine, are found in the chapters devoted to them.

THE SKELETON

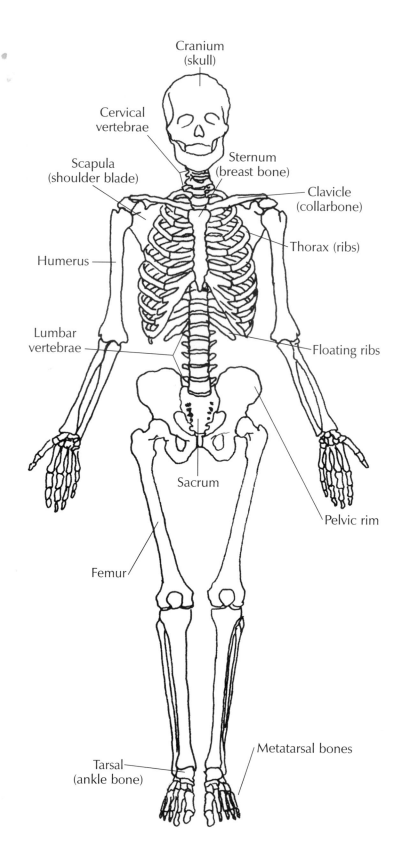

Cranium (skull)

Cervical vertebrae

Sternum (breast bone)

Scapula (shoulder blade)

Clavicle (collarbone)

Thorax (ribs)

Humerus

Lumbar vertebrae

Floating ribs

Sacrum

Pelvic rim

Femur

Metatarsal bones

Tarsal (ankle bone)

MUSCLES AND OTHER PARTS OF THE BODY YOU'LL NEED TO KNOW

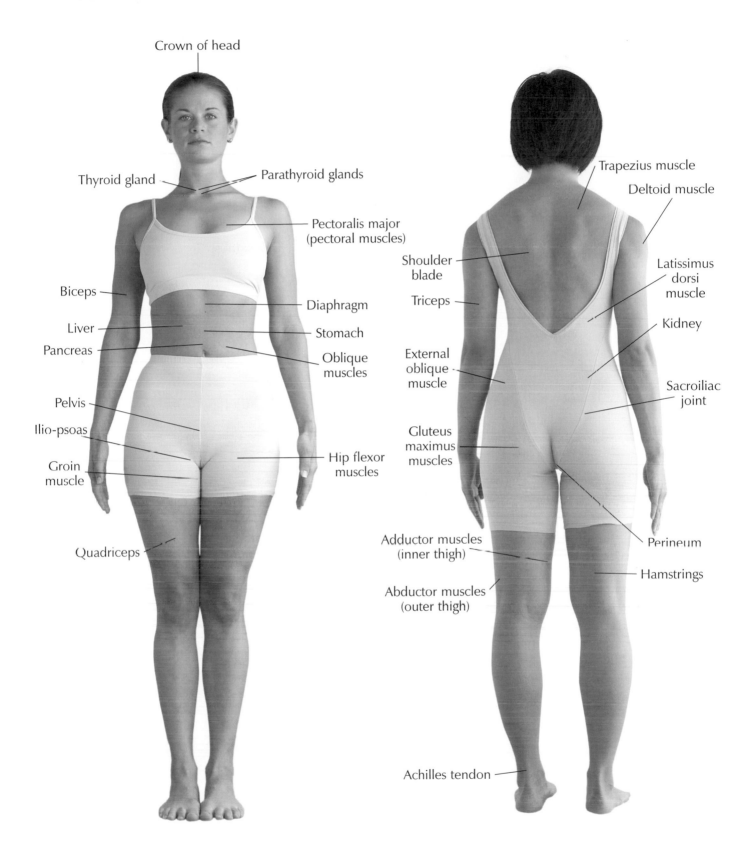

Crown of head

Thyroid gland

Parathyroid glands

Pectoralis major
(pectoral muscles)

Biceps

Diaphragm

Liver

Stomach

Pancreas

Oblique
muscles

Pelvis

Ilio-psoas

Groin
muscle

Hip flexor
muscles

Quadriceps

Trapezius muscle

Deltoid muscle

Shoulder
blade

Latissimus
dorsi
muscle

Triceps

Kidney

External
oblique
muscle

Sacroiliac
joint

Gluteus
maximus
muscles

Adductor muscles
(inner thigh)

Perineum

Abductor muscles
(outer thigh)

Hamstrings

Achilles tendon

PART ONE

Essential Yoga Sequences

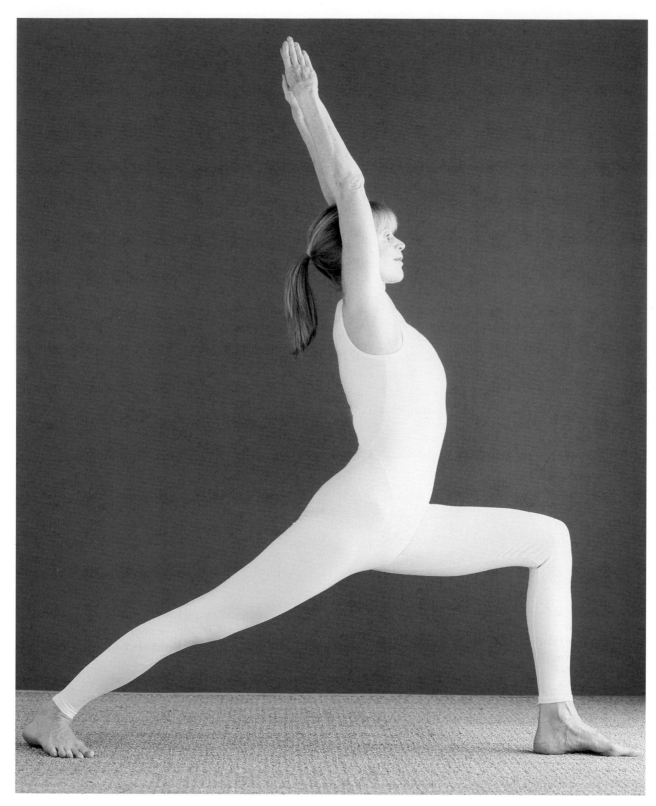

Warrior I Pose (Virabhadrasana I)

Chapter 1 — *The Woman's Essential Sequence*

by Patricia Walden

THE POSES

1. Bound Angle Pose (Baddha Konasana)
2. Wide-Angle Seated Pose I
   (Upavistha Konasana I)
3. Mountain Pose (Tadasana)
4. Mountain Pose with Arms Overhead
   (Urdhva Hastasana in Tadasana)
5. Extended Triangle Pose
   (Utthita Trikonasana)
6. Warrior II Pose (Virabhadrasana II)
7. Extended Side-Angle Pose
   (Utthita Parsvakonasana)
8 Half-Moon Pose (Ardha Chandrasana)
9. Standing Forward Bend (Uttanasana)
10. Warrior I Pose (Virabhadrasana I)
11. Revolved Triangle Pose
    (Parivrtta Trikonasana)
12. Intense Side Stretch Pose
    (Parsvottanasana)
13. Wide-Angle Standing Forward Bend
    (Prasarita Padottanasana)
14. Hero Pose with Cow-Face Arms
    (Virasana with Gomukhasana Arms)
15. Simple Seated Twist Pose
    (Bharadvajasana)
16. Spinal Twist Pose (Marichyasana III)
17. Head-on-Knee Pose (Janu Sirsasana)
18. Seated Forward Bend
    (Paschimottanasana)
19. Downward-Facing Dog Pose
    (Adho Mukha Svanasana)
20. Headstand (Sirsasana)
21. Child's Pose (Adho Mukha Virasana)
22. Shoulderstand (Sarvangasana)
23. Plough Pose (Halasana)
24. Bridge Pose
    (Setu Bandha Sarvangasana)
25. Legs-Up-the-Wall Pose
    (Viparita Karani) and Cycle
26. Corpse Pose (Savasana)

I DESIGNED THE WOMAN'S ESSENTIAL SEQUENCE TO PUT YOUR body through its full range of motion—using forward bends and backbends, inversions and twists.† The first two poses particularly benefit older women; younger women may skip them and begin with Mountain Pose (Tadasana). For full benefits, do this sequence at least three times a week.

As you practice, learn to distinguish between muscular discomfort and pain. Newcomers to yoga may feel sore for a day or two. However, if the soreness persists—or if you experience pain at any time—ease up, do the suggested modifications, or seek guidance from an experienced yoga teacher.

This sequence is preventive in nature and I've created it to support your endocrine, nervous, digestive, and reproductive systems so you'll stay healthy and strong. But don't forget that a conscious and consistent yoga practice is as much internal as it is external. Creating a balanced and healthy body allows your mind and heart to open more readily to the joyful possibilities of life. Yoga is a vehicle for experiencing deeper and deeper levels of self-awareness.

†CAUTION Don't do unsupported backbends if you suffer from heart problems or other serious illnesses, or if you are menstruating or pregnant. Avoid inversions if you are menstruating or have a headache. If you have knee, back, or neck problems, seek help from an experienced teacher.

1. BOUND ANGLE POSE (Baddha Konasana) Sit with your back straight and your abdomen lifted. Bending your legs, open your knees out and bring the soles of your feet together. Hold the tops of your feet and draw your heels in toward your perineum or pubic bone. The outer edges of your feet should remain on the floor. Lengthen your spine upward, leading with the crown of your head. Stretching your inner thighs from groin to knee, gently lower your knees as far as possible. Place your hands on the floor behind you to sit up straighter, and lift your abdomen. Stay in this position for 30 seconds, breathing normally. (If you are menstruating or your hips are tight and you can't lengthen your spine, sit against the wall on a block or blanket about 4 inches thick.) To come out, relax your arms and bring your knees up one at a time. Stretch your legs out in front of you.

EFFECTS This is a wonderful pose for women of all ages. It tones your kidneys; strengthens your bladder and uterus; and eases menstrual disorders, such as cramps, heavy bleeding, heaviness in your abdomen, and PMS or perimenopausal symptoms.

2. WIDE-ANGLE SEATED POSE I (Upavistha Konasana I) Sit in the middle of your sticky mat and spread your legs wide apart; flex your feet. Adjust the flesh of your buttocks by drawing it behind you and out to the sides. (If you find it hard to sit up straight in this position, sit on two or more blankets or a block positioned against the wall.) Place your hands on the floor behind you, draw your abdomen and floating ribs up toward your chest, and move your shoulder blades into your back. Sit up tall, pressing down through your legs and extend up through your spine. Hold the pose for 30 to 60 seconds. To come out, relax your arms and release your legs.

EFFECTS This pose improves circulation in and around your and pelvic area, stimulates your ovaries, and helps lift and tone your uterus.

3. MOUNTAIN POSE (Tadasana)

Stand up straight, your legs together (with big toes touching, if that's comfortable). Distribute your weight evenly between the front of your feet and your heels. Tighten your knees by pulling up with your quadricep (front thigh) muscles. Raise your sternum (breastbone) and broaden your chest by rolling your shoulders back and drawing your shoulder blades in. Lift your abdomen up and draw your tail-bone in without pushing your thighs forward. Extend your arms downward with palms facing your thighs and fingers together. Keep your shoulders moving away from your ears. It is normal to have some curvature in your lumbar area (lower back). Stand in this posture for 20 to 30 seconds—or longer—breathing normally and keeping your face, neck, and throat relaxed.

EFFECTS This pose strengthens and tones your whole body, keeps your mind alert, and helps create balance. Standing in this pose (especially against a wall) is a wonderful way to notice and correct postural problems.

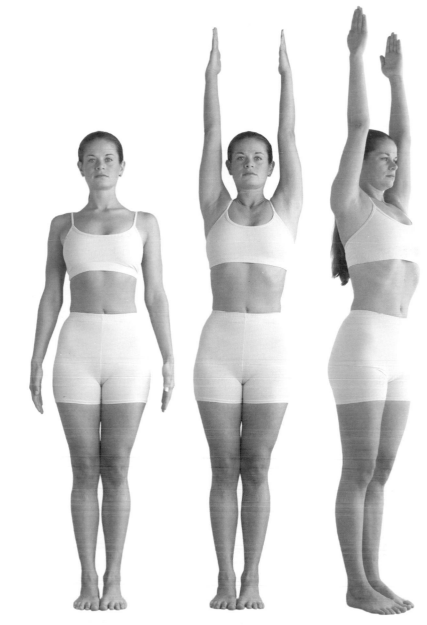

4. MOUNTAIN POSE WITH ARMS OVERHEAD (Urdhva Hastasana in Tadasana)

Stand in Mountain Pose (Tadasana). Turn your palms outward and slowly lift your arms to the side and over your head, keeping your shoulders down and away from your ears. Lift your chest and draw your shoulder blades deep into your back. Breathe normally and stay in this position for 15 to 20 seconds. To come out, release your arms down to your sides.

EFFECTS This pose awakens your whole body, toning your arms, legs, feet, and ankles. It also helps alleviate stiffness in your shoulders, arms, and upper and lower back, and improves circulation throughout your body.

5. EXTENDED TRIANGLE POSE (Utthita Trikonasana) Stand in Mountain Pose (Tadasana). Step your feet about 3½ feet apart; turn your left foot out 90 degrees and your right foot slightly inward. The heel of your left foot should line up with the arch of your right. (Place a block beside the outside edge of your left foot if you need to.) Stretch your arms out to the sides, draw up through your quadriceps, and lift your abdomen and chest. On an exhalation, keeping your back straight, extend your trunk to the left and bring your left hand down to the floor or the block. Press your hand into the floor or block, stretch across your chest and up through your right arm. Draw your shoulder blades in, turn your chest toward the ceiling, and look straight ahead or up at your right hand. Turn your abdomen to the right. Breathe normally and hold this pose for 20 to 30 seconds. On an inhalation, lift up and straighten your torso. Repeat the pose on your right side, then turn your toes forward and step your feet back toward each other, returning to Mountain Pose.

EFFECTS This pose elongates and strengthens your spine, brings flexibility to your back muscles, increases circulation to your pelvic region, and tones and improves functioning of your reproductive and digestive organs. It also calms your mind and relieves anxiety and nervous tension.

Modification

6

6. WARRIOR II POSE (Virabhadrasana II)
Stand in Mountain Pose (Tadasana). Step your feet as far apart as is comfortable (about 4½ feet); turn your left foot out 90 degrees and your right foot slightly inward. The heel of your left foot should line up with the arch of your right. Stretch your arms out to the sides so they're parallel to the floor. As you exhale, bend your left knee so your thigh is parallel and your shin is perpendicular to the floor. (If your knee extends beyond your ankle, you need to widen your stance.) Turn your head to look over your right arm just past your fingertips. Imagine both arms are engaged in a tug-of-war. Hold this pose for about 20 to 30 seconds, if possible. To come out of the pose, straighten your left leg as you inhale and turn your feet so they're parallel to each other. Repeat the pose on the other side.

EFFECTS This pose promotes stability, strength, and balance. It opens your chest, improves respiration and circulation, and helps alleviate depression and fatigue. It is also good for strengthening your legs and abdominal region.

7. EXTENDED SIDE-ANGLE POSE (Utthita Parsvakonasana) Stand in
Mountain Pose (Tadasana). Step your feet out as wide as possible
(about 4½ feet apart, if you can); turn your left foot out 90 degrees
and your right foot slightly inward. The heel of your left foot should
line up with the arch of your right. Stretch your arms out to the sides
so they are parallel to the floor. As you exhale, bend your left knee so
your thigh is parallel and your shin perpendicular to the floor. (If your
knee extends beyond your ankle, you need to widen your stance.)
Keeping your back straight, exhale and extend your trunk to the left,
bring your left hand down to the floor (or a block), and stretch your
right arm up over your right ear. Draw your shoulder blades in, turn
your chest toward the ceiling, and look straight ahead or up toward
the ceiling. Turn your abdomen to the right. Breathe normally and
hold this pose for 20 to 30 seconds, if possible. Inhale as you lift up,
come to standing, and straighten your torso. Repeat the pose on your
right side, then turn your toes forward and step your feet back to
Mountain Pose.

EFFECTS This pose elongates and strengthens your spine, brings
flexibility to your back muscles, increases circulation to your pelvic
region, and tones and improves functioning of your digestive and
reproductive organs. It also calms your mind; relieves anxiety
and nervous tension; and helps relieve pain from sciatica
and joint stiffness, particularly in your hips, groin, and
hamstring muscles (behind your knees).

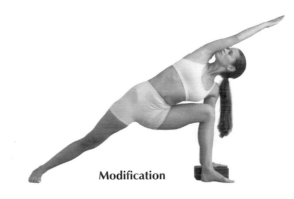

Modification

8. HALF-MOON POSE (Ardha Chandrasana)

Do Extended Triangle Pose (Utthita Trikonasana) to the left (see page 6). Bending your left leg so your knee extends beyond your ankle, place the fingertips of your left hand on the floor (or a block) about a foot in front of your left leg. Raise your right heel off the floor and come up onto your toes. With an exhalation, simultaneously straighten your left leg and raise your right up until it is parallel to the floor (or slightly higher). Turn your pelvic area and chest toward the ceiling. Stretch your right arm up in line with your shoulders and open your chest and pelvis more. Draw your shoulder blades into your back and expand your chest. Look up at your right hand or straight ahead. Hold this position for 10 to 15 seconds, breathing normally.

To come down, bend your left leg, while reaching your right leg back. Return to Extended Triangle Pose. Inhale, lift up to standing, repeat the pose on the other side, and return to Mountain Pose.

EFFECTS This pose helps slow heavy bleeding and it's excellent for countering symptoms of fatigue, PMS, depression, and morning sickness. It allows your belly to stay soft, while opening your chest, improving respiration and increasing circulation to your chest and pelvis.

Modification

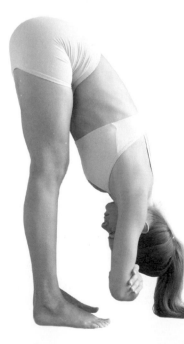

9. STANDING FORWARD BEND (Uttanasana)

Stand in Mountain Pose (Tadasana). Balance the weight evenly between your feet, lengthen up through your inner thighs, and roll your thighs in. Keep your legs and knees firm as you lift your arms overhead, stretching up through your waist and ribs. Fold your arms and cup your elbows with your hands. As you exhale, bend forward from your hips with straight legs, and release your side body down. Continue to hold your elbows and release your spine. Breathe normally for 30 to 60 seconds. To come out, release your arms, keep your legs active, and lift up slowly. Your head should come up last.

EFFECTS This pose brings a sense of peace when you feel agitated or anxious. It relieves a jittery stomach, lifts and tones your uterus, and improves circulation to your pelvic area. It can be effective in helping to lower high blood pressure by relieving mental and physical tension.

10. WARRIOR I POSE (Virabhadrasana I) Stand in Mountain Pose (Tadasana). Step your feet as far apart as possible (about 4½ feet) with your toes pointing forward. Stretch your arms out to the sides, turn your palms up, and raise both arms until they are in line with your ears and parallel to each other; your elbows should be straight. Draw up through your quadriceps and lift your abdomen and chest. As you exhale, simultaneously turn your torso and left leg 90 degrees to the left and your right foot about 60 degrees to the left. Inhale and stretch through your upper arms; exhale and bend your left knee so your thigh and shin form a right angle. (If your knee extends beyond your ankle, widen your stance.) Put your palms together if you can do so without bending your elbows or collapsing your chest. Stretch your torso up toward the ceiling as you look up at your hands or straight ahead. Hold this pose for 10 to 15 seconds, breathing evenly.

To come out of the pose, release your arms out to the sides and straighten your knee. Return to center and repeat on the other side. Then step your feet together and return to Mountain Pose.

EFFECTS This pose is excellent for stability, strength, balance, and flexibility. Women feel powerful and strong in this pose. It's great for relieving joint stiffness in older women.

11. REVOLVED TRIANGLE POSE (Parivrtta Trikonasana) Stand in Mountain Pose (Tadasana). Step your feet about 3 to 3½ feet apart; turn your right foot out 90 degrees and your left foot slightly inward. The heel of your right foot should line up with the arch of your left. (Place a block parallel to the outside edge of the right foot if you need to.) As you exhale, rotate your torso so you are facing right; your left leg and knee should turn inward. Place the fingertips of your left hand on either the floor next to the outside of your right foot or on a block. Tighten both legs and keep your chest expanded by drawing your left shoulder blade into your back. Extend your right arm up, turn your head, and look up. (If you have trouble balancing, keep your right hand on your hip as you expand your chest and look straight ahead.) Breathe normally for 10 to 15 seconds. Come up on an inhalation by raising your left hand off the floor. Repeat the pose on the other side and return to Mountain Pose.

EFFECTS This pose increases the blood flow to your abdomen, pelvis, and legs. It strengthens your body, bringing stability and flexibility to your bones and muscles. Because of the twisting action, this pose also tones your kidneys, liver, and spleen.

Modification

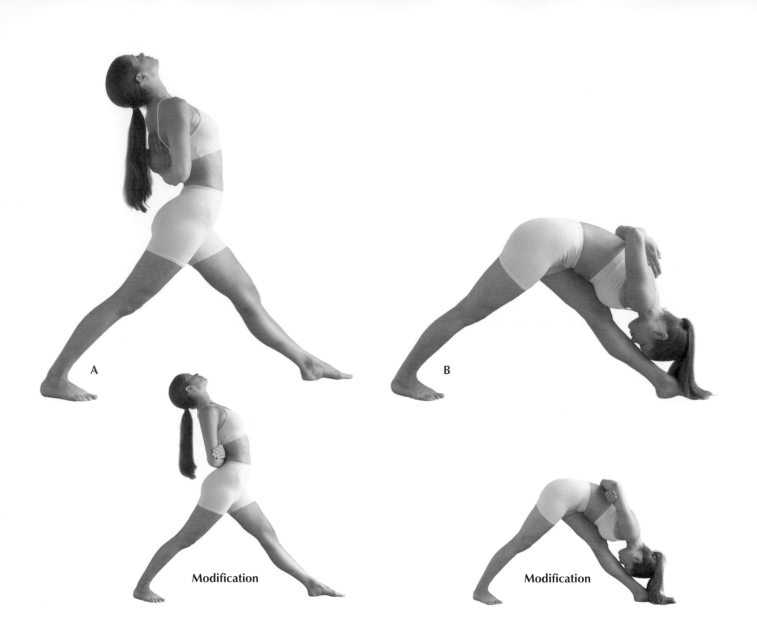

A

B

Modification

Modification

12. INTENSE SIDE STRETCH POSE (Parsvottanasana)

Stand in Mountain Pose (Tadasana). Put your palms together behind your back with your fingertips toward the floor. Rotate your wrists so your fingertips point toward the ceiling and your hands are in prayer position. Move your joined hands up to just between your shoulder blades, or as far as you can. (If this is too difficult, simply fold your arms behind your back, fingertips touching your elbows, if possible.) Roll your shoulders back and press your palms together to open your chest and broaden your shoulders. Raise your sternum. Step your feet about 3 to 3½ feet apart, so your weight is distributed equally between your legs. Turn your left foot 90 degrees and your right foot about 75 degrees to the left. Turn your torso to face the left, arching your back slightly and looking up toward the ceiling (if that is comfortable). Stay in this position for a full breath or two (A). As you exhale, lift

your head up, extend your spine, and bend forward so your head rests below your left knee (B). Keep both legs straight throughout the pose. Remain like this for 15 to 20 seconds, breathing normally. (If you have trouble balancing, put your hands on the floor or rest them on your leg below the knee.) Lift your head and torso as you inhale as you return to a standing position. Look up and arch your back slightly before releasing your arms. Now turn your right foot 90 degrees and your left foot about 75 degrees to the right, and repeat the pose on the other side before returning to Mountain Pose.

EFFECTS This pose is especially good for stiffness in your neck, shoulders, elbows, and wrists and for helping ease the pain of arthritis, scoliosis, and kyphosis. It also tones your abdomen, calms your mind, and helps relieve anxiety and nervous tension.

13. WIDE-ANGLE STANDING FORWARD BEND

(Prasarita Padottanasana) Step your feet apart about 4 feet (or as wide as possible), keeping the outer edges of your feet parallel. Tighten your quadriceps to draw your kneecaps up and keep your thighs well lifted. On an exhalation, bend forward from your hips and place your hands on the floor—in line with your shoulders—between your feet. (If you feel strain in your lower back, place your hands on blocks.) Lift your hips toward the ceiling, draw your shoulder blades into your back, and extend your chest forward (A). Look up and extend your trunk forward, keeping your entire spine concave. Remain this way for 10 to 15 seconds.

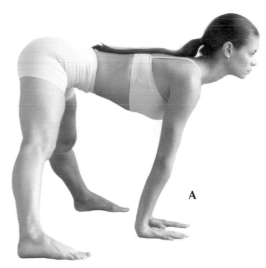

Keeping your trunk extended, exhale, bend your elbows, and release the crown of your head toward the floor—resting it on the floor, if possible (B). Keep your legs firm, but relax your shoulders and neck. Breathe deeply and let your trunk release downward. Stay in this pose for 1 minute, if possible. To come out, return to the concave back position, bring your hands to your hips, and raise your trunk. Step your feet together.

EFFECTS The effects of this pose are similar to those of Standing Forward Bend (Uttanasana). Besides increasing flexibility in your hamstrings, it combats fatigue, calms anxious or jittery nerves, lifts and tones your uterus, and improves circulation in your pelvic area. It helps ease heavy bleeding and a feeling of heaviness during menstruation, and it can be effective in helping to lower high blood pressure by relieving mental and physical tension. It may also be effective for most headaches.

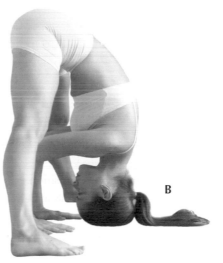

14. HERO POSE† WITH COW-FACE ARMS (Virasana with Gomukhasana Arms)

Kneel on the floor with your knees together, your feet pointing straight back, and your calves slightly wider than hip-width apart. Sit between your feet on the floor (or on a block or bolster if you feel any pressure on your knees). Put your left arm behind you and stretch the forearm up your back as far as you can, with the back of your hand against your back. Reach your right arm over your head, bend it at the elbow, and reach down your back toward your left hand. Grasp the fingers of both hands together (or lower a strap in your right hand if your hands won't meet). Keep your right elbow pointing toward the ceiling and your head up. Roll your shoulders back and open your chest. Breathe normally and hold this pose for 30 seconds to 1 minute. Repeat the arm position on the other side.

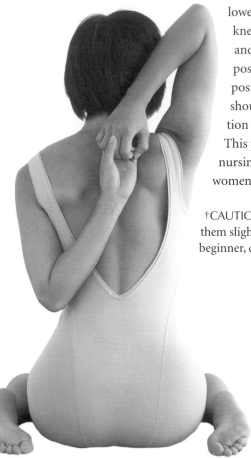

EFFECTS Sitting this way stretches the muscles of your lower body, particularly your calves, quadriceps, knees, and feet, bringing flexibility to those muscles and joints. It is a wonderful way to practice good posture and improve circulation to your pelvis. The positioning of your arms opens your chest and shoulder area, improving respiration and circulation and helping alleviate depression and fatigue. This pose is very beneficial to pregnant women and nursing mothers, as well as peri- and postmenopausal women who suffer from joint stiffness and arthritis.

†CAUTION If you feel any strain in your knees, separate them slightly and sit on a bolster or block. If you are a beginner, don't stay in this pose longer than 1 minute.

15. SIMPLE SEATED TWIST POSE† (Bharadvajasana) Sit up straight with your legs stretched out in front of you. Bend both legs to the left so your feet are next to your left hip. Keeping your thighs and knees facing forward, make sure your left ankle rests on the arch of your right foot and that your buttocks are on the floor, not on your foot. Draw your shoulder blades into your back, broaden your chest, and extend your spine upward. On an exhalation, turn your abdomen, ribs, chest, and shoulders (in that order) to the right; place your left hand on the outside of your right thigh and your right hand on the floor behind you (or on a block). Take several breaths, holding the posture for 20 to 30 seconds. Relax your face, neck, and throat. Come back to the center position, straighten your legs, and change sides.

EFFECTS This pose keeps your spine and hips flexible and your back pain-free, while releasing tension in your neck and shoulders. The gentle twist massages your reproductive organs, energizes your adrenal glands, and tones your kidneys. It also helps firm your waist and tone your abdominal region.

†CAUTION Do not practice twists if you have diarrhea or feel nauseous. Do not do this pose if you have arthritis in your knees. If you suffer from sacroiliac pain, release your pelvis whenever you twist.

16. SPINAL TWIST POSE (Marichyasana III) Sit with your legs stretched out in front of you. Bend your right leg up, with your foot resting flat on the floor near your perineum and your calf tight against your thigh. Keep your left leg outstretched and active. Take a deep breath. As you exhale, extend your spine and rotate your torso toward your right leg, so that your abdomen is close to your thigh. Place your right hand on the floor (or a block) behind you, several inches away from your buttocks; open your chest. Raise your left arm and bend your elbow, placing the outside of the elbow on the outside of your right knee. Your fingertips should point toward the ceiling. Turn your head to look over your left shoulder. Hold the pose, breathing normally, for 10 to 20 seconds. Release your head, arms, and legs, and sit with your legs outstretched before repeating on the other side.

EFFECTS This pose brings flexibility to your spine; tones and strengthens your abdominals; and rejuvenates your liver, kidneys, and spleen. Done gently, it opens your chest—improving respiration and circulation and helping alleviate depression and fatigue—and increases mobility in your shoulders and upper back.

17. HEAD-ON-KNEE POSE† (Janu Sirsasana) Sit on the floor with your legs stretched out in front of you. Bend your right knee to the side so it is at a 45-degree angle to your left leg and your right heel is near the right side of your groin. Push your right knee as far back as you comfortably can; keep your left leg straight.

Turn your abdomen and chest so your sternum is in line with the center of your left leg. With an exhalation, bend forward from your hips and catch the sides of your left foot with your hands; keep your head and back lifted (A). (If this is difficult to do without bending your left knee, use a strap looped around the ball of your foot.) Inhale and lift your trunk up from the base of your pelvic area. Remain like this for 15 to 20 seconds, if possible.

As you exhale, bend your elbows, draw your trunk forward, and rest your head on your left knee, without straining (B). (If you can't reach your head to your knee, stretch as far as you can along your leg and hold on to your knee, shin, or ankle. Release your head toward your leg.) Stay in this pose for 30 seconds, resting your head, the base of your skull, your eyes, and your mind. To come out, lift your head and torso slightly, release your hands, and sit up. Straighten your right leg, and repeat the pose on the other side.

EFFECTS This pose counteracts the effects of stress on the body and mind and relieves stiffness in the hips. In addition, because of its twisting action, it has a toning and activating effect on your liver, spleen, kidneys, and reproductive organs.

†CAUTION Do not do this pose if you have diarrhea.

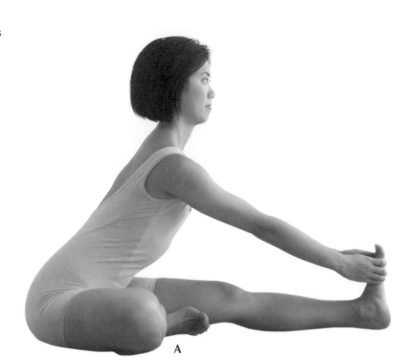

A

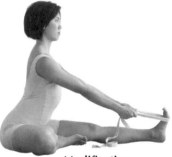

Modification

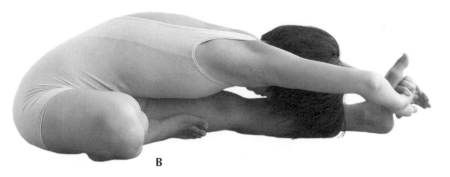

B

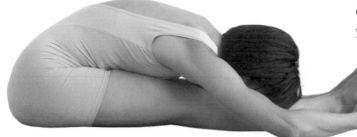

18. SEATED FORWARD BEND† (Paschimottanasana)

Sit on your mat or on one or two folded blankets with your legs stretched out in front of you. Take a full, deep breath; as you exhale, bend forward and extend your arms beyond your feet, clasping your wrist, if you can. On an inhalation, stretch up through your spine and lift your sternum and head, keeping your back slightly concave. Exhale and extend your torso over your legs; rest your head just beyond your knees, if you can. Do not allow your buttocks to come off the floor. Stay in this pose for 20 to 30 seconds, then slowly return to an upright position.

EFFECTS This pose is beneficial for women who suffer from high blood pressure, the free-floating anxiety of PMS or perimenopause, or bad menstrual cramps. Geeta Iyengar says it is good for the digestive system because it massages and strengthens your abdominal organs and tones your kidneys and liver. It helps instill a sense of safety and peace.

†CAUTION Do not do this pose if you have diarrhea or feel nauseous.

19. DOWNWARD-FACING DOG POSE (Adho Mukha Svanasana)
To find the correct distance between your hands and feet for this pose, lie facedown. Place your palms on the floor by each side of your chest with your fingers well spread and pointing straight ahead. Come up on your hands and knees, and turn your toes under.

Exhale, press your hands firmly into the mat and extend up through your inner arms. Exhale again as you raise your buttocks high in the air and move your thighs up and back. Keep stretching through your legs and bring your heels toward the floor. Keep the legs firm and the elbows straight as you lift your buttocks upward. The action of the arms and legs serves to elongate your spine and release your head. Hold this pose for 30 seconds to

1 minute, breathing deeply. Let your head rest completely and release the base of your neck. To come out, either return to your hands and knees and sit back on your heels or step your feet forward into Standing Forward Bend (Uttanasana) and slowly stand up.

EFFECTS This pose increases the blood supply to your brain and offers many of the same benefits as Headstand (Sirsasana) if you don't do that pose as part of your practice. This is a wonderful pose to combat depression because it helps increase circulation to your chest and calms your mind, especially when you support your head with blankets or a bolster.

20. HEADSTAND† (Sirsasana) Place a folded blanket against the wall. Kneel in front of it with your feet and knees together. Interlace your fingers firmly, thumbs touching and hands cupped. Position your hands no more than 3 inches from the wall with your elbows no wider than shoulder-width apart and your wrists perpendicular to the floor. Your wrists, forearms, and elbows form the foundation for this pose.

Lengthen your neck and place the crown of your head on the blanket. The back of your head should be in contact with your hands. Press your forearms into the floor and lift your shoulders away from the floor. Maintain this action throughout the pose. Straighten your legs, raise your hips toward the ceiling, and walk your feet in until your spine is almost perpendicular to the floor. As you exhale, lift one leg at a time, and bring your feet to the wall. (Or you can bend both legs at once, bring your knees to your chest, lift your toes off the floor, and slowly move your knees up toward the ceiling. Then stretch your legs straight up.)

Keep your heels and buttocks against the wall. Roll your thighs in, lift your tailbone, lengthen your legs upward, and keep your feet together. Remember to balance on the crown of your head, support yourself by pressing your forearms into the floor, and continue to lift your shoulders away from your ears. Keep your breathing even, your eyes and throat soft, and your abdomen relaxed. With regular practice, you can slowly learn to bring your buttocks and heels away from the wall. Hold the pose as long as you can, up to 5 minutes.

To come out, exhale, bend your knees, and bring your feet to the floor one at a time. Rest for a few breaths before raising your head. Move away from the wall, stretch your arms out in front of you, and rest in Child's Pose (Adho Mukha Virasana), described next.

EFFECTS Like all inversions, this pose balances your neuroendocrine system. In particular, it stimulates the blood flow to your brain, activates your pituitary gland and pineal body, and energizes your entire body. Regular practice of this pose can help regulate menstruation and digestion and relieve urinary problems. Many women find it beneficial when they feel depressed, anxious, or spacey from premenstrual or perimenopausal symptoms.

†CAUTION Do this pose only if it is already part of your yoga practice. Do not do this pose if you have high blood pressure, have your period, or suffer from neck or back problems or migraines.

A

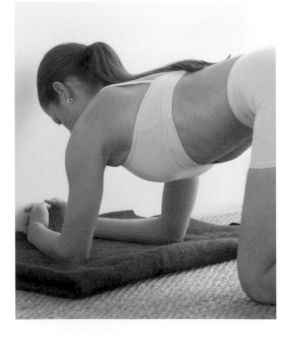

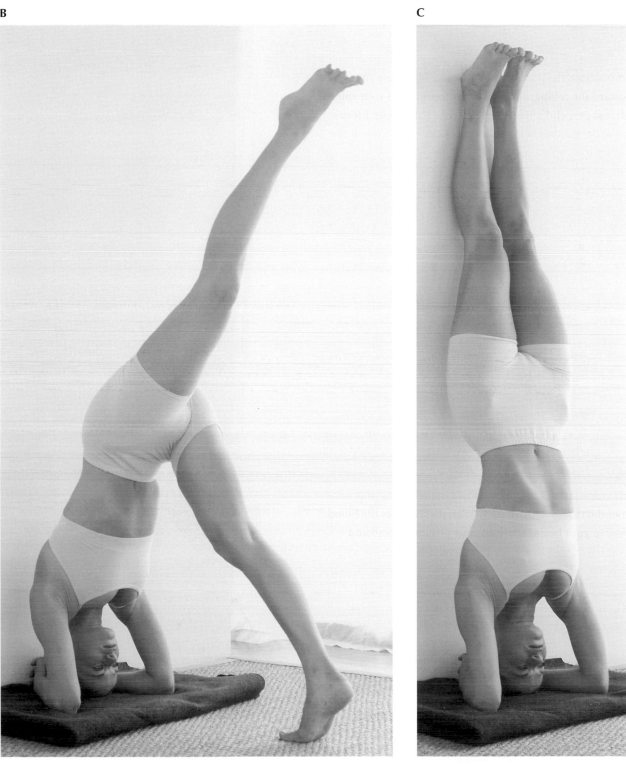

21. CHILD'S POSE (Adho Mukha Virasana) Kneel on the floor with your knees slightly wider than your hips and bring your big toes together. Bend forward and stretch your arms and trunk forward. Rest your head on the floor or a blanket.

EFFECTS This pose calms your nervous system, helps lower blood pressure, and relaxes your body and mind. Done as part of an active practice, it lengthens and tones your spine and releases tension in your back and neck.

22. SHOULDERSTAND† (Sarvangasana) Lie on your back with two folded blankets ➤ supporting your shoulders, your head resting on the floor. Stretch your arms out to the sides with palms down, close to your body. Roll your outer shoulders back and press them into your blanket, away from your ears. On an exhalation, bend your knees and raise your legs toward your chest. Pressing your hands into the floor, swing your bent legs over your head. Support your back with your hands, elbows pressed firmly into the blankets. Raise your torso up until it is perpendicular to the floor and your knees are close to your chest (A). Continue to support your back and raise your legs until your thighs are parallel to the floor (B). Breathe evenly. Now begin to straighten your legs until your knees point up toward the ceiling (C). On an exhalation, straighten your legs completely and extend up through your heels until your whole body is perpendicular to the floor (D). Move your tailbone up and use your hands to lift your back ribs. (If you have trouble keeping your elbows in, come down and secure a strap around both arms just above your elbows, and go back up.) Feel that your whole body is long and straight—stretching from your armpits up through the balls of your feet. Keep your shoulders moving into the blanket and away from your ears. Hold this pose as long as you can, preferably at least 2 minutes.

To come out, exhale as you bend your knees. Slowly roll down onto your back. Lie still for several breaths.

EFFECTS Sometimes called "the Queen of all Poses," this posture supplies fresh, oxygenated blood to your thyroid and parathyroid glands, soothes your nerves, stimulates your kidneys, and calms your mind. It can help ease premenstrual disorders, digestive complaints, and uterine dysplasia (such as fibroids). It can also bring peace, strength, and new resolve when you feel tired, listless, unstable, or nervous.

†CAUTION Do not do this pose if you suffer from neck or shoulder problems, if you have high blood pressure, if you are menstruating, or if you have a headache.

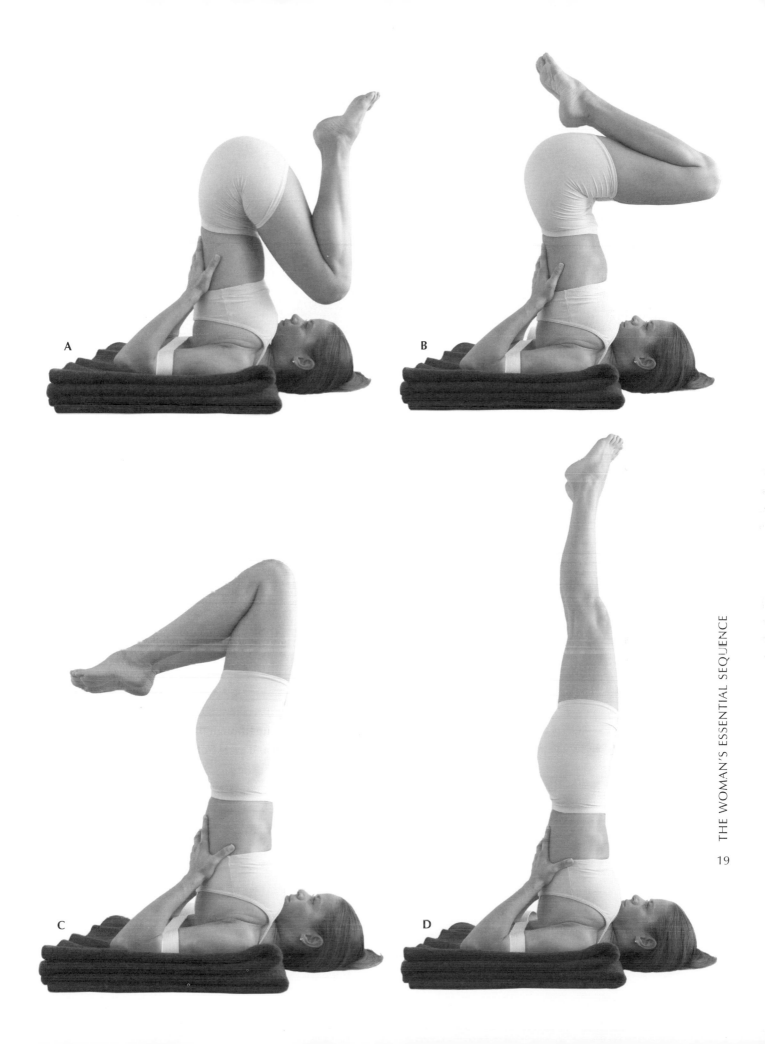

23. PLOUGH POSE† (Halasana) Lie on your back with two folded blankets supporting your neck and shoulders; your head should rest on the floor. Place your arms by your sides, palms pressed into the floor. Your legs should be straight out in front of you, feet together and knees tightened. As you exhale, bend your knees and bring your thighs in to your chest. Pressing your palms into the floor, roll your shoulders away from your ears and open your chest. Exhale again as you swing or lift your buttocks and legs toward the ceiling, supporting your back with your hands (fingers pointing toward your spine and elbows parallel to each other), and extend your legs over your head. Your bent knees should reach just beyond your forehead as you place your toes on the floor behind you. (If you have trouble keeping your elbows in toward your body, come out of the pose and secure a strap around both arms, just above your elbows, then go back into the pose.) Keep your thighs active by tightening your knees to create space between your face and your legs. Your back should be perpendicular to the floor, if possible. Raise your sternum toward your chin (not the other way around) so your neck remains long and relaxed. Stay in this pose, breathing deeply and slowly, for several minutes or as long as you're comfortable. To come out, slowly roll down one vertebra at a time. Rest with your back flat on the floor, breathing deeply, for several breaths.

EFFECTS This pose balances your endocrine system and quiets your sympathetic nervous system so your mind feels uncluttered and deeply relaxed. Resting in this pose lifts your spirits, relieves tension headaches, and helps tame irritability and anxiety. Regular practice of this pose improves posture and helps lengthen your spine.

†CAUTION Do not do this pose if you have neck problems or if you are menstruating.

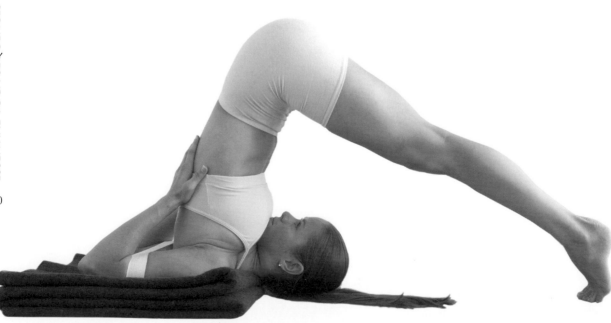

24. BRIDGE POSE (Setu Bandha Sarvangasana) Place a block vertically against the wall and have another one beside you. Lie on your back with your knees bent and your arms stretched out by your sides, palms up. Roll your shoulders back and away from your head, expanding your chest. Raise your hips and chest as high as possible and support your back with your hands, fingers pointing toward your spine. Keeping your head and shoulders flat on the floor, lift your spine even farther, increasing the arch, and place the other vertical block under the fleshy part of your buttocks. Stretch out one leg at a time, resting your heels on the block against the wall. Release your arms so your hands reach just beyond the block under your buttocks. Clasp your hands together, if you can. Hold this pose for at least 1 minute, breathing normally.

To come out, bend your knees and place your feet on the floor. Then release the block under your sacrum and slowly roll down one vertebra at a time. Hug both knees to your chest and rest for several breaths.

EFFECTS This is an active, energizing pose that tones your kidneys and adrenal glands and helps regulate your menstrual cycle.

MODIFICATION If this pose is too difficult (or you feel tired), use bolsters instead of blocks. Position one bolster horizontally at the wall and a second one vertically in front of it to form a T shape. Place a folded blanket on the floor for your head. Sit on the end of the vertical bolster that is closest to the wall. Keeping your knees bent, lie back over the bolster. Slide down until the end of the bolster is in the middle of your back and your shoulders just reach the floor. Rest your head and shoulders on the blanket. With your feet and heels together, stretch your legs toward the wall and place your heels on the horizontal bolster so your toes touch the wall. Rest your arms by your sides, close your eyes, and relax completely. Stay in this position for 5 to 10 minutes, or as long as you like.

To come out, bend your knees and slowly roll to one side. Using your hands, push yourself up to a seated position.

EFFECTS This modification helps relieve anxiety and high blood pressure and can benefit women suffering from depression or nervous exhaustion.

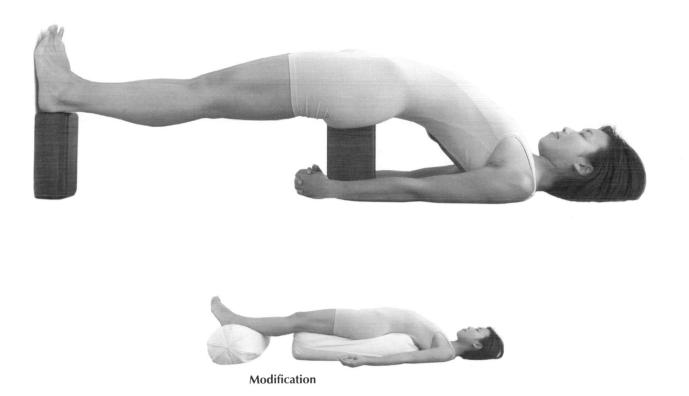

Modification

A

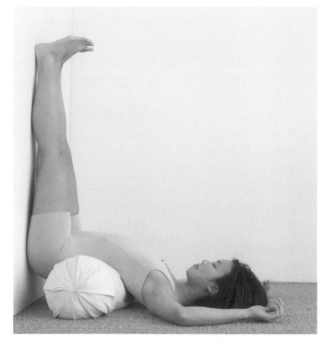

B

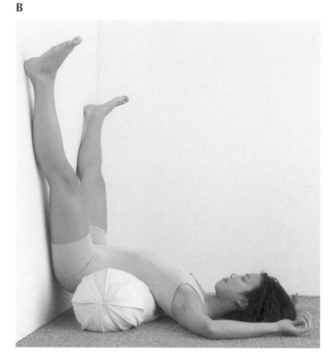

25. LEGS-UP-THE-WALL POSE† (Viparita Karani) AND CYCLE Place a bolster about 3 inches from the wall. (If you are tall, you may need a higher support, such as a folded blanket on top of the bolster.) Sit on the bolster so your right hip and side are touching the wall. Using your hands to support you, lean back and swivel your body around, taking your right leg and then your left leg up the wall. Keep your buttocks close to or against the wall; if they moved away from the wall as you lifted your legs, place your feet on the wall and use your hands for support to lift your hips and move your buttocks back into position. (If you feel discomfort in your legs or back, push your buttocks slightly away from the wall.) Lie down so your lower back and ribs are supported by the bolster, your tailbone is descending toward the floor, and your shoulders and head are resting on the floor (A). (If your neck is uncomfortable, put a folded towel or blanket under it.) Extend through your legs and place your arms out at your sides, elbows bent and palms up. Rest in this position, eyes closed, for 5 minutes.

CYCLE Without moving your torso, allow your legs to open out to the sides (B). Remain in this position, breathing normally, for 3 to 5 minutes.

Again keeping your torso in the same position, bend your knees, cross your legs at the ankles, and continue in the pose for another 3 to 5 minutes (C).

Gently push away from the wall until your buttocks are just off the bolster and resting on the floor; the backs of your thighs and legs should rest on the bolster (D). Rest in this position for 5 minutes, or as long as you like.

To come out of the pose, uncross your legs, push away from the bolster, and roll to one side. Breathe quietly for a few breaths, then use your arms to help you to a seated position.

EFFECTS The poses in this cycle help calm your nerves, balance your endocrine system, relieve fatigue, and increase blood flow to your pelvic region. They also offer your body complete relaxation.

†CAUTION Do not do this pose when you are menstruating.

C

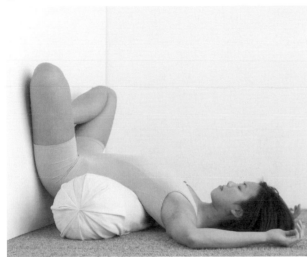

D

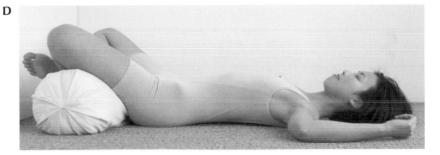

26. CORPSE POSE (Savasana) Lie on your back with your legs stretched out in front of you. (Put a blanket under your head and neck if you wish.) Place your arms comfortably at your sides, slightly away from your torso, with your palms facing upward. Actively stretch your arms and legs away from you, then allow them to release completely. Close your eyes and let everything relax. Take a few deep breaths, inhaling into your chest without tensing your throat, neck, or diaphragm. Exhale your body into the floor, releasing your shoulders, neck, and facial muscles. Keep your abdomen soft and relaxed, and release your lower back. As your eyes relax, breathe normally for at least 5 to 10 minutes. To come out of the pose, bend your knees, roll slowly to one side, and after a few breaths, gently push yourself to a seated position.

EFFECTS This is a wonderfully restful pose. Deeply relaxing and soothing to your sympathetic nervous system, it relieves fatigue and anxiety and restores balance.

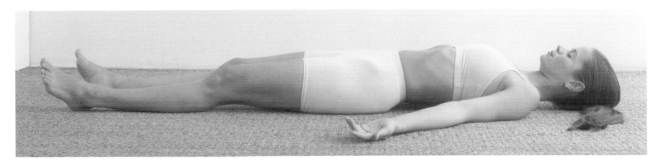

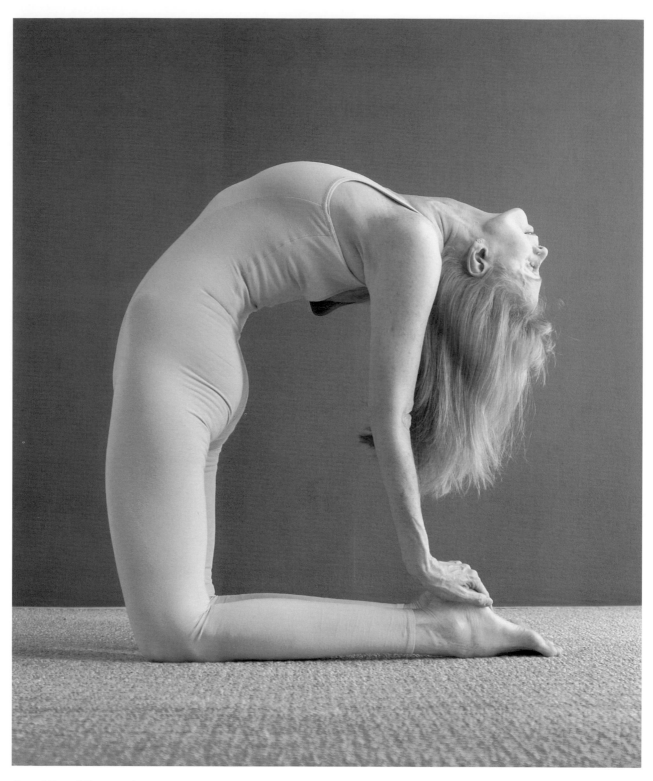

Camel Pose (Ustrasana)

Chapter 2 *The Woman's Energizing Sequence*

by Patricia Walden

THE POSES

1. Mountain Pose (Tadasana)
2. Mountain Pose with Arms Overhead (Urdhva Hastasana in Tadasana)
3. Extended Triangle Pose (Utthita Trikonasana)
4. Warrior II Pose (Virabhadrasana II)
5. Extended Side-Angle Pose (Utthita Parsvakonasana)
6. Warrior I Pose (Virabhadrasana I)
7. Intense Side Stretch Pose (Parsvottanasana)
8. Hero Pose with Cow-Face Arms (Virasana with Gomukhasana Arms)
9. Downward-Facing Dog Pose (Adho Mukha Svanasana)
10. Headstand (Sirsasana)
11. Child's Pose (Adho Mukha Virasana)
12. Downward Facing Dog Pose (Adho Mukha Svanasana)
13. Inverted Staff Pose (Viparita Dandasana)
14. Camel Pose (Ustrasana)
15. Upward-Facing Dog Pose (Urdhva Mukha Svanasana)
16. Upward-Facing Bow Pose (Urdhva Dhanurasana)
17. Downward-Facing Dog Pose (Adho Mukha Svanasana)
18. Standing Forward Bend (Uttanasana)
19. Standing Forward Bend with a Twist (Parsva Uttanasana)
20. Shoulderstand (Sarvangasana)
21. Plough Pose (Halasana)
22. Bridge Pose (Setu Bandha Sarvangasana)
23. Legs-Up-the-Wall Pose (Viparita Karani) and Cycle
24. Corpse Pose (Savasana)

THIS SERIES OF POSES—WHICH INCLUDES SEVERAL BACKBENDS†— is designed to complement The Woman's Essential Sequence. This energizing series increases circulation throughout your body, opens your chest, and allows your breath to flow more freely. Backbends also help tone your spine, strengthen your bladder, and bring vitality and lightness to your body and mind.

I recommend doing this sequence at least three times a week, alternating with the more forward-bending Essential Sequence. Keep your eyes open during the poses, and don't worry if you can't do all of them when you first begin—they get easier with practice.

†CAUTION Don't do unsupported backbends if you suffer from heart problems or other serious illnesses, or if you are menstruating or pregnant. Also avoid inversions if you are menstruating or have a headache. If you have knee, back, or neck problems, seek help from an experienced teacher.

1. MOUNTAIN POSE (Tadasana)

Stand up straight, your legs together (with big toes touching, if that's comfortable). Distribute your weight evenly between the front of your feet and your heels. Tighten your knees by pulling up with your quadricep (front thigh) muscles. Raise your sternum (breastbone) and broaden your chest by rolling your shoulders back and drawing your shoulder blades in. Lift your abdomen up and draw your tailbone in without pushing your thighs forward. Extend your arms downward with palms facing your thighs and fingers together. Keep your shoulders moving away from your ears. It is normal to have some curvature in your lumbar area (lower back). Stand in this posture for 20 to 30 seconds—or longer—breathing normally and keeping your face, neck, and throat relaxed.

EFFECTS This pose strengthens and tones your whole body, keeps your mind alert, and helps create balance. Standing in this pose (especially against a wall) is a wonderful way to notice and correct postural problems.

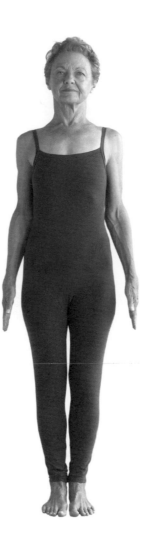

2. MOUNTAIN POSE WITH ARMS OVERHEAD (Urdhva Hastasana in Tadasana)

Stand in Mountain Pose (Tadasana). Turn your palms outward and slowly lift your arms to the side and over your head, keeping your shoulders down and away from your ears. Lift your chest and draw your shoulder blades deep into your back. Breathe normally and stay in this position for 15 to 20 seconds. To come out, release your arms down to your sides.

EFFECTS This pose awakens your whole body, toning your arms, legs, feet, and ankles. It also helps alleviate stiffness in your shoulders, arms, and upper and lower back, and improves circulation throughout your body.

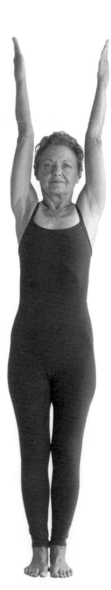

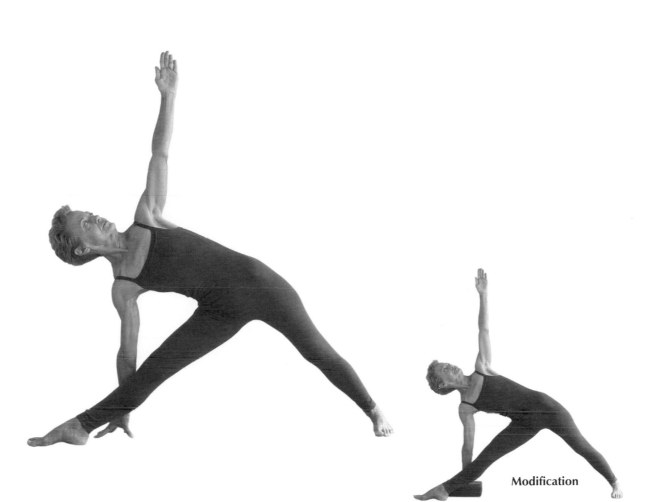

Modification

3. EXTENDED TRIANGLE POSE (Utthita Trikonasana)

Begin in Mountain Pose (Tadasana). Step your feet 3½ to 4 feet apart; keep them parallel to each other. Stretch your arms out to the sides, draw up through your quadriceps, lift your chest, and look straight ahead. Turn your left foot slightly inward and your right foot out 90 degrees; the heel of your left foot should line up with the arch of your right. (Place a block beside the outer edge of your right foot if you need to.) On an exhalation, keeping your back straight, extend your trunk to the right and bring your right hand down to the floor or the block. Press your hand into the floor or block; stretch across your chest and up through your left arm as you extend it toward the ceiling. Your left arm should be in line with your shoulders and your right arm. Draw your shoulder blades in, turn your chest toward the ceiling and your abdomen to the left, and look straight ahead or up at your left hand. Both of your legs should remain active and strong. (If you have trouble balancing, keep your left hand on your left hip and hold on to your shin or ankle with your right hand until you feel steady.) Breathe normally and hold this pose for 20 to 30 seconds, if possible. On an inhalation, lift up and straighten your torso, turning your feet back to a parallel position. Repeat the pose on your left side, then turn your toes forward and step your feet back to Mountain Pose.

EFFECTS This pose elongates and strengthens your spine, brings flexibility to your back muscles, increases circulation to your pelvic region, and tones and improves functioning of your reproductive and digestive organs. It also calms your mind and relieves anxiety and nervous tension.

4. WARRIOR II POSE (Virabhadrasana II) Stand in Mountain Pose (Tadasana). Step your feet out as wide as possible (about 4 to 4½ feet apart, if you can); they should be parallel. Stretch your arms out to the sides, palms down and fingers straight, so they're in line with your shoulders and parallel to the floor. As you exhale, turn your right foot slightly inward and your left foot out 90 degrees. The heel of your left foot should line up with the arch of your right. To maintain your balance, keep your right leg and knee straight and strong, and press your weight into the last two toes of your right foot. On an exhalation, bend your left knee so your thigh is parallel and your shin is perpendicular to the floor; your knee should be in line with your middle toe. (If your knee extends beyond your ankle, you need to widen your stance.) Turn your head and look over your left arm, just past your fingertips. Imagine both arms are engaged in a tug-of-war. Hold this pose for about 20 to 30 seconds, if possible. Otherwise, come in and out of the pose two or three times.

To come out of the pose, straighten your left leg as you inhale and turn your feet so they're parallel again. Keeping your arms outstretched, slowly turn your left foot slightly inward and your right foot out 90 degrees. Repeat the pose on the other side.

EFFECTS This pose promotes stability, strength, and balance. It opens your chest, improving respiration and circulation, and helps relieve depression and fatigue. It is also good for strengthening your legs, reducing fat around your hips and waist, and toning your abdominal region.

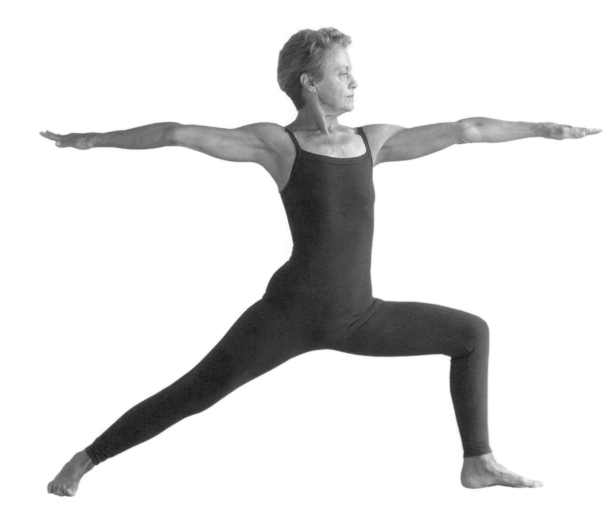

5. EXTENDED SIDE-ANGLE POSE (Utthita Parsvakonasana) Stand in Mountain Pose (Tadasana). Step your feet out as wide as possible (about 4½ feet apart, if you can); turn your left foot out 90 degrees and your right foot slightly inward. The heel of your left foot should line up with the arch of your right. Stretch your arms out to the sides so they're parallel to the floor. As you exhale, bend your left knee so your thigh is parallel and your shin is perpendicular to the floor. (If your knee extends beyond your ankle, you need to widen your stance.) Keeping your back straight, exhale and extend your trunk to the left, bring your left hand down to the floor (or a block), and stretch your right arm up over your right ear. Draw your shoulder blades in, turn your chest toward the ceiling, and look straight ahead or up toward the ceiling. Turn your abdomen to the right. Breathe normally and hold this pose for 20 to 30 seconds, if possible. Inhale as you lift up and straighten your torso. Repeat the pose on your right side, then turn your toes forward and step your feet back to Mountain Pose.

EFFECTS This pose elongates and strengthens your spine, brings flexibility to your back muscles, increases circulation to your pelvic region, and tones and improves functioning of your digestive and reproductive organs. It also calms your mind; relieves anxiety and nervous tension; and helps relieve pain from sciatica and joint stiffness, particularly in your hips, groin, and hamstring muscles (behind your knees).

Modification

6. WARRIOR I POSE (Virabhadrasana I) Stand in Mountain Pose (Tadasana). Step your feet out as wide as possible (about 4 to 4½ feet apart, if you can), with your toes pointing forward. Stretch your arms out to the sides so they're in line with your shoulders and parallel to the floor. Your palms should face the floor; keep your fingers together and stretched out long. Turn your palms up and raise both arms until they are in line with your ears (parallel to each other); keep your elbows straight. Draw up through your quadriceps (upper thigh muscles) and lift your abdomen and chest. As you exhale, turn your torso and right leg to the right 90 degrees as you simultaneously rotate your left foot inward about 60 degrees. Inhale and stretch up through your arms; on an exhalation, bend your right knee so your thigh and shin form a right angle and your thigh is parallel to the floor. (If your knee extends beyond your ankle, you need to widen your stance.) Put your palms together if you wish, but only if you can do so without bending your elbows or collapsing your chest. Stretch your torso up toward the ceiling as you look either up at your hands or straight ahead. Hold this pose for 10 to 15 seconds, breathing normally. If you have trouble holding the pose, come into and out of it two or three times.

To come out of the pose, release your arms out to the sides, stopping at shoulder height, and straighten your right knee. Turn your torso and feet forward. Raise both arms over your head until they are again in line with your ears. On an exhalation, turn your torso and left leg to the right 90 degrees, rotate your right foot in about 60 degrees, and repeat the pose on the left side. Then step your feet together and return to Mountain Pose.

EFFECTS This pose is excellent for stability, strength, balance, and flexibility. Women feel powerful and strong in this pose. It's great for relieving joint stiffness in older women (see modifications throughout the book). If you take your head back, this pose massages and tones your thyroid and parathyroids, bringing oxygenated blood to the area.

7. INTENSE SIDE STRETCH POSE

(Parsvottanasana) Stand in Mountain Pose (Tadasana). Join your palms in prayer position behind your back. (If this is too difficult, simply fold your arms behind your back, fingertips touching your elbows, or raise your arms over your head.) Roll your shoulders back and press your palms together to open your chest. Raise your sternum. Step your feet about 3 to 3½ feet apart, so your weight is distributed equally between your legs. Turn your left foot 90 degrees and your right foot about 75 degrees to the left. Turn your torso to face the left, arching your back slightly and looking up toward the ceiling (if that is comfortable) (A). Stay in this position for a few breaths. As you exhale, lift your head up, extend your spine, and bend forward so your head rests on your left knee (B). Keep both legs straight throughout the pose. Remain like this for 15 to 20 seconds, breathing normally. (If you have trouble balancing, put your hands on the floor, on blocks, or on your leg below the knee.) Lift your head and torso as you inhale and return to a standing position. Look up and arch your back slightly before releasing your arms. Return to center and repeat the pose on the other side.

EFFECTS This pose is especially good for stiffness in your neck, shoulders, elbows, and wrists and for helping ease the pain of arthritis, scoliosis, and kyphosis. It also tones your abdomen, calms your mind, and helps relieve anxiety and nervous tension.

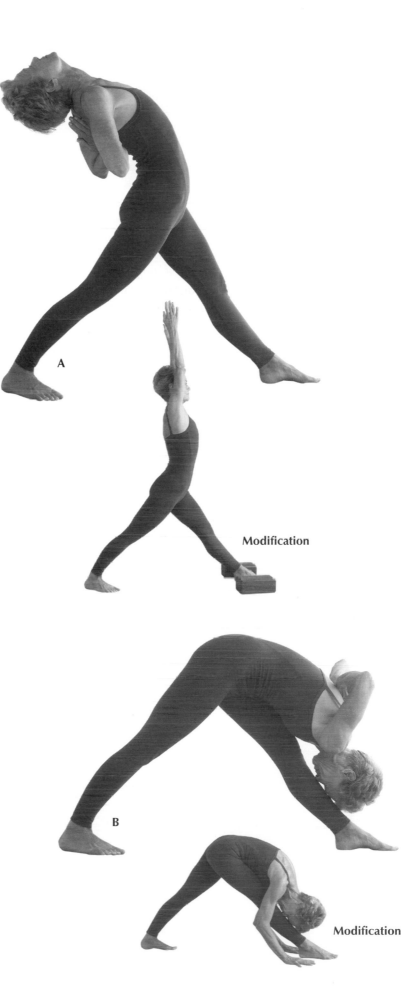

A

Modification

B

Modification

8. HERO POSE† WITH COW-FACE ARMS (Virasana with Gomukhasana Arms) Kneel on the floor with your knees together, your feet pointing straight back, and your calves slightly wider than hip-width apart. Sit between your feet on the floor (or on a block or bolster if you feel any pressure on your knees). Put your left arm behind you and stretch the forearm up your back as far as you can, with the back of your hand against your back. Reach your right arm over your head, bend it at the elbow, and reach down your back toward your left hand. Grasp the fingers of both hands together (or lower a strap in your right hand if your hands won't meet). Keep your right elbow pointing toward the ceiling and your head up. Roll your shoulders back and open your chest. Breathe normally and hold this pose for 30 seconds to 1 minute. Repeat the arm position on the other side.

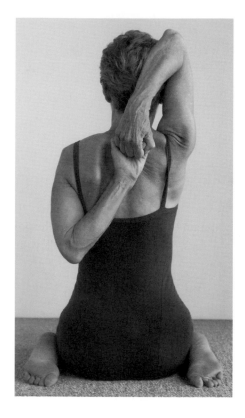

EFFECTS Sitting this way stretches the muscles of your lower body, particularly your calves, quadriceps, knees, and feet, bringing flexibility to those muscles and joints. It is a wonderful way to practice good posture and improve circulation to your pelvis. The positioning of your arms opens your chest and shoulder area, improving respiration and circulation and helping alleviate depression and fatigue.

†CAUTION If you feel any strain in your knees, separate them slightly and sit on a bolster or block. If you are a beginner, don't stay in this pose longer than 1 minute.

9. DOWNWARD-FACING DOG POSE (Adho Mukha Svanasana) Begin on your hands and knees; turn your toes under. Exhale, press your hands into the mat and extend up through your inner arms. Exhale again and raise your buttocks high into the air. Move your thighs up and back, keep stretching through your legs, and bring your heels toward the floor as you lift your buttocks higher. The action of the arms and legs serves to elongate the spine and release your head. Stay in this pose for 30 seconds to 1 minute, breathing deeply. Let your head rest completely and release the base of your neck. Return to your hands and knees and sit back on your heels and lift your head up.

EFFECTS This pose increases the blood supply to your brain and offers many of the same benefits as Head-stand (Sirsasana). It's also a good preparatory pose for backbends.

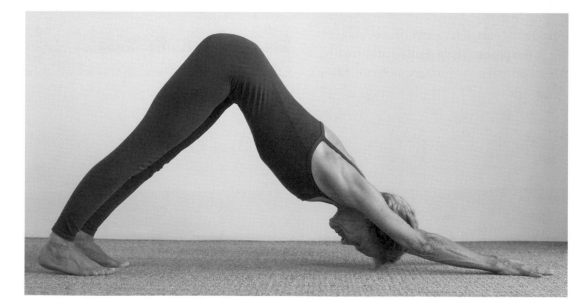

10. HEADSTAND† **(Sirsasana)** (Before beginning, see pages 16–17.) Place a folded blanket against the wall. Kneel in front of it with your feet and knees together. Interlace your fingers firmly, thumbs touching and your hands cupped. Position your hands no more than 3 inches from the wall with your elbows shoulder-width apart and wrists perpendicular to the floor. Your wrists, forearms, and elbows form the foundation for this pose.

Lengthen your neck and place the crown of your head on the blanket. The back of your head should be in contact with your hands. Press your forearms into the floor and lift your shoulders away from the floor. Maintain this action throughout the pose. Straighten your legs, raise your hips, and walk your feet in until your spine is almost perpendicular to the floor. As you exhale, lift one leg at a time, and bring your feet to the wall.

Straighten your legs, and keep your heels and buttocks against the wall. Roll your thighs in, lift your tailbone, lengthen your legs upward, and keep your feet together. Keep your breathing even, your eyes and throat soft, and your abdomen relaxed. With regular practice, you can slowly learn to bring your buttocks and heels away from the wall. Hold the pose as long as you can, up to 5 minutes.

To come out, exhale, bend your knees, and bring your feet to the floor one at a time. Rest for a few breaths before raising your head. Move away from the wall, stretch your arms out in front of you, and rest in Child's Pose (Adho Mukha Virasana), described next.

EFFECTS Like all inversions, this pose balances your neuroendocrine system. In particular, it stimulates the blood flow to your brain, activates your pituitary gland and pineal body, and energizes your entire body. Regular practice of this pose can help regulate menstruation and digestion and relieve urinary problems. Many women find it beneficial when they feel depressed, anxious, or spacey from premenstrual or perimenopausal symptoms.

†CAUTION Do this pose only if it is already part of your yoga practice. Do not do this pose if you have high blood pressure, have your period, or suffer from neck or back problems or migraines.

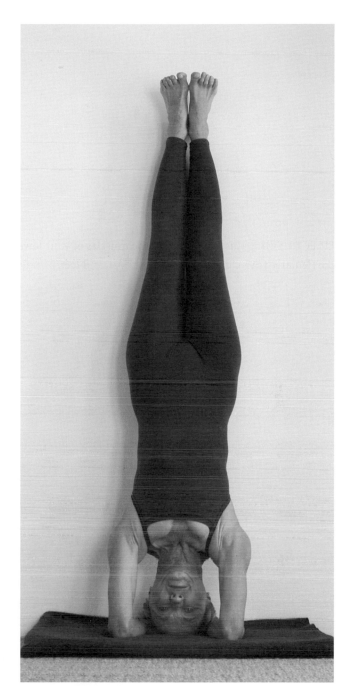

11. CHILD'S POSE (Adho Mukha Virasana) Kneel on the floor with your knees slightly wider than your hips and bring your big toes together. Bend forward and stretch your arms and trunk forward. Rest your head on the floor or a blanket.

EFFECTS This pose calms your nervous system, helps lower blood pressure, and relaxes your body and mind. Done as part of an active practice, it lengthens and tones your spine and releases tension in your back and neck.

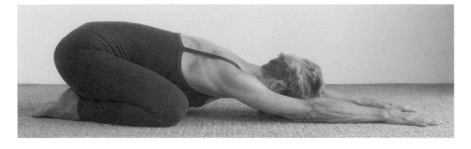

12. DOWNWARD-FACING DOG POSE (Adho Mukha Svanasana) If you did Headstand, repeat Downward Dog here to prepare your back and shoulders for backbends (see page 32).

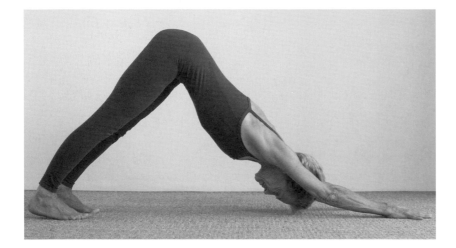

13. INVERTED STAFF POSE† ➤
(Viparita Dandasana) Although the classic version of this pose is for advanced practitioners, you can reap the same benefits by doing this variation. Place a folded blanket on a chair that has been placed about 2 feet from the wall—far enough away so your feet can press into the wall when your legs are outstretched. Sit backward on the chair, facing the wall, with your feet through the chair back (A). Letting your hands slide down the sides of the chair and supporting yourself on your elbows, lean back slowly so your head and neck extend past the front of the chair.

Still holding the sides of the chair, arch back so your shoulder blades are at the front edge of the seat (B). (You may need to scoot your buttocks farther toward the back edge of the seat.) Take your feet to the wall, legs slightly bent, and hold the back legs or sides of the chair. Lengthen your legs, pressing the chair away from the wall, roll your thighs in toward each other and release your head back (C). Keep your hands on the chair sides or legs. (If you have neck problems, rest your head on a bolster. If you feel any pain in your lower back, elevate your feet on a block or bolsters placed against the wall.) Breathe quietly for 30 to 60 seconds.

To come out, bend your knees and place your feet flat on the floor. Hold on to the sides of the chair back and carefully come up, lifting from your sternum. Lean over the chair back for a few breaths to release your back.

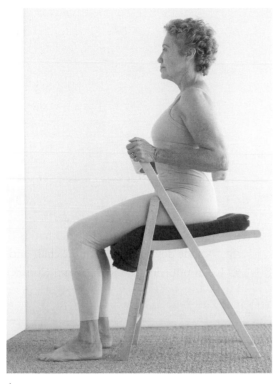

A

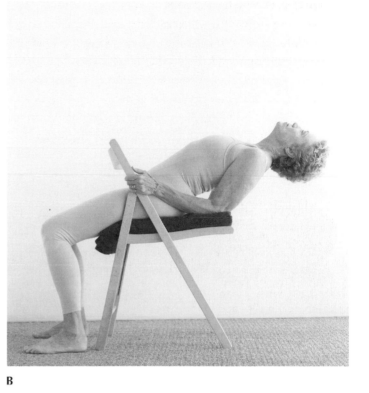

B

EFFECTS This is an excellent pose if you are suffering from depression. It opens your chest, improves respiration and circulation, and invigorates your whole body.

†CAUTION Seek the advice of an experienced teacher if you have neck problems. Do not do this pose if you have a migraine or tension headache or diarrhea.

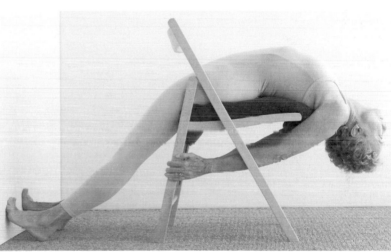

C

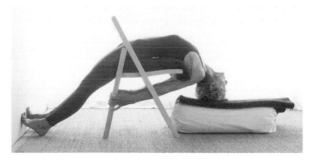

Modification

14. CAMEL POSE† (Ustrasana) Kneel on the floor with your knees and feet hip-width apart. Place your palms on your buttocks and as you exhale, move your thighs slightly forward and raise your side ribs. Gradually bend back as far as possible, lift your chest, and broaden your shoulders. Move your hands from your buttocks to your feet, and take hold of your heels. (If you can't reach your heels, place your hands on blocks positioned next to each ankle with fingers pointing in the same direction as your feet.) Your thighs should be perpendicular to the floor. Take your head back, if that's comfortable, and breathe steadily for 10 to 15 seconds, if you can.

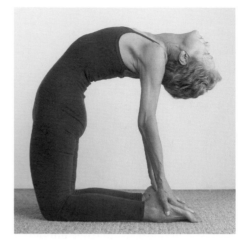

To come out, release your hands one at a time. As you exhale, slowly lift up from your sternum, using your thigh muscles. Your head should come up last.

EFFECTS This pose is good for increasing lung capacity, increasing circulation throughout your body, and strengthening your back muscles.

†CAUTION Do not do this pose if you have a migraine or tension headache, or if you suffer from hypertension.

15. UPWARD-FACING DOG POSE (Urdhva Mukha Svanasana) Lie facedown with your feet about hip-width apart, your toes pointing back, and legs active. Bend your elbows and place your hands next to your floating ribs, fingers pointing straight ahead, and chin resting on the mat. Roll your inner thighs toward each other, and leading with your sternum and the crown of your head, raise the upper part of your body off the mat. Press your hands firmly into the mat and raise your sternum as high as you can, while bringing your pelvis toward your hands. Lift your hips off the mat, keep your thighs strong and your knees pulled up so they don't rest on the floor. Move your shoulder blades into your back ribs, expand your chest, and take your head back, looking up at the ceiling. (If you have trouble with your neck, look straight ahead.) Remain in this position for 15 to 20 seconds. (Put your hands on blocks if you can't lift your thighs off the floor or open your chest.) To come out, exhale as you bend your elbows, resting the hips, thighs, and chest on the mat. Lower your head and relax.

EFFECTS This pose is especially good for sciatic pain, stiffness in your shoulders and upper back, and lower back tension. Opening your chest can lift your spirits when you are depressed and helps calm agitated or nervous energy. (If you have back problems, see the variation on page 184.)

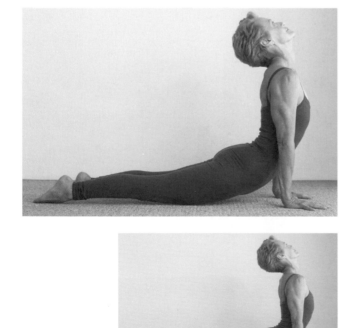

Modification

16. UPWARD-FACING BOW POSE†

(**Urdhva Dhanurasana**) Lie on your back with your knees bent, your feet hip-width apart, and your heels close to your buttocks. Bend your elbows and place your hands alongside your head with your fingers pointing toward your feet. As you exhale, raise your hips and chest, straighten your arms, and stretch your legs. Lift your tailbone and move the backs of your thighs toward your buttocks. To come out of the pose, bend your knees and elbows, and slowly lower your body to the floor. Hold this pose for 5 to 10 seconds, if you can. If not, come in and out of the pose two or three times.

MODIFICATION If you have trouble pushing up into a backbend, try this pose with blocks and a bolster. Position two blocks against the wall, shoulder-width apart, with a vertical bolster between them, touching the wall (A). Lie on your back on the bolster, with your head closest to the wall. Bend your elbows and place your hands on the blocks, fingers pointing toward your feet. Push up as instructed above (B).

EFFECTS This pose improves circulation throughout your body, stimulates your entire nervous system, and generates an overall feeling of elation and well-being.

†CAUTION Do the unsupported version of this pose only if it is already part of your yoga practice. Seek the advice of an experienced teacher if you have neck problems. Do not do this pose if you have a migraine or tension headache, suffer from heart trouble or any serious illness, or are pregnant.

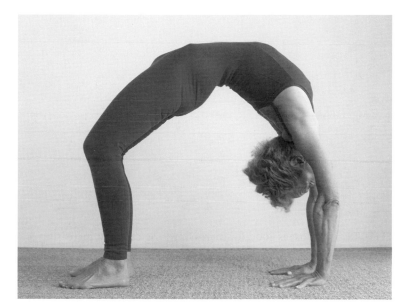

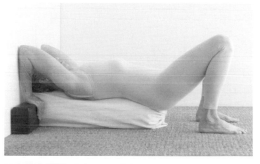

Modification A

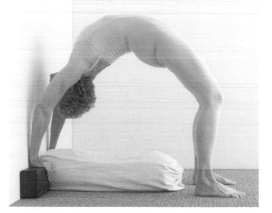

Modification B

17. DOWNWARD-FACING DOG POSE (Adho Mukha Svanasana)
Repeat Downward-Facing Dog (see page 32) to stretch out your
back if you've just finished Upward-Facing Bow Pose (Urdhva
Dhanurasana) or Upward-Facing Dog (Urdhva Mukha Svanasana).

18. STANDING FORWARD BEND (Uttanasana) Stand in
Mountain Pose (Tadasana). Balancing the weight evenly
between your feet, lengthen up through your inner
thighs, and roll your thighs in. Keep your legs and knees
firm as you lift your arms overhead, stretching up
through your waist and ribs. As you
exhale, bend forward from your
hips and release your side body
and head down. Press your hands
into the floor next to your feet.
(If you can't touch the floor, place
your hands on blocks or on your
shins.) Breathe normally for 30
to 60 seconds. To come out, keep
your legs active, and slowly lift
up to standing.

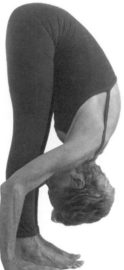

EFFECTS This pose brings a sense of peace when you feel
agitated or anxious. It calms your mind, relieves a jittery
stomach, lifts and tones your uterus, and improves
circulation to your pelvic area. It can be effective in
helping to lower high blood pressure by relieving mental
and physical tension. It may also be effective for most
headaches.

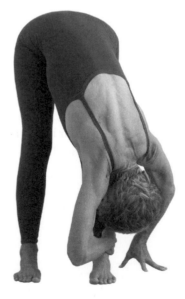

**19. STANDING FORWARD BEND WITH A TWIST (Parsva
Uttanasana)** Stand with your feet hip-width apart. Turn
your palms outward and, as you inhale, lift your arms up
over your head, stretching your whole body. As you
exhale, twist from your lower abdominals so your upper
torso is facing your left leg. Inhale, extend your spine and
then exhale, bend forward, placing your right hand on
your left ankle and your left hand on the floor next to
your left foot. Move your head toward your left knee and
breathe normally for 30 to 60 seconds. To come out,
release your right hand to the floor and turn your torso
to the front. Lift up slowly, your head coming up last.

EFFECTS Like Standing Forward Bend (Uttanasana), this
pose calms your mind and nerves. It gives the added bonus
of calming and engaging your adrenal glands, and toning
and massaging your kidneys and reproductive organs.

ESSENTIAL YOGA SEQUENCES

20. SHOULDERSTAND† **(Sarvangasana)** (Before beginning, see pages 18–19.) Lie on your back with two folded blankets supporting your shoulders and your arms stretched out beside your body. On an exhalation, bend your knees and raise your legs toward your chest. Pressing your hands into the floor, swing your bent legs over your head; support your back with your hands and press your elbows firmly into the blankets. Raise your torso up until it is perpendicular to the floor and your knees are close to your chest. Supporting your back, raise your legs until your thighs are parallel to the floor; raise them some more until your knees point toward the ceiling. Now raise your legs completely and extend up through your heels until your whole body is perpendicular to the floor. Move your tailbone up and in and use your hands to lift your back ribs. Feel that your whole body is long and straight. Move your shoulders away from your ears. Hold this pose as long as you can, preferably at least 2 minutes. To come out, exhale as you bend your knees. Slowly roll down. Lie still for several breaths.

EFFECTS Shoulderstand regulates your thyroid and parathyroid glands, stimulates your kidneys, and soothes your nerves. It can help ease premenstrual disorders, digestive complaints, and uterine dysplasia (such as fibroids). It can also bring peace, strength, and new resolve when you feel tired, listless, unstable, or nervous.

†CAUTION Do not do this pose if you suffer from neck or shoulder problems, if you have high blood pressure, if you are menstruating, or if you have a migraine or tension headache.

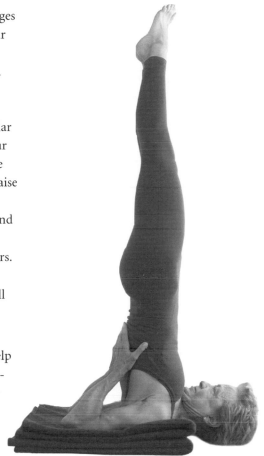

21. PLOUGH POSE† **(Halasana)** Lie on your back with two folded blankets supporting your neck and shoulders; your head is on the sticky mat and your arms are down by your sides. Bend your knees and bring your thighs in to your chest. On an exhalation, swing or lift your buttocks and legs up, supporting your back with your hands, and extend your legs over your head, placing your toes on the floor behind you. Keep your thighs active by tightening your knees to create space between your face and your legs. Stay in this pose, breathing deeply and slowly, for several minutes. To come out, slowly roll down one vertebra at a time. Rest with your back flat on the floor, breathing deeply, for several breaths.

EFFECTS This pose balances your endocrine system and quiets your sympathetic nervous system so your mind feels uncluttered and deeply relaxed. Resting in this pose lifts your spirits and helps tame irritability and anxiety. It is also excellent for tension headaches.

†CAUTION Do not do this pose if you have neck problems or if you are menstruating.

22. BRIDGE POSE (Setu Bandha Sarvangasana) Place one bolster horizontally against the wall and the other vertically, forming a T shape. Spread a folded blanket on the floor for your head. Sit on the end of the vertical bolster that is closest to the wall. Keeping your knees bent, lie back over the bolster. Slide down until the end of the bolster is in the middle of your back and your shoulders just reach the floor. Rest your shoulders and head on the blanket. Keeping your feet and heels together, stretch your legs toward the wall and put your heels on the horizontal bolster so your feet touch the wall. Your legs should be straight out in front of you. Rest your arms in any comfortable position. Close your eyes and relax completely, softening your abdomen and breathing deeply. Stay in this position for 5 to 10 minutes, or as long as you like.

To come out, bend your knees and slowly roll to one side. Using your hands, push yourself up to a seated position.

EFFECTS When modified with bolsters, this is a resting pose. It helps relieve anxiety, erratic mood swings, hot flashes, and high blood pressure. Since it is a slight backbend, it can relieve depression and nervous exhaustion as well.

23. LEGS-UP-THE-WALL POSE† (Viparita Karani) AND CYCLE Place a bolster about 3 inches from the wall. Sit on the bolster so your right hip and side are touching the wall. Using your hands to support you, lean back and swivel your body around, taking your right leg and then your left leg up the wall. Keep your buttocks close to or against the wall; if they moved away from the wall as you lifted your legs, place your feet on the wall and use your hands for support to lift your hips and move your buttocks back into position. (If you feel stiffness or discomfort in your legs, push your buttocks slightly away from the wall.) Lie down so your lower back and ribs are supported by the bolster, your tailbone is descending toward the floor, and your shoulders and head are on the floor (A). (If your neck is uncomfortable, put a folded towel or blanket under it.) Extend through your legs and place your arms out at your sides, elbows bent and palms up. Rest in this position, eyes closed, for 5 minutes.

CYCLE Without moving your torso, allow your legs to open out to the sides (B). Remain in this position, breathing normally, for 3 to 5 minutes.

Again keeping your torso in the same position, bend your knees, cross your legs at the ankles, and continue in the pose for another 3 to 5 minutes (C).

Gently push away from the wall until your buttocks are just off the bolster and resting on the floor; the backs of your thighs and legs rest on the bolster. Stay in this position for 5 minutes, or as long as you like (D).

To come out of the pose, uncross your legs, push gently away from the bolster, and roll to one side. Breathe quietly for a few breaths, then use your arms to help you to a seated position.

EFFECTS The poses in this cycle help calm your nerves, balance your endocrine system, relieve fatigue, and increase blood flow to your pelvic region. They also offer your body complete relaxation.

†CAUTION Do not do this pose if you are menstruating.

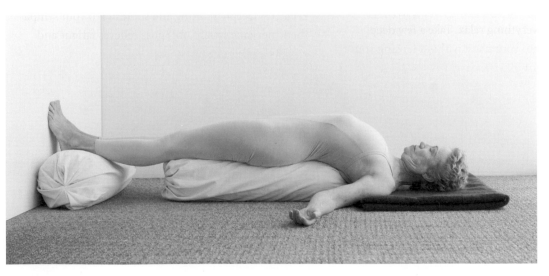

A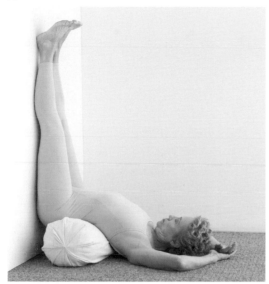

B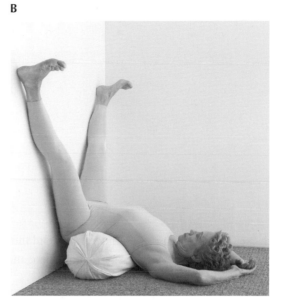

C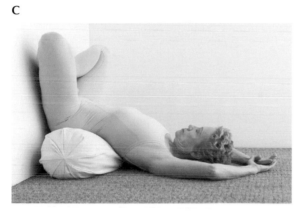

D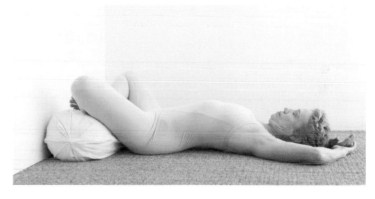

24. CORPSE POSE (Savasana) Lie on your back with your legs stretched out in front of you. (Put a blanket under your head if you wish.) Place your arms comfortably at your sides, slightly away from your torso, with your palms facing upward. Actively stretch your arms and legs away from you, then release completely. Close your eyes and let everything relax. Take a few deep breaths, inhaling into your chest without tensing your throat, neck, or diaphragm. Exhale your body into the floor, releasing your shoulders, neck, and facial muscles. Keep your abdomen soft and relaxed, and release your lower back. Breathe normally for at least 5 to 10 minutes. To come out, bend your knees, roll slowly to one side, and gently push yourself to a seated position.

EFFECTS Deeply relaxing and soothing to your sympathetic nervous system, this pose relieves fatigue and anxiety and restores balance.

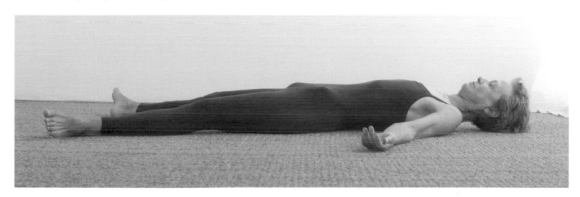

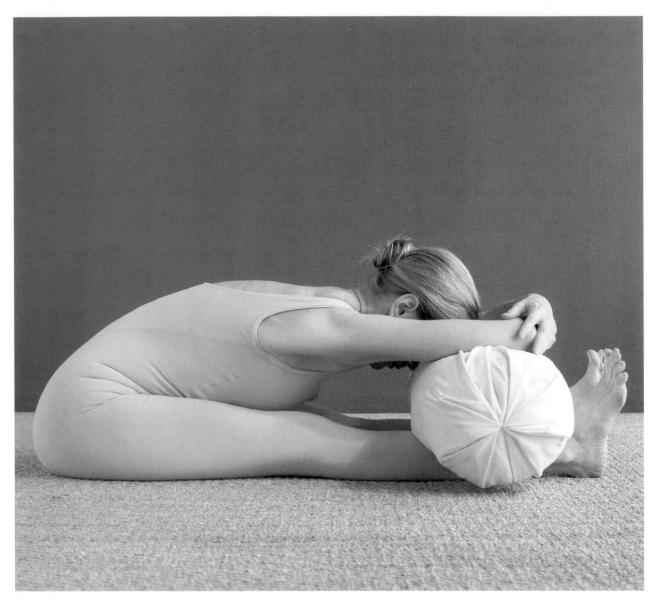

Seated Forward Bend (Paschimottanasana)

Chapter 3 *The Woman's Restorative Sequence*
by Patricia Walden

THE POSES

1. Reclining Bound Angle Pose
   (Supta Baddha Konasana)
2. Reclining Easy Seated Pose
   (Supta Sukhasana)
3. Reclining Big Toe Pose I
   (Supta Padangusthasana I)
4. Reclining Big Toe Pose II
   (Supta Padangusthasana II)
5. Downward-Facing Dog Pose
   (Adho Mukha Svanasana)
6. Headstand (Sirsasana)
7. Child's Pose (Adho Mukha Virasana)
8. Head-on-Knee Pose (Janu Sirsasana)
9. Seated Forward Bend
   (Paschimottanasana)
10. Shoulderstand (Sarvangasana)
11. Half-Plough Pose (Ardha Halasana)
12. Bridge Pose
    (Setu Bandha Sarvangasana)
13. Legs-Up-the-Wall Pose (Viparita Karani)
    and Cycle

DO THIS NURTURING AND SOOTHING PRACTICE AT THE END OF A long day, in the middle of a stressful week, or whenever you want to restore balance to your life. This sequence provides gentle backbends, supported forward bends, and modified inversions to calm your nerves and recharge your batteries. But its rewards go beyond the physical. It uses conscious breathing—the direct link between your body and mind—to move you into deeper and deeper levels of relaxation. As your body lets go of stress and your mind quiets its constant chatter, you come closer to understanding who you truly are and connecting with your true self. Incorporate this ancient discipline into your life at least two or three times a week, or choose two or three poses to practice each day.

†CAUTION Don't do unsupported backbends if you suffer from heart problems or other serious illnesses, or if you are menstruating or pregnant. Avoid inversions if you are menstruating or have a headache. If you have knee, back, or neck problems, seek help from an experienced teacher.

1. RECLINING BOUND ANGLE POSE (Supta Baddha Konasana) Place a bolster vertically behind you and sit just in front of it with your knees bent and your sacrum touching the bolster's edge. Place a strap behind your back, at your sacrum; draw it forward over your hips, across your shins, and under your feet (see page xv). Put the soles of your feet together and let your knees and thighs fall to the sides. Cinch the strap securely under your feet. Lie back so your head and torso rest comfortably on the bolster and your buttocks and legs are on the floor. (If you feel any discomfort in your lower back, add some height to your support with a folded blanket or two. If you feel any strain in your neck, place a folded blanket under your head and neck. If you feel any muscle tension in your legs, roll two blankets vertically and place one under the top of each thigh.) Rest in this pose for as long as you like, breathing deeply.

To come out, draw your knees together, slip the strap off, and slowly roll to one side. Use your hands to push yourself up to a seated position.

EFFECTS This pose can help relieve menstrual cramps, spasms, and heaviness in your uterus. It also takes pressure off your pelvic area, opens your chest, quiets your mind, and calms your nerves. Try it to ease anxiety during times of stress and for headache relief. It's even good for hemorrhoids and indigestion.

2. RECLINING EASY SEATED POSE (Supta Sukhasana) Place a bolster vertically on the floor behind you and sit just in front of it with your knees bent and your sacrum touching the bolster's edge (just like in Reclining Bound Angle Pose). You may put a folded blanket on the bolster to support your head. Cross your legs comfortably at your shins and extend up through your spine. Using your hands to support you, lie back on the bolster. Rest your arms out to the sides, bring your shoulder blades into your back ribs, and lift your chest. This should be a restful pose and you should feel no discomfort anywhere. (If you feel any strain in your back, add more height to your support.) To come out, uncross your legs, place your feet flat on the floor, and roll slowly to one side. Use your hands to push yourself up to a sitting position.

EFFECTS This pose helps relieve headaches, menstrual cramps, and abdominal heaviness; softens your belly; opens your chest; and stimulates your thyroid and adrenal glands. Thus, it's a beneficial pose for depression and anxiety.

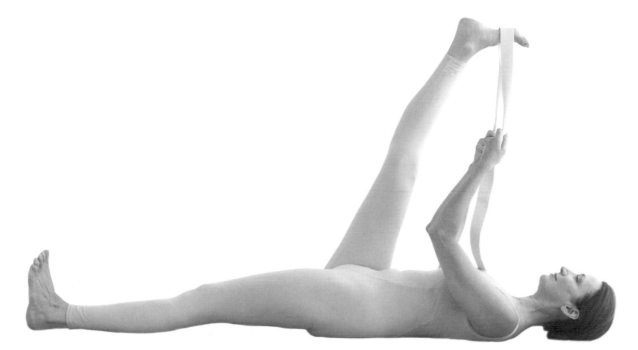

3. RECLINING BIG TOE POSE I (Supta Padangusthasana I)
Lie flat on the floor with your legs outstretched and together. As you inhale, draw your right knee up to your chest and place a strap around the ball of your foot. Exhale as you extend your leg straight up to the ceiling. With both hands pulling the strap, ease your leg closer to your head (if possible), keeping your right buttock firmly on the floor. Keep your left leg on the floor, actively pressing it into the ground, with your toes toward the ceiling. (If you suffer from joint stiffness or arthritis, move your right leg gently back and forth in its socket to increase mobility and to keep the joints fluid.) Repeat the pose with your left leg.

EFFECTS This pose can relieve stiffness in your lower back and the backs of your legs, as well as your hip joints. It can also help ease menstrual discomfort.

4. RECLINING BIG TOE POSE II (Supta Padangusthasana II)
Place a bolster on the floor about 6 inches to your right so the bottom edge is in line with your right hip. Loop a strap around your right foot as shown in the photo, holding the long end with your left hand. Raise your leg straight up to the ceiling, run the long end of the strap behind your head, and straighten your left arm out to the side. On an exhalation, ease your right leg out to the side and down onto the bolster. Pull gently on the strap with your left hand to add a little resistance. Rest comfortably for at least 1 to 2 minutes. Repeat this pose with your left leg.

EFFECTS Some women find that this pose relieves menstrual cramps. It is also beneficial for peri- and postmenopausal joint stiffness, hot flashes, back pain, and prevention of osteoporosis.

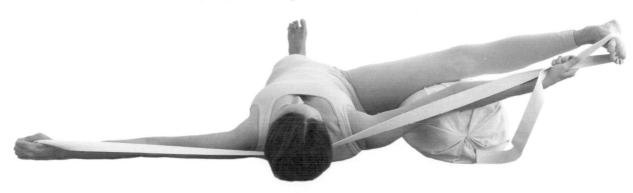

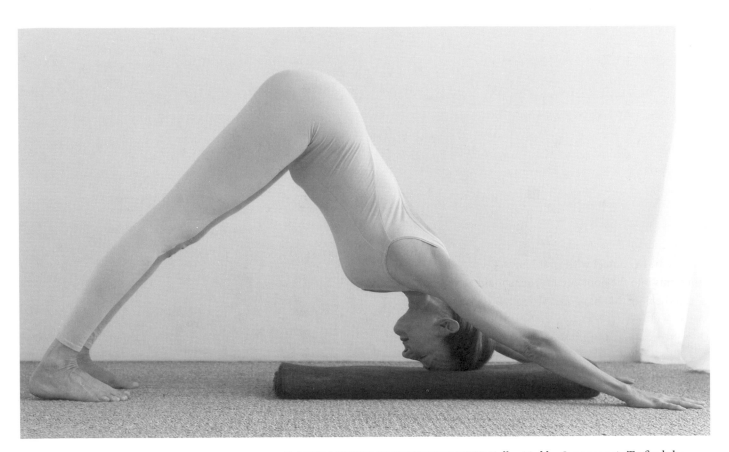

5. DOWNWARD-FACING DOG POSE (Adho Mukha Svanasana) To find the correct distance between your hands and feet for this pose, lie facedown on your sticky mat. Place your palms on the floor by each side of your chest with your fingers well spread and pointing straight ahead. Come up on your hands and knees. That's your position. Now place a bolster or one or two folded blankets vertically, so your support is in line with your sternum. Your support should be high enough to support your head, but low enough to lengthen your neck. Return to your hands-and-knees position, and turn your toes under.

Exhale, press your hands firmly into the mat and extend up through your inner arms. On your next exhalation, raise your buttocks high into the air and move your thighs up and back. Keep stretching through your legs and bring your heels toward the floor. Keep your legs firm and your elbows straight as you lift your buttocks upward and release your head onto your support. The action of the arms and legs serves to elongate your spine and release your head. Hold this pose for 30 seconds to 1 minute, breathing deeply. Let your head rest completely and release the base of your neck. To come out, either return to your hands and knees and sit back on your heels or step your feet forward into Standing Forward Bend (Uttanasana) and slowly stand up.

EFFECTS This pose increases the blood supply to your brain and offers many of the same benefits as Headstand (Sirsasana). This modification combats depression because it helps increase circulation to your chest, improve respiration, and calm your mind, especially when you support your head with a blanket or bolster. Downward-Facing Dog also stretches your calf muscles, back, and achilles tendon and relieves arthritic stiffness in your shoulders, wrists, and fingers.

6. HEADSTAND† **(Sirsasana)** (Before beginning, see pages 16–17.) Place a folded blanket against the wall. Kneel in front of it with your feet and knees together. Interlace your fingers firmly, thumbs touching and your hands cupped. Position your hands no more than 3 inches from the wall with your elbows shoulder-width apart and wrists perpendicular to the floor. Your wrists, forearms, and elbows form the foundation for this pose.

Lengthen your neck and place the crown of your head on the blanket. The back of your head should be in contact with your hands. Press your forearms into the floor and lift your shoulders away from the floor. Maintain this action throughout the pose. Straighten your legs, raise your hips toward the ceiling, and walk your feet in until your spine is almost perpendicular to the floor. As you exhale, lift one leg at a time, and bring your feet to the wall.

Keep your heels and buttocks against the wall. Roll your thighs in, lift your tailbone, lengthen your legs upward, and keep your feet together. Balance on the crown of your head, press your forearms into the floor, and continue to lift your shoulders away from your ears. Keep your breathing even, your eyes and throat soft, and your abdomen relaxed. With regular practice, you can learn to bring your buttocks and heels away from the wall. Hold the pose as long as you can, up to 5 minutes.

To come out, exhale and bring your feet to the floor one at a time. Bend your knees, sit back on your heels, and rest for a few breaths before raising your head. Move away from the wall, stretch your arms out in front of you, and rest in Child's Pose (Adho Mukha Virasana), described next.

EFFECTS Like all inversions, this pose balances your neuroendocrine system. It stimulates the blood flow to your brain and activates your pituitary gland and pineal body. Regular practice of this pose can help regulate menstruation and digestion and relieve urinary problems. Many women find it beneficial when they feel depressed, anxious, or spacey.

†CAUTION Do this pose only if it is already part of your yoga practice. Do not do this pose if you have high blood pressure, have your period, or suffer from neck or back problems or migraines.

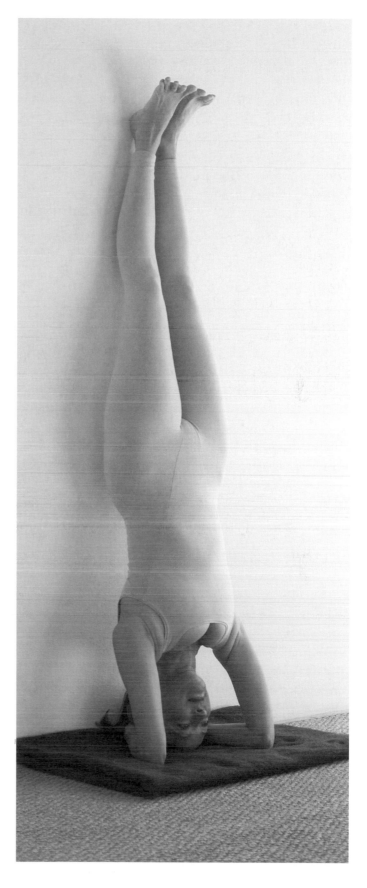

7. CHILD'S POSE (Adho Mukha Virasana) Kneel on the floor with a vertical bolster directly in front of you, the short end between your knees. Spread your knees wide, straddling the bolster, and bring your toes together. Bend forward and stretch your arms and trunk up and over the bolster, pressing it into your abdomen. Fold your arms to cradle your head, turn your head to one side, and relax completely for a minute or two. Push yourself up with your hands to release the pose.

EFFECTS This pose calms your nervous system, helps lower blood pressure, and relaxes your body and mind. It's basically good for everyone!

8. HEAD-ON-KNEE POSE† (Janu Sirsasana) Sit on the floor with your legs stretched out in front of you. Bend your right knee to the side so it is at a 45-degree angle to your left leg and your right heel is near the right side of your groin. Push your right knee as far back as you comfortably can; keep your left leg straight.

Place a folded blanket or a bolster on your outstretched leg, and turn your abdomen and chest so your sternum is in line with the center of your left leg. As you inhale, lift your trunk up from the base of your pelvis; as you exhale, reach your arms out in front of you as you lean your trunk forward. Fold your arms on your support and cradle your head on your arms. (If you still feel strain, add more height to your support or rest your head on a padded chair. If you feel any pressure or strain in your back or legs, simply cross your legs in front of you.)

Stay in this pose for at least 3 minutes, resting your head, the base of your skull, your eyes, and your brain. Inhale while coming up, straighten your right leg, and reverse sides by bending your left knee.

EFFECTS This pose brings a sense of peace when you feel agitated or anxious. It calms your mind, relieves a jittery stomach, and tones your reproductive organs and the supporting muscles. It can be effective in helping to lower high blood pressure by relieving mental and physical tension. It may also be effective for most headaches.

†CAUTION Do not do the full pose if you have diarrhea.

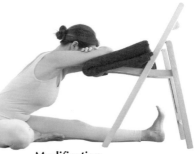

Modification

9. SEATED FORWARD BEND† **(Paschimottanasana)** Sit on the floor with your legs stretched out in front of you. Your big toes, ankles, knees, and thighs should be close together. (If you're unable to sit in this position without rounding your back or slumping, sit on a block or on two folded blankets.) Place a folded blanket or two (or a bolster, depending on your flexibility) across your lower legs. Take a full, deep breath and lift your arms over your head, stretching up through your spine and lifting your sternum (breastbone) and head. Keep your back slightly concave as you bend forward on an exhalation and extend your torso over your legs. You should feel the extension all the way from your groin to your navel, but your abdominals should remain soft. Cross your arms over your support and cradle your head on your arms; close your eyes. (If you feel strain in your back or legs, add more height to your support or rest your head on a padded chair.) Do not allow your buttocks to come off the floor or blankets. Press your shoulders away from your ears and elongate your neck. Breathe evenly and consciously relax your neck, face, shoulders, and eyes. Stay in this pose for 3 to 5 minutes, then slowly roll up to a seated position, lifting your head last.

EFFECTS This pose is beneficial for women who suffer from high blood pressure, the free-floating anxiety of PMS or perimenopause, or bad menstrual cramps. It may also be helpful in relieving symptoms of uterine fibroids, and chronic tension and migraine headaches, activating your adrenals, and toning your thyroid gland. Geeta Iyengar says it is good for the digestive system because it massages and strengthens your abdominal organs and tones your kidneys and liver. It also helps instill a sense of safety and peace.

†CAUTION Do not do the full pose if you have diarrhea.

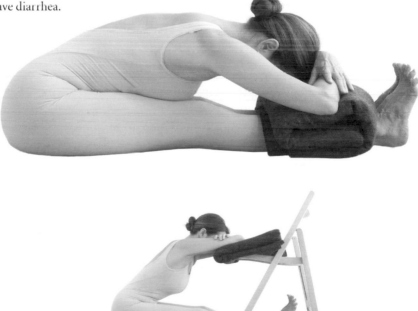

Modification

A

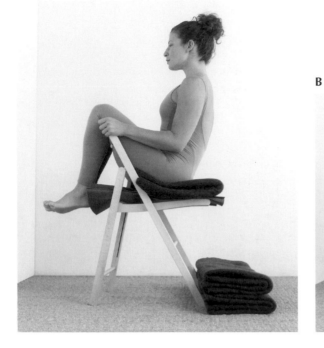

B

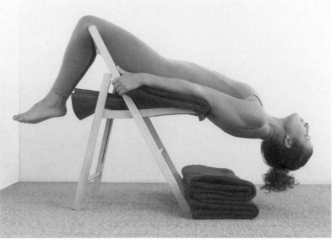

10. SHOULDERSTAND† **(Sarvangasana)** Place a chair about 8 to 10 inches away from the wall. Put a folded blanket on the chair seat, and two or three folded blankets in front of the chair. Sit backward on the chair with your legs bent over the top of the back; move your buttocks into the center of the chair seat (A).

Holding the sides and then the front legs of the chair, slowly lower your torso so your shoulders are on the blankets and your head is on the floor (B). You must extend your spine and open your chest while doing this to get the proper position. Move your hands, one at a time, to hold the back legs of the chair; your arms should be between the front legs. Stretch your legs straight up, keeping your sacrum on the chair seat. Rotate your thighs in and extend from your groin to your heels. Close your eyes, bring your chest to your chin (C), and breathe normally for 3 to 5 minutes, or as long as you're comfortable.

To release from the pose, bend your knees, place your feet on the chair back, release your hands, and slide down until your sacrum rests on the blankets and your calves are on the chair seat. Rest here a moment, then roll to your side and sit up slowly.

EFFECTS Sometimes called "the Queen of all Poses," this posture supplies fresh, oxygenated blood to your thyroid and parathyroid glands, stimulates your kidneys, and soothes your nerves. It can help ease premenstrual disorders, digestive complaints, and uterine dysplasia (such as fibroids). It can also bring peace, and new resolve when you feel tired, listless, or nervous.

†CAUTION Do not do this pose if you suffer from neck or shoulder problems, if you have diarrhea, if you are menstruating, or if you have a migraine or tension headache.

C

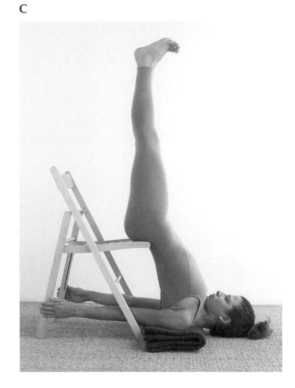

11. HALF-PLOUGH POSE† (Ardha ➤ Halasana) Place two folded blankets on top of your sticky mat with the rounded edges near the legs of a chair. Lie on your back with your legs outstretched, your shoulders on the blanket, and your head beneath the chair seat. As you exhale, bend your knees and swing or lift your buttocks and legs, so your thighs rest completely on the chair seat. (Pad the seat with blankets if you need more height for your legs to be parallel to the floor.) Move your chest in toward your chin (not your chin toward your chest). Bend your elbows at right angles to your body and relax with your palms up and your eyes closed. Rest here for as long as you like—at least 3 to 5 minutes, if possible—breathing deeply to relax and quiet your mind. To come out, place your hands on your back and slowly roll down, one vertebra at a time. Roll to one side and sit up.

EFFECTS This pose balances your endocrine system and quiets your sympathetic nervous system so your mind feels uncluttered and your whole body can relax deeply. It helps relieve throat problems and congestion and may improve thyroid and parathyroid function. Resting in this pose lifts your spirits and helps tame irritability and anxiety. It is also excellent for headaches.

†CAUTION Do not do this pose if you suffer from neck or shoulder problems, or if you have your period.

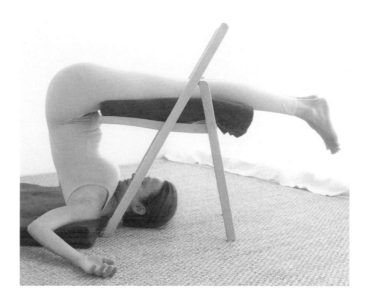

12. BRIDGE POSE (Setu Bandha Sarvangasana) Have two bolsters and a blanket on hand. Place one bolster horizontally against the wall and the other vertically, forming a T shape. Spread a folded blanket on the floor at the end of the vertical bolster that is farthest from the wall (for your head). Sit on the end of the vertical bolster that is closest to the wall. Keeping your knees bent, lie back over the bolster. Slide down until the end of the bolster is in the middle of your back and your shoulders just reach the floor. Rest your shoulders and head on the blanket. Keeping your feet and heels together, stretch your legs toward the wall and put your heels on the horizontal bolster so your feet touch the wall. Your legs should be straight out in front of you. Rest your arms in any comfortable position—over your head or out by your sides. Close your eyes and relax completely, softening your abdomen, releasing your vaginal walls, and breathing deeply. Stay in this position for 5 to 10 minutes, or as long as you like.

To come out, bend your knees and slowly roll to one side. Using your hands, push yourself up to a seated position.

EFFECTS This modified pose helps relieve anxiety, erratic mood swings, hot flashes, tension headaches, and depression. It is also beneficial for regulating blood pressure.

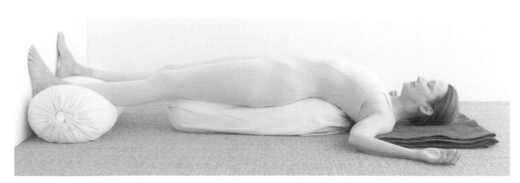

13. LEGS-UP-THE-WALL POSE†
(Viparita Karani) AND CYCLE

Place a bolster about 3 inches from the wall. (If you are tall, you may need a higher support, such as a folded blanket on top of the bolster.) Sit on the bolster so your right hip and side are touching the wall. Using your hands to support you, lean back and swivel your body around, taking your right leg and then your left leg up the wall. Keep your buttocks close to or against the wall; if they moved away from the wall as you lifted your legs, place your feet on the wall and use your hands for support to lift your hips and move your buttocks back into position. (If you feel stiffness or discomfort in your legs, push your buttocks slightly away from the wall.) Lie down so your lower back and ribs are supported by the bolster, your tailbone is descending toward the floor, and your shoulders and head are on the floor (A). (If your neck is uncomfortable, put a folded towel or blanket under it.) Extend through your legs and place your arms out at your sides, elbows bent and palms up. Rest in this position, eyes closed, for 5 minutes.

CYCLE Without moving your torso, allow your legs to open out to the sides (B). Remain in this position, breathing normally, for 3 to 5 minutes.

Again keeping your torso in the same position, bend your knees, cross your legs at the ankles, and continue in the pose for another 3 to 5 minutes (C).

Gently push away from the wall until your buttocks are just off the bolster and resting on the floor; the tops of your thighs and legs remain on the bolster (D). Rest in this position for 5 minutes, or as long as you like.

To come out of the pose, uncross your legs, push gently away from the bolster, and roll to one side. Breathe quietly for a few breaths, then use your arms to help you to a seated position.

EFFECTS This pose helps calm your nerves, balance your endocrine system, relieve fatigue, and increase blood flow to your pelvic region. It also offers your body complete relaxation.

†CAUTION Do not do this pose if you are menstruating.

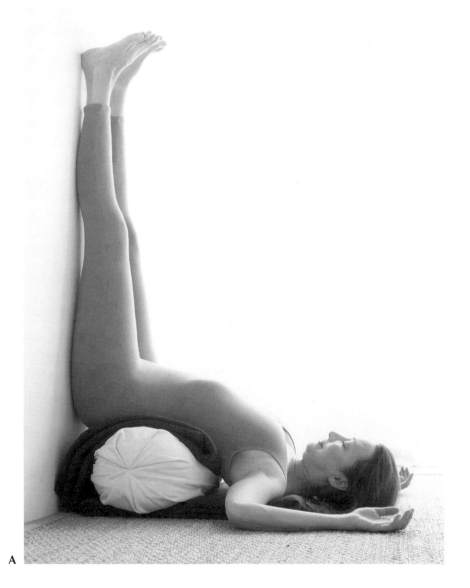

A

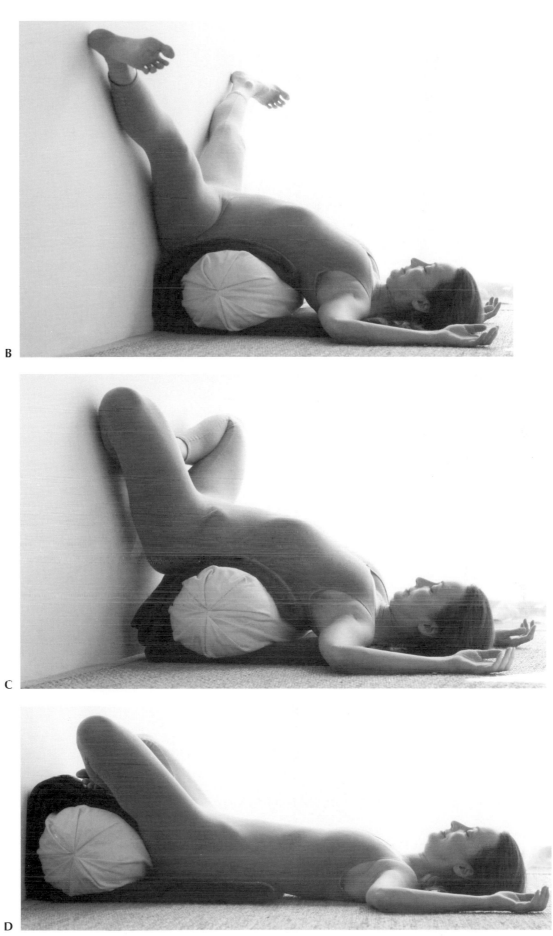

B

C

D

PART TWO

The Time of Awakening

Introduction

When my daughters were growing up, our house was like Grand Central Station. They and their friends saw it as a place to eat, hang out, laugh, and even cry when things just weren't going their way. Because I wasn't their mom, most of my daughters' friends liked talking to me and trusted me with tales of love gone sour, daring escapades, friends who betrayed them, and enemies who befriended them. I learned when to ask questions, when to give advice, and when to shut my mouth and just listen. And I saw anew that the teenage/young adult years can be as frustrating as they are exhilarating.

Pubescence is filled with societal pressures, wildly erratic hormones, and conflicting messages from family and friends. I'm sure you're well aware of how the media shape (and warp) your sense of self, how it bombards you with unrealistic images of sticklike women who have perfect skin, teeth, and hair. All of this makes the new body you're discovering—with its acne, braces, and sometimes expanding hips—that much harder to handle. You sometimes feel like you're on an emotional roller-coaster.

Although the conditions explored in the next three chapters apply to women in other stages of life, too, Patricia and I have chosen to place them within this stage because this is when they're likely to surface for the first time. You'll discover that yoga works in many wonderful ways. Whether you're a teenager or a college student, yoga can help ease the horrendous cramps you get every month, calm you down when you have PMS (or final-exam jitters), jump-start a sluggish period or regulate an overly active one, and even prevent colds and flus.

While these physical benefits are all well and good, the greatest gifts yoga brings you are those of strength, awareness, and self-love or self acceptance. No matter how awkward you feel in "real" life, a yoga class offers you a safe haven from your own insecurities and the judgments of others. The poses teach you to stand firm in your power, to reach out to the world from the core of your body. The strength you derive from yoga is emotional as well as physical.

During yoga class, you are free to explore your own body, your own emotional needs, and your own thoughts, unencumbered by the outside world. Moving from pose to pose, allowing your breath to take you deeper into your body, you learn to pay attention to what's going on inside. This gift of awareness can be a powerful ally. After all, it's a great lesson to learn that feelings can change from moment to moment; it's even more exciting to discover that you can survive them!

Many teenagers and young women I spoke with expressed their gratitude for yoga. Ellen and Sophia, two sixteen-year-olds from Massachusetts, couldn't stop talking about how much they love it. They started taking classes when they were 12, and they agree that yoga is about more than just poses—it's about community, trusting and loving the teacher, and feeling safe. Sophia, who became severely

57

depressed and suffered from anxiety disorders when she hit puberty, explained, "Yoga helps me stay with and in my body like nothing else does. I think it's partly because of the supportive environment of the class, and partly because yoga itself transcends this stuff." Ellen said she wanted other young women to know that yoga can be anything you want it to be—invigorating, dreamy, strengthening, opening. But more than anything else, she said, "Whether or not you can do the poses is not the issue. It's not about doing the poses exactly right, but that you allow your body to be where it needs to be. After all, wherever you are in your poses, in your body, or in your life, you're safe right there. Yoga is about being present to yourself, facilitating whatever you do in your life."

Chapter 4   *Befriending Your Body*

KAREN IS A SELF-PROCLAIMED DIET JUNKIE. SHE'S TRIED WEIGHT Watchers at least a dozen times. She's been on the Zone, the Akins diet, the Pritikin plan, and the Fit-or-Fat solution. She's even popped diet pills. Desperate to lose thirty pounds, she once went on a ten-day grape fast. She lost the weight, but gained it right back again. In fact, Karen admits, over the last five years of on-again, off-again dieting, she's "probably lost the same thirty pounds every year!" Exercising is akin to torture in her mind, but she knows it speeds up her metabolism and helps her lose weight. So, she's joined her local gym and she's taken up jogging, which she hates. "I can't stand going to the gym— there are so many mirrors in that place, constant reminders of how ugly my body looks. And, working out with all those already-beautiful bodies makes me feel worse, so I go home and console myself with a bowl of ice cream or a plate of chocolate-chip cookies. Then I hate myself even more for being so weak."

Karen's predicament is far from unusual. One expert wryly commented that 99 percent of all women suffer from a distorted body image. Judging from the popularity of today's innumerable weight-loss programs, that comment may not be far off the mark. Most women have been obsessed with some part of their anatomy at one time in their lives—their hips, breasts, double chins, or waistlines. According to the Council on Size and Weight Discrimination, statistics tell a discouraging story: 75 percent of all American women are dissatisfied with their appearance; 50 percent of all American women are on a diet, including 50 percent of nine-year-old girls and 80 percent of ten-year-olds. Ninety percent of U.S. high school juniors and seniors diet, even though only between 10 and 15 percent of them are overweight.

With numbers like that, you'd think American women would be trimmer than ever before. Unfortunately, according to the Council, 90 to 99 percent of all reducing diets fail and over two-thirds of dieters regain what they've lost within a year. Even so, the diet industry is a multibillion-dollar-a-year conglomerate, which continues to feed (pardon the pun) off society's unhealthy obsession with thinness.

Besides being bombarded with media images that show thin, beautiful women as the paradigm for health and fitness, young women are taught that excess weight invites major health risks—high blood pressure, heart disease, and cancer. But, in fact, women who spend their lives going from one diet to another risk more health problems from extreme weight fluctuations than those women who are consistently overweight. According to Genia Pauli Haddon, creator of the *Yoga for Round Bodies* video series, "much of the health risk from obesity may be the result of stress and self-rejection, due to repeated failed efforts to reduce weight, and internalized messages that round bodies are both unattractive and dangerous to our health." She certainly knows what she's talking about. As a "hefty person who kept 'failing' to become thin," Genia decided a dozen years ago that "if I could accept myself as I am, if I could find a way to enjoy being in my body as it is, then I should be healthier than if I kept trying to lose weight."

ANOREXIA NERVOSA

Unfortunately, for many women, enjoying their body "as it is" doesn't feel like an option. In fact, their fixation with thinness becomes more than an unhealthy desire to lose weight; it turns into an obsession that can lead to death. Clearly no one embarks on a diet with anorexia nervosa in mind. But, nonetheless, this dangerous condition, in which victims literally starve themselves to death, claims approximately 1 percent of all adolescent girls and 5 percent of all young college women, according to statistics released by the National Association of Anorexia Nervosa and Associated Disorders (ANAD). Many experts say the numbers could be as high as three out of every hundred young women. If you suffer from this disease, you know how insidious it is and how utterly and completely it can take hold of your life. If you compete as a gymnast, are a ballet dancer, or train in any sport or discipline that places a strict limitation on weight, you stand an even greater chance of succumbing to anorexia.

Generally speaking, the disease begins when your desire to be thin conflicts with your body's natural size. Let's say that you normally weigh 115 pounds, but you want to weigh 105, so you go on a diet to lose those 10 pounds. Since your body feels perfectly healthy at 115, it resists your attempts to impose that lower goal. It slows down its metabolism, storing fat more efficiently, and increases its appetite for fatty, sugary foods. Your frustration with and hatred toward your body escalate, and you respond by withholding even more nourishment.

Specialists have, in fact, identified what they call an anorexic personality. According to literature from the National Eating Disorders Organization (NEDO), anorexics tend toward perfectionism, bordering on obsessive-compulsive behavior. These good girls, who rarely disobey their teachers or their parents, make excellent students and athletes, but tend to keep their feelings to themselves. Because they have followed the wishes of others most of their lives, they are ill equipped to handle the typical problems and stresses of growing up. What they eat and what they deny themselves give them a way of controlling at least one aspect of their lives—their own bodies.

If you are like most anorexics, you have a hard time admitting you have a problem. In fact, the newfound sense of control and power you feel when you can make yourself lose weight is not an easy thing to give up, so you are not likely to seek out therapy to stop your behavior.

This mind-set makes anorexia nervosa one of the hardest mental illnesses to cure.

Unfortunately, anorexia nervosa can be life-threatening. According to the National Institute of Mental Health (NIMH), this obsessive-compulsive disorder claims the lives of up to 20 percent of its victims and has a cure rate of only 50 percent. Long-lasting effects include heart irregularities, reduced muscle mass, low blood pressure, osteoporosis, decreased sexual appetite, cessation of ovulation (which prevents the anorexic from ever getting pregnant), and permanent brain damage.

BULIMIA NERVOSA

Researchers at NIMH say that at least 2 to 3 percent of all adolescent girls suffer from bulimia, a destructive ritual of overeating followed by vomiting, laxative abuse, or obsessive exercise to purge their bodies of calories and control their weight. Other experts say those numbers are too conservative, and that one in five young college women purges regularly.

Outgoing, adventurous, and impulsive, a young bulimic girl often looks like an all-American teenager of average weight. But underneath the facade, her obsession with food and dieting rivals that of her sister anorexic. However, unlike the anorexic who refuses to eat, a bulimic binges on enormous amounts of food before she forces herself to vomit (often several times a day) or uses laxatives or enemas to rid her body of excess calories. Anorexics may feel strong in their resolve to conquer their bodies, but if you suffer from bulimia you are more apt to battle shame and confusion about the behavior you keep hidden from your family, roommates, and friends. Interestingly enough, most bulimics begin bingeing and purging in their teens, but they don't seek help until well into their thirties or forties. By then the behavior is so ingrained that it's almost impossible to treat. To make matters worse, if you suffer from bulimia, you often fight other compulsive disorders such as alcoholism, drug abuse, or sexual addiction.

If you are bulimic, you run the risk of serious health problems associated with binging and purging. Heart failure from loss of vital minerals is common; so are kidney stones and even kidney failure. Violent and frequent bingeing and purging can even cause the stomach to rupture in rare instances. Other less deadly effects include damage to the esophagus and the intestinal lining, hemorrhages in the blood vessels of the eyes through excessive and forceful vomiting, and swollen neck glands. The acid from excessive vomiting can cause tooth enamel to erode, and the stress you put your body through can cause ovulation to stop.

COMPULSIVE OR BINGE EATING

If you are a compulsive or binge eater, you're not alone. The National Institute of Mental Health estimates that at least 2 percent of the teenage population suffers along with you. Much like a bulimic, if you have a compulsive eating disorder, you crave and consume large amounts of food, sometimes as often as six or seven times a day. The difference between you and your bulimic sister, however, is that you don't finish the ritual by purging your body of the calories you've consumed. According to NIMH, most compulsive eaters are obese and have a history of wild weight fluctuations, which leaves them prone to high blood pressure, high cholesterol, diabetes, heart disease, and gallbladder problems. To compound these physical ailments, most struggle to overcome depression and anxiety, making them a high risk for suicide.

WHAT CAUSES EATING DISORDERS?

Specialists agree that Western society's fixation on excessively thin models and celebrities causes many young girls to despise and punish themselves for the curves puberty has brought to their adolescent bodies. But why do some young women react so violently to these messages, while others appear to take them in stride?

The fact is no one knows for sure. Most eating disorder specialists agree that a combination of social, biological, and environmental factors contribute to the disease. In a conversation I had a couple of years ago with Jody Yeary, Ph.D., a San Francisco psychologist specializing in eating disorder therapy, she stated the obvious: "Eating disorders begin when people go on diets; you don't get an eating disorder if you don't start dieting." Gretchen Newmark, a licensed dietitian and clinical nutritionist whose practice focuses on weight management and eating disorders, blames our society's demand that women be thin for many a teenager's descent into anorexia, bulimia, and compulsive eating disorders. In fact, she says, she often wonders why more girls don't succumb to the disease.

It's no coincidence that most eating disorders begin shortly after puberty, a stressful time in itself, when your hormone levels start to fluctuate, making your body curvier. Your parents may insist that the weight gain is temporary, but you're not so sure; your body has betrayed you and you no longer feel in control of how you look. Besides, "temporary" can seem like forever when your peers—and society as a whole, for that matter—judge you strictly on how you look. Even if you know in your head that this obsession with thinness isn't healthy for you, it's sometimes hard to ignore when you're inundated with examples of how thin, "beautiful" bodies seemingly lead to happiness, friends, dates, and all the good things in life.

Of course, longing to fit in and be popular with boys isn't the only reason young girls abuse their bodies this way. For some, the idea of being sexually attractive to boys is actually traumatic and shameful; these girls may try to starve their bodies back to a more childlike appearance. For others, family dynamics (alcoholism, physical or emotional abuse, divorce) push them to use food as a way of blocking out pain or gaining a sense of control in a world that increasingly fails to make sense. One such girl, now recovering from anorexia, told me she would have sought therapy much earlier had her mother actually noticed her sudden weight loss and showed some concern.

Because eating disorders appear to run in families, Dr. Yeary believes successful treatment depends on involving the whole family. Researchers at NIMH cite one study that found that a young girl whose mother is overly concerned with her daughter's weight and attractiveness, and whose father is overly critical of her appearance, is more likely to develop an eating disorder. Still other researchers note that mothers who obsessively and vocally worry about their own weight and body image send a strong message to their daughters that equates physical appearance to self-worth and personal success. And, of course, girls involved in activities like gymnastics, cheerleading, dance, and track and field—all of which prescribe an ideal weight— often suffer from eating problems.

BIOCHEMICAL INDICATORS

One research study funded by NIMH has begun to focus on the biochemical malfunctions of those suffering from eating disorders, looking particularly at the neuroendocrine system, a combination of the central nervous system and the body's hormones. This system controls a multitude of activities in the body and the mind, including sexual function, physical development, appetite and digestion, sleep patterns, heart and kidney function, emotions, thinking, and memory. Scientists already know that people suffering from depression exhibit low levels of serotonin and norepinephrine; since many people with eating disorders also battle depression, their systems may lack adequate amounts of these neurotransmitters as well.

The same research group also found higher levels of cortisol—a hormone released during times of stress—in the brains of both anorexics and people with clinical depression, which may be caused by a malfunction in the hypothalamus. (The hypothalamus is a tiny gland near the emotional center of the brain that is responsible for regulating the body's basic needs such as hunger, thirst, sexual desire, and body temperature.) Other hormones found to be outside normal limits include vasopressin, released during times of acute physical and emotional stress, and cholecystokinin (CCK), a hormone that causes the body to feel full after eating. Scientists have found very low levels of CCK in bulimics, leading them to wonder whether that's what prevents these young women from feeling sated as they consume large amounts of food.

THE AYURVEDIC THEORY

Nancy Lonsdorf, M.D., a Western physician and Ayurvedic healer, and her coauthors offer the Ayurvedic explanation for eating disorders in their book *A Woman's Best Medicine: Health, Happiness, and Long Life through Ayurveda*. In keeping with India's three-thousand-year-old healing system, the authors explain that everything you experience through your senses and your mind affects you physiologically. In fact, they write that you "ingest and digest everything" from the air you breathe to the behavior of the people around you. Teenage life is difficult enough, but if you're suddenly faced with additional stresses—you have to lose weight for ballet, your boyfriend dumps you, your grandmother dies—it all becomes too much for you to process; you may even blame yourself for all the stress you feel. Some young women then punish themselves by withholding nourishment, which Lonsdorf calls a form of self-loathing. The more you deny yourself, of course, the further away from yourself you travel and the less likely you will be able to hear or feel what your body really needs.

CONVENTIONAL TREATMENT

Physicians and therapists specializing in eating disorders don't always agree on the best course of treatment, but they unanimously say that early intervention is critical. In Kristin Leutwyler's article published in the women's health issue of *Scientific American,* Katherine Halmi, M.D., professor of psychiatry at Cornell University and director of the Eating Disorders Clinic at New York Hospital, offers the following sobering statistics: 7.7 percent of anorexics will die within the first ten years; a whopping 25 percent will succumb after suffering for thirty years. Specialists also agree that anorexics must reach 90 percent of their normal weight to have the best chance of a full recovery, something most anorexics are loath to do. Some therapists have had good results by first giving anorexics just enough food to maintain their current weight and then increasing the caloric amounts gradually, no more than two hundred additional calories a week. But to succeed, therapy must address the psychological issues of any eating disorder, not just the physical ones. Furthermore, Dr. Yeary says it's counterproductive to wait until these young women hit rock bottom to intervene, because once the eating disorder becomes a part of "their developmental evolvement, it becomes a part of them. They completely lose their identity into the eating disorder" and they can no longer separate themselves from their behavior.

Conventional treatment includes medical intervention, psychotherapy with the patient and her family, nutritional counseling, and often hospitalization. Some doctors have had limited success with antidepressants such as Zoloft and Prozac, especially in treating bulimics and binge eaters who suffer from depression as well. Few therapists see these drugs as a panacea; in fact, they rarely work for anorexics.

Some therapists believe that food allergies play a role, especially for compulsive eaters. Overeaters Anonymous encourages its members to refrain from using white sugar, white flour, and processed foods, and many say those simple dietary changes have kept them symptom-free. Some bulimics and binge eaters actually suffer from candidiasis, a condition that causes yeast to run rampant in the intestines and provoke strong food cravings, so it doesn't hurt to get a complete physical to rule that out.

Unfortunately, if you are battling anorexia, you know that it's really hard to admit you have a problem, which is a vital step for treatment to work; even if you do want to get better, the idea of gaining weight can be frightening at best. If you struggle with bulimia or compulsive overeating, the good news is that you may benefit from group therapy and cognitive behavioral therapy.

HOW YOGA CAN HELP

Whether you struggle with your weight like Karen in the opening story or suffer from a full-blown eating disorder, yoga can help. Hatha yoga and gentle pranayama exercises can provide relief for those struggling with any kind of eating disorder or body image fixation. Gretchen Newmark says that yoga is a good therapeutic agent because "it focuses on the body from the inside. It centers on strength, flexibility, balance, and breath rather than on appearance."

Genia Pauli Haddon, of *Yoga for Round Bodies*, agrees. Yoga, she says, helps many young women focus less on weight loss as a goal and more on being as healthy as possible with the bodies they have. She finds that allowing yoga to ease her beyond her old limitations was far more effective than trying to change her body (its weight, flexibility, or strength) through sheer willpower. Although the first two years of her practice did trim fifty pounds off her figure, without dieting, the biggest change for Genia was that she felt good about her round body for the first time. She claims, "I've learned by experience that the yogic way to reach my goals is to let go of them and simply enjoy yoga every day." She recommends that instead of fixing your attention on the ways in which you want your body to be different, you become acutely observant of your body as it is. Observe it anew every time you enter a posture, becoming absorbed in the sensations of each present moment. "Yoga has taught me that the most powerful agent for transformation is this kind of conscious, loving attention."

The best advice Genia shares with her students is to reassess their goals. "The goal should never be to look like a picture of someone else doing the posture or to criticize yourself for not being different than you are," she cautions. "Let your intention be to discover how each posture lives within your own unique body, even as you pay careful attention to your teacher's instructions for good alignment." Whatever your struggles may be, whatever issues you have about your figure and self-image, Genia's advice serves as a constant reminder to trust your own body and its ability to teach you the nuances of what is best for you.

The biggest challenge therapists face in recommending yoga to their clients is getting them to do it. Many anorexics reject yoga because it's not aerobic and

Patricia Says

Besides offering emotional and spiritual support, yoga provides physiological help to reverse or minimize the long-lasting effects of starving or bingeing on food.

• Inversions are a young girl's best friend. They work by helping to balance your endocrine (glandular) system and stabilize blood pressure (which can fall dangerously low if you're anorexic) and jump-starting delayed menstruation.

• Shoulderstand (Sarvangasana), a favorite among many teenage yoga students, calms your nervous system and arrests the fight-or-flight response that chronic stress triggers in your body (see chapter 6 for more information). Because it employs a chin lock, Shoulderstand stabilizes your thyroid as well.

• Forward bends calm your adrenal glands, which work overtime when your body is under stress.

• Standing and balancing poses build strength.

• Twists and backbends activate your adrenal glands and help them perform properly.

they can't burn enough calories. Amie, a client of Gretchen Newmark's who has both anorexia and bulimia, says yoga wasn't easy at the beginning. She resisted because she felt she wasn't accomplishing anything. In the first three classes, when she lay in a resting pose, all she could think about was how many calories she'd ingested that day and how many she had burned so far. But by her fourth class, she began to really enjoy it. She not only felt accomplished in many of the stronger poses, but as she settled into Corpse Pose (Savasana), she felt a sense of calm she hadn't experienced before.

By the time she had completed a month of classes, Amie realized something else: Yoga had replaced her habit of bingeing and purging. She was used to performing that ritual in the evening, but she no longer has time because that's when her yoga class meets. Yoga became the new habit that shook up and eventually will replace the old one. Marion Woodman, Jungian therapist and author of *Addiction to Perfection*, emphasizes this point. She says that addicts are masters at creating ritual and women suffering from eating disorders are no different. The key to recovery, according to Woodman, is "finding a creative outlet to break the old pattern. You have to find your own way of expressing who you are."

Those who are bulimic, as Amie attested, are not always eager to give up their nightly bingeing and purging. Compulsive eaters often feel such shame and self-loathing that they can't conceive of their bodies doing anything like yoga postures. In fact, one woman admitted she was reluctant to go to a yoga class designed especially for round bodies, because she feared that other students would be horrified to see just how round she really was. And what if she got into a pose and couldn't get out of it? She'd be too mortified to ask for help.

No matter what type of eating disorder you suffer from, doing only the more rigorous forms of yoga like Ashtanga or Bikram is not the answer. If you are anorexic, you don't really need active, flowing sequences to feel more capable or more powerful, because you don't really experience yourself as weak or helpless. Calorie-burning poses are what you seek; after all, how can a restorative yoga practice make your hips smaller? If you are bulimic or a binge eater, you certainly don't want to get too close to your emotions, either. However, what you really need to help you heal are the restorative poses, which allow you to turn your attention inward and make friends with your body.

Unfortunately, it's not easy to introduce the more meditative poses to women suffering with eating disorders. According to Newmark, a yoga teacher herself, the impulsive, agitated state of bulimics and compulsive eaters, as well as the underdeveloped nervous system and electrolyte imbalance of anorexics, make lying still in Corpse Pose (Savasana) or sitting in meditation almost impossible at first. Most yoga teachers who work with anorexics or bulimics believe that you can succeed more often with a well-rounded, though not rigorous, practice. As an anorexic, in particular, you gain a lot of power by denying your body nourishment. Yoga, in contrast, can show you a way to gain that sense of power in partnership with your body rather than against it.

Yoga and Your Emotions

Yoga can also challenge you by bringing you face-to-face with your emotions—not always an easy place to be. On a physical level, an anorexic works very hard not to experience hunger pangs, dizziness, and fatigue. On an emotional level, she separates herself from any sensations that crop up; they may prove too painful for her to deal with. Lying still on your yoga mat with no place to go, nothing to achieve, and no one to impress, there's nothing to stop your emotions, sensations, and feelings from coming to the surface. It can be exhilarating or it can be frightening, but as Patricia says, you soon learn that you are not your feelings, that you can survive them, and that you can empower yourself in healthful ways.

If you suffer from bulimia or compulsive eating, you also may be divorced from your emotions. In fact, the very nature of your bingeing is unconscious. As Jungian analyst Marion Woodman points out, food has a way of "keeping the pain down and the fear away." Newmark says that when many of her clients (like Amie) first begin therapy and yoga, they often feel a lot worse. "They start to notice they're really unhappy," she says. "That they're really in a lot of emotional pain." And they get scared. For some women, yoga may be too internal, too close to the heart, and they're reluctant to go there.

But for others, yoga offers a safe place to explore their feelings, because it starts on a physical level with the body. Amie is a good example. By discovering that she could stay in a pose and be fine—even when it felt uncomfortable, even when she wanted to run away—she learned a few valuable lessons: She doesn't have to act on every impulse (including her desires to binge or withhold food); she can be patient; and she can trust her body to tell her what it needs. She even admits that she now looks forward to her thrice-weekly class, because it's the only time in her day that she doesn't wonder, "Am I fat? Am I thin? Am I attractive or not?" Instead she wonders, "Can I hold this pose? Can I balance?"

But, most important, yoga teaches young women like Amie that if they can survive the discomfort of a difficult pose, they can survive their feelings, too. Carla, a compulsive binger, remembers the day she discovered that her body could actually move into a modified Warrior Pose II (Virabhadrasana II) without getting stuck or falling over. "It was the first day I can ever remember feeling proud of myself." Genia Pauli Haddon echoes this sentiment: "As I learned to stay present through yoga, I used food less as a substitute way of feeling better." And Rosie, a young bulimic from Wisconsin, found that a consistent

Yoga Practice Dos and Don'ts

• If you are a compulsive eater or bulimic, you may experience vomit reflux (the feeling that you need to throw up) when you first try inversions or standing forward bends. If so, begin with easier, supported inversions like Legs-Up-the-Wall Pose (Viparita Karani) and forward bends like Wide-Angle Standing Forward Bend (Prasarita Padottanasana), but keep your head up. These poses will get easier rather quickly.

• If lying in Corpse Pose (Savasana) agitates you, don't force yourself to remain in this position. Stay there for just a few breaths. Try sitting up, breathing with your eyes closed, and then returning to the pose, or even standing in Mountain Pose (Tadasana) for a few breaths.

• Look for a local yoga class where the atmosphere is supportive, not competitive, and where the teacher is comfortable working with props so you can adjust poses to fit your body's needs. Practicing yoga with like-minded/like-bodied women makes a difference.

• Everyone's body is unique. What works for one woman may not be right for you. Trust that your body can teach you the nuances of what is best for you.

yoga practice helped calm her jittery, nervous energy and gave her a way of focusing on her body that wasn't negative or destructive.

All of the teenagers I spoke with agreed that while yoga definitely helps them physiologically and emotionally, the key to its power lies in the safety of the class, the sense of kinship they feel with the other members of the group. None felt judged on how she looked or what she said. One young girl said that her teacher always has a pose for "anything we may be going through." Another one said that the group of girls doing yoga together is so nurturing that it "allows us to be whoever we want to be and the class becomes whatever we need it to be on any given day."

Jill Minye, my friend and yoga teacher from northern California, has worked with countless young women suffering from obsessive-compulsive disorders, including anorexia, bulimia, and alcohol and drug addiction. She's told me amazing stories of young women whose lives have been turned around through therapy that includes a consistent, well-rounded yoga practice. What does she recommend? Do standing poses to help you feel strong and grounded. Through asanas like Warrior (Virabhadrasana) or Extended Triangle Pose (Utthita Trikonasana), you can learn how to stand on your own two feet; practice being in your power and in the world. For an anorexic or a bulimic, standing poses teach that power is not confined to what you deny yourself or what you allow yourself to do. For a compulsive eater, it is not confined to how you protect yourself. No matter what your eating challenges, you can learn to hold power in a single moment—as in Mountain Pose (Tadasana)—and it will feel wonderful. These tiny moments of success bring the realization that "Hey, I did the pose, I didn't fall over, and I got to the next moment intact!" Jill also recommends balancing poses to help you "get out of your head" by focusing attention on your center.

Patricia includes backbends, which she says open up the chest and can have a remarkable effect on well-being, and inversions, which can be emotionally balancing. Restorative poses, including Corpse Pose (Savasana), offer deep relaxation and surrender, qualities that Gretchen Newmark says are markedly different from the need to control that young women with eating disorders cling to.

The attention to breathing in yoga class brings women even more in touch with their emotions. Amie remembers the relief—and joy—she felt when she first discovered that her breath happened all by itself, naturally. She didn't have to control it, and she learned that if she just paused and waited, the breath would come again. For many women, it's their first lesson in letting go. For others, just learning how to breathe properly proves to be a great stress reliever. The deep, relaxed state that yoga brings helps you become receptive to positive suggestions from your yoga teacher and ultimately your own body.

Patricia Says

I've given two types of sequences here. The first one begins more vigorously and offers plenty of poses to make you feel powerful and capable, as well as a few to help you relax completely—an essential part of yoga. Use the wall as a support in the standing poses if you need to, or modify any of the poses as described in the Woman's Restorative Sequence in chapter 3. Don't get discouraged if you can't do some of the poses; there is definitely value in trying—you'll be amazed at how quickly your body will respond to your efforts.

The second sequence begins with restorative poses and works up to the more challenging poses. This is a nice sequence if you feel depressed or just low in energy, because the first few postures are designed to open your chest and heart (which serves to open your mind and enliven your spirits). These are followed by forward bends that calm your nervous system and cool your brain.

A SEQUENCE FOR EATING DISORDERS: STRENGTHEN AND ENERGIZE

Many young women who suffer from poor body image, even if they don't have acute eating disorders, benefit from this strengthening and energizing sequence. The standing and balancing poses will bring a sense of strength and accomplishment that is not connected to the foods you eat (or don't eat). And the final poses offer a relaxing treat for your whole body and mind.

1. Mountain Pose (Tadasana)
2. Mountain Pose with Arms Overhead (Urdhva Hastasana in Tadasana)
3. Extended Triangle Pose (Utthita Trikonasana)
4. Warrior II Pose (Virabhadrasana II)
5. Extended Side-Angle Pose (Utthita Parsvakonasana)
6. Half-Moon Pose (Ardha Chandrasana)
7. Wide-Angle Standing Forward Bend (Prasarita Padottanasana)
8. Downward-Facing Dog Pose (Adho Mukha Svanasana)
9. Standing Forward Bend (Uttanasana)
10. Child's Pose (Adho Mukha Virasana)
11. Simple Seated Twist Pose (Bharadvajasana)
12. Headstand (Sirsasana)
13. Inverted Staff Pose (Viparita Dandasana)
14. Upward-Facing Bow Pose (Urdhva Dhanurasana)
15. Shoulderstand (Sarvangasana)
16. Plough Pose (Halasana)
17. Bridge Pose (Setu Bandha Sarvangasana)
18. Legs-Up-the-Wall Pose (Viparita Karani)
19. Corpse Pose (Savasana)

1. MOUNTAIN POSE (Tadasana) Stand up straight, your legs together (with big toes touching, if that's comfortable). Distribute your weight evenly between the front of your feet and your heels. Tighten your knees by pulling up with your quadricep (front thigh) muscles. Raise your sternum (breastbone) and broaden your chest by rolling your shoulders back and drawing your shoulder blades in. Lift your abdomen up and draw your tailbone in without pushing your thighs forward. Extend your arms downward with palms facing your thighs and fingers together. Keep your shoulders moving away from your ears. It is normal to have some curvature in your lumbar area (lower back). Stand in this posture for 20 to 30 seconds—or longer—breathing normally and keeping your face, neck, and throat relaxed.

EFFECTS This pose opens your chest, improves respiration and circulation, and helps you to correct postural problems. It can also help you feel strong and grounded.

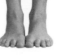

2. MOUNTAIN POSE WITH ARMS OVERHEAD (Urdhva Hastasana in Tadasana) Stand in Mountain Pose (Tadasana). Lift your arms to the side and over your head, palms facing each other. Keep your shoulders down and away from your ears. Lift your chest and draw your shoulder blades deep into your back. Breathe normally for 20 to 30 seconds. To come out, release your arms down to your sides.

EFFECTS This pose enlivens your whole body, eases stiffness in your shoulders and upper back, and helps correct postural alignment.

3. EXTENDED TRIANGLE POSE (Utthita Trikonasana) Stand in Mountain Pose (Tadasana). Step your feet about 3½ feet apart; turn your left foot out 90 degrees and your right foot slightly inward. The heel of your left foot should line up with the arch of your right. (Place a block beside the outside edge of your left foot if you need to.) Stretch your arms out to the sides, draw up through your quadriceps, and lift your abdomen and chest. On an exhalation, keeping your back straight, extend your trunk to the left and bring your left hand down to the floor or the block. Press your hand into the floor or block, stretch across your chest and up through your right arm. Draw your shoulder blades in, turn your chest toward the ceiling, and look straight ahead or up at your right hand. Breathe normally for 20 to 30 seconds. On an inhalation, lift up and straighten your torso. Repeat the pose on your right side before returning to Mountain Pose.

EFFECTS This pose elongates and strengthens your spine; brings flexibility to back muscles; tones your legs; and helps balance your liver, kidney, and spleen function. It's a powerful pose that can help you learn to stand your ground and build strength and determination.

Modification

4. WARRIOR II POSE (Virabhadrasana II) Stand in Mountain Pose (Tadasana). Step your feet as far apart as is comfortable (about 4½ feet); turn your left foot out 90 degrees and your right foot slightly inward. The heel of your left foot should line up with the arch of your right. Stretch your arms out to the sides so they're parallel to the floor. As you exhale, bend your left knee so your thigh is parallel and your shin is perpendicular to the floor. (If your knee extends beyond your ankle, you need to widen your stance.) Turn your head to look over your left arm just past your fingertips. Imagine both arms are engaged in a tug-of-war. Remain in the pose for 20 to 30 seconds, if possible. If not, come in and out of the pose several times.

EFFECTS This pose helps you build strength, confidence, and a feeling of power. It also tones your legs, hips, and thighs.

5. EXTENDED SIDE-ANGLE POSE (Utthita Parsvakonasana) Follow the instructions for Warrior II Pose (Virabhadrasana II), bending your left knee so your thigh is parallel and your shin is perpendicular to the floor. (If your knee extends beyond your ankle, you need to widen your stance.) Keeping your back straight, exhale and extend your trunk to the left, bring your left hand down to the floor (or a block), and stretch your right arm up over your right ear. Draw your shoulder blades in, turn your chest toward the ceiling, and look straight ahead or up toward the ceiling. Turn your abdomen to the right. Breathe normally and hold this pose for 20 to 30 seconds, if possible. Inhale as you lift up and straighten your torso. Repeat the pose on your right side, then turn your toes forward and step your feet back to Mountain Pose (Tadasana).

EFFECTS This pose elongates and strengthens your spine and helps relieve joint stiffness, particularly in your hips, groin, hamstrings, and shoulders. It can also help you build strength, confidence, and determination.

Modification

6. HALF-MOON POSE (Ardha Chandrasana) Do Extended Triangle Pose (Utthita Trikonasana) to the left (see page 70). Bending your left leg so your knee extends beyond your ankle, place the fingertips of your left hand on the floor (or a block) about a foot in front of your left leg. Raise your right heel off the floor and come up onto your toes. With an exhalation, simultaneously straighten your left leg and raise your right up until it is parallel to the floor (or slightly higher). Turn your pelvic area and chest toward the ceiling. Stretch your right arm up in line with your shoulders and open your chest and pelvis further. Draw your shoulder blades into your back and expand your chest. Look up at your right hand or straight ahead. Hold this position for 10 to 15 seconds, breathing normally.

To come down, bend your left leg, while reaching your right leg back. Return to Extended Triangle Pose (Utthita Trikonasana). Inhale, lift up to standing, repeat the pose on the other side, and return to Mountain Pose.

EFFECTS This pose helps strengthen your legs, energize your body, and promote balance. Many girls and women find it helps to alleviate depression and ease heavy bleeding.

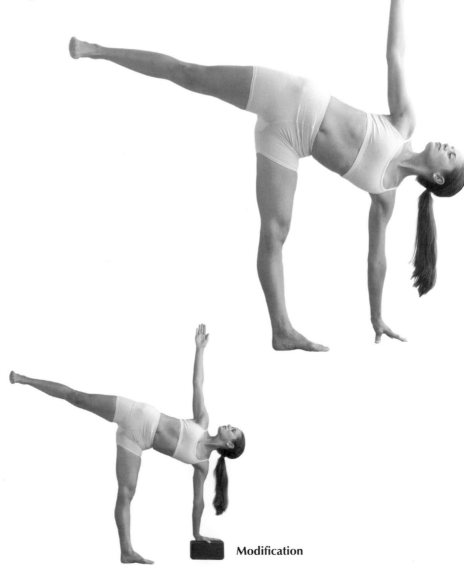

Modification

7. WIDE-ANGLE STANDING FORWARD BEND (Prasarita Padottanasana) Step your feet apart about 4 feet (or as wide as possible), keeping the outer edges of your feet parallel. Tighten your quadriceps to draw your kneecaps up and keep your thighs well lifted. On an exhalation, bend forward from your hips and place your hands on the floor—in line with your shoulders—between your feet. (If you feel strain in your lower back, place your hands on blocks.) Lift your hips toward the ceiling, draw your shoulder blades into your back, and extend your chest forward (A). Look up and extend your trunk forward, keeping your entire spine concave. Remain this way for 10 to 15 seconds.

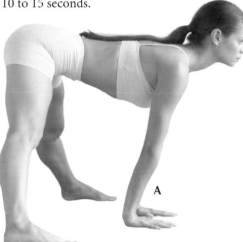

Keeping your trunk extended, exhale, bend your elbows, and release the crown of your head toward the floor—resting it on the floor, if possible (B). Keep your legs firm, but relax your shoulders and neck. Breathe deeply and let your trunk release downward. (If you experience vomit reflux or are concerned about keeping your balance, keep your head lifted or support your head on a bolster or a folded blanket or two.) Breathe normally for 30 to 60 seconds.

To come out, return to the concave back position, bring your hands to your hips, and raise your trunk. Step your feet together.

EFFECTS This pose can help calm your nerves and mind, increase flexibility in the backs of your legs, and ease a heavy period.

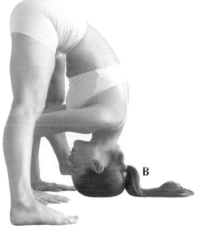

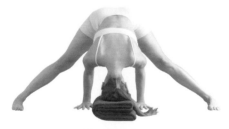

Modification

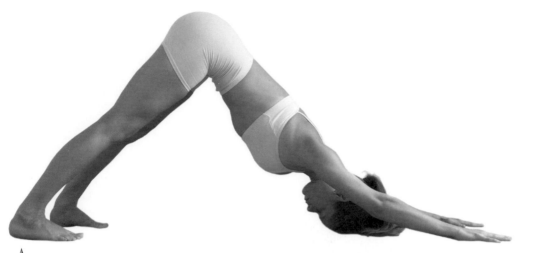

8. DOWNWARD-FACING DOG POSE (Adho Mukha Svanasana) To find the correct distance between your hands and feet for this pose, lie facedown on your sticky mat. Place your palms on the floor by each side of your chest with your fingers well spread and pointing straight ahead. Come up on your hands and knees, and turn your toes under.

Exhale, press your hands firmly into the mat and extend up through your inner arms. Inhale, and as you exhale again, raise your buttocks high into the air and move your thighs up and back. Keep stretching through your legs and bring your heels toward the floor. Keep the legs firm and the elbows straight as you lift your buttocks upward. The action of the arms and legs serves to elongate your spine and release your head. Hold this pose for 30 seconds to 1 minute, breathing deeply. Let your head rest completely and release the base of your neck. To come out, either return to your hands and knees and sit back on your heels or step the feet forward into Standing Forward Bend (Uttanasana) and slowly stand up.

EFFECTS This is a wonderful pose for fighting depression. It can increase your circulation and calm your mind. It also strengthens and elongates your back, shoulders, and legs.

9. STANDING FORWARD BEND (Uttanasana) Stand in Mountain Pose (Tadasana). Balance the weight evenly between your feet, lengthen up through your inner thighs, and roll your thighs in. Keep your legs and knees firm as you lift your arms out to the sides and overhead, stretching up through your waist and ribs. Fold your arms and cup your elbows with your hands. As you exhale, bend forward from your hips, and release your side body down. Continue to hold your elbows and release your spine. (If you experience vomit reflux when you bend forward, keep your head up and your back slightly concave.) Breathe normally for 30 to 60 seconds. To come out, release your arms, put your hands on your hips, keeping your legs active. Then lift up slowly. Your head should come up last.

EFFECTS This pose brings a sense of peace when you feel agitated or anxious. It calms your mind and relieves a jittery stomach, and can even help tone your reproductive organs.

10. CHILD'S POSE (Adho Mukha Virasana) Kneel on the floor with your knees slightly wider than your hips and bring your big toes together. Bend forward and stretch your arms and trunk forward. Rest your head on the floor or a blanket. (Alternatively, you may rest your head on a bolster for more height.) Rest completely for several breaths.

EFFECTS This is a wonderful pose to help calm your nerves and rejuvenate your body, mind,

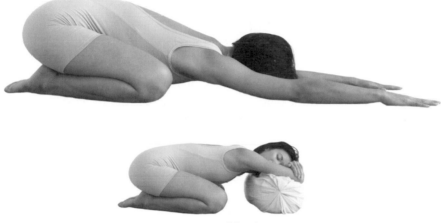

Modification

11. SIMPLE SEATED TWIST POSE† (Bharadvajasana) Sit up straight with your legs stretched out in front of you. Bend both legs to the left so your feet are next to your left hip. Keeping your thighs and knees facing forward, make sure your left ankle rests on the arch of your right foot and that your buttocks are on the floor, not on your foot. Draw your shoulder blades into your back, broaden your chest, and extend your spine upward. On an exhalation, turn your abdomen, ribs, chest, and shoulders (in that order) to the right; place your left hand on the outside of your right thigh and your right hand on the floor behind you (or on a block). Take several breaths, holding the posture for 20 seconds. Relax your face, neck, and throat. Come back to the center position, straighten your legs, and change sides.

EFFECTS This gentle twist massages your reproductive organs, energizes your adrenal glands, and tones and massages your kidneys. It also helps firm your waist and tone your abdominal region.

†CAUTION Do not practice twists if you have diarrhea or feel nauseous.

12. HEADSTAND† **(Sirsasana)** (Before beginning, see pages 16–17.) Place a folded blanket against the wall. Kneel in front of it with your feet and knees together. Interlace your fingers firmly, thumbs touching and your hands cupped. Position your hands no more than 3 inches from the wall, your elbows shoulder-width apart. Your wrists, forearms, and elbows form the foundation for this pose.

Lengthen your neck and place the crown of your head on the blanket. The back of your head should be in contact with your hands. Press your forearms into the floor and lift your shoulders away from the floor. Maintain this action throughout the pose. Straighten your legs, raise your hips toward the ceiling, and walk your feet in until your spine is almost perpendicular to the floor. As you exhale, lift one leg at a time, and bring your feet to the wall. (Or bend your knees, slowly bring your feet to the wall, and straighten your legs.)

Keep your heels and buttocks against the wall. Roll your thighs in, lift your tailbone, lengthen your legs upward, and keep your feet together. Remember to balance on the crown of your head, support yourself by pressing your forearms into the floor, and continue to lift your shoulders away from your ears. Keep your breathing even, your eyes and throat soft, and your abdomen relaxed. With regular practice, you can slowly learn to bring your buttocks and heels away from the wall. Hold the pose as long as you can, up to 5 minutes.

To come out, exhale and bring your legs down to the floor one at a time. Bend your knees, sit back on your heels, and rest for a few breaths before raising your head.

EFFECTS This pose helps balance your endocrine system, increase your circulation, and energize your whole body. Completing it can give you a fabulous sense of accomplishment.

†CAUTION Do this pose only if it is already part of your yoga practice. Seek the advice of an experienced teacher if you have neck problems. Do not do this pose if you have your period or suffer from back problems or migraines.

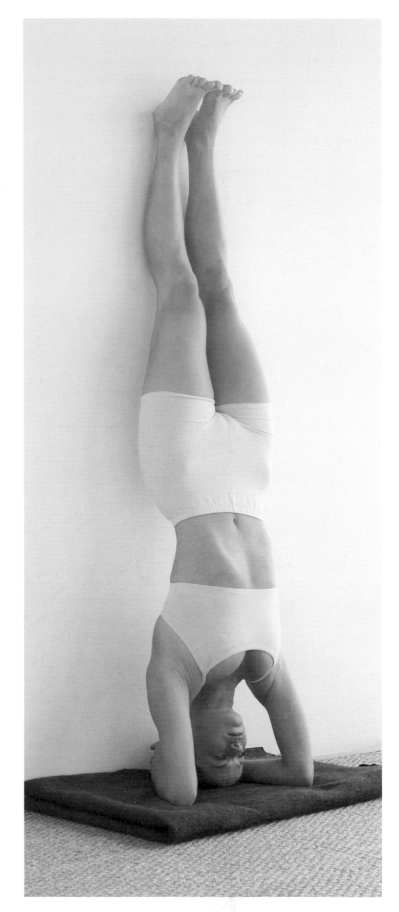

13. INVERTED STAFF POSE† (Viparita Dandasana)
(Before begining, see pages 34–35.) Place a folded blanket on a chair that has been placed about 2 feet from the wall—far enough away from the wall so your feet can press into the wall when your legs are outstretched. Sit backward on the chair, facing the wall, with your feet through the chair back. Letting your hands slide down the sides of the chair and supporting yourself on your elbows, lean back slowly so your head and neck extend past the front of the chair seat.

Still holding the sides of the chair, arch back so your shoulder blades are at the front edge of the seat. (You may need to scoot your buttocks farther toward the back of the seat.) Take your feet to the wall, legs slightly bent, and hold the back legs or sides of the chair. Lengthen your legs, pressing the chair away from the wall, and roll your thighs in toward each other as you release your head back. Keep your hands on the chair sides or legs. (If you have neck problems, rest your head on a bolster. If you feel any pain in your lower back, elevate your feet on a block or bolsters placed against the wall.) Breathe quietly for 30 to 60 seconds. (If you find this pose too difficult, don't stay too long; instead, come into and out of the pose two or three times. See page 104 for a modification.)

To come out, bend your knees and place your feet flat on the floor. Hold on to the sides of the chair back and carefully come up, lifting from your sternum. Lean over the chair back for a few breaths to release your back.

EFFECTS This exhilarating pose can promote a feeling of happiness by opening your chest, improving respiration, and increasing the circulation in and around your heart. It also helps build emotional stability and self-confidence.

†CAUTION Seek the advice of an experienced teacher if you have neck problems. Do not do this pose if you have a migraine or tension headache or diarrhea.

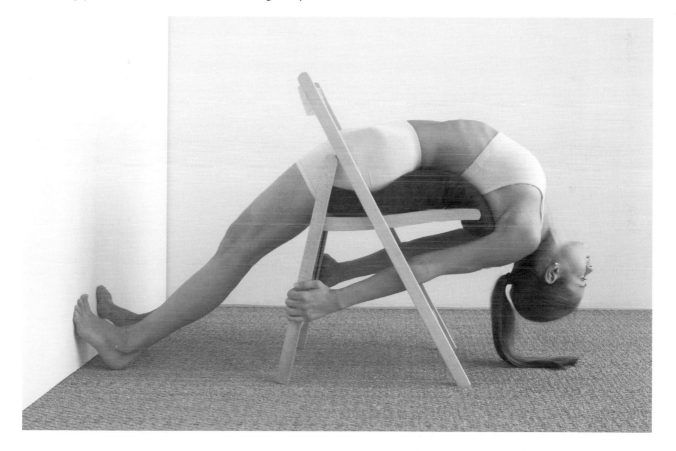

14. UPWARD-FACING BOW POSE† (Urdhva Dhanurasana)

Lie on your back with your knees bent, your feet hip-width apart, and your heels close to your buttocks. Bend your elbows and place your hands alongside your head with your fingers pointing toward your feet. As you exhale, raise your hips and chest, straighten your arms, and stretch your legs. Lift your tailbone and move the backs of your thighs toward your buttocks. Hold this pose for 5 to 10 seconds, if you can, or come in and out of the pose two or three times.

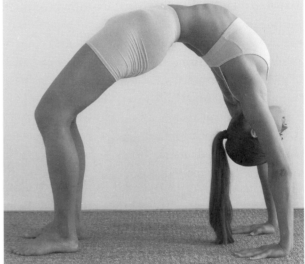

To come out of the pose, bend your knees and elbows, and slowly lower your body to the floor. (If you find this pose too difficult, do the modification in the Woman's Energizing Sequence on page 37.) Even if the pose seems too difficult at first, keep trying—just the attempt can be exhilarating.

EFFECTS This pose opens your chest and improves respiration and circulation, helping to bring you a sense of lightness and self-confidence and a wonderful feeling of power. It's also good for strengthening and toning the area around your waist.

†CAUTION Do not do this pose if you have a migraine or tension headache, suffer from heart trouble or any serious illness, or are pregnant.

15. SHOULDERSTAND† (Sarvangasana)

(Before beginning see pages 18–19.) Lie on your back with two folded blankets supporting your shoulders and your arms stretched out beside you. On an exhalation, bend your knees and raise your legs toward your chest. Pressing your hands into the floor, swing your bent legs over your head; support your back with your hands and press your elbows firmly into the blankets. Raise your torso up until it is perpendicular to the floor and your knees are close to your chest. Supporting your back, raise your legs until your thighs are parallel to the floor; raise them some more until your knees point toward the ceiling. Now raise your legs completely and extend up through your heels until your whole body is perpendicular to the floor. Move your tailbone up and in and use your hands to lift your back ribs. Feel that your whole body is long and straight. Move your shoulders away from your ears. Hold this pose as long as you can, at least 2 minutes. To come out, bend your knees and slowly roll down. Lie still for several breaths.

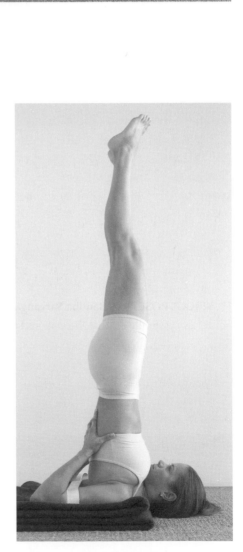

EFFECTS This pose is a favorite among teenagers because it helps develop patience and emotional stability. Practice this pose when you feel irritable, anxious, or fatigued.

†CAUTION Do not do this pose if you suffer from neck or shoulder problems, if you have high blood pressure, if you are menstruating, or if you have a migraine or tension headache.

16. PLOUGH POSE† **(Halasana)** Lie on your back with two folded blankets supporting your neck and shoulders; your head is on the floor and your arms are down by your sides. Bend your knees and bring your thighs in to your chest. On an exhalation, swing or lift your buttocks and legs up, supporting your back with your hands, and extend your legs over your head, placing your toes on the floor behind you. (To keep your elbows in, you can use a strap around both arms, just above your elbows, before you begin.) Keep your thighs active by tightening your knees to create space between your face and your legs. Stay in this pose for at least 30 seconds and up to 2 minutes. To come out, slowly roll down

one vertebra at a time. Rest with your back flat on the floor for several breaths.

EFFECTS This pose can be helpful when you need to balance your endocrine system or relax deeply. It is also good for lifting your spirits, restoring a sense of calm, taming irritability and anxiety, and building self-confidence.

†CAUTION Do not do this pose if you have neck problems, without the help of an experienced teacher, or if you are menstruating.

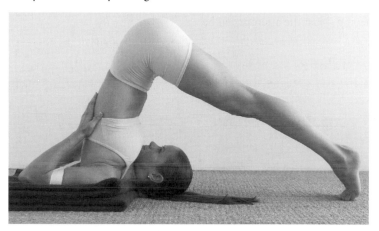

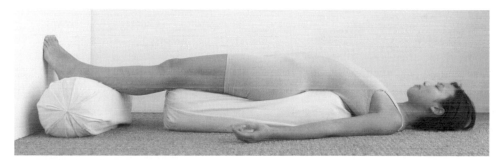

17. BRIDGE POSE (Setu Bandha Sarvangasana) Place one bolster horizontally against the wall and another vertically, forming a T shape. Sit on the end of the vertical bolster that is closest to the wall. Keeping your knees bent, lie back over the bolster. Slide down until the end of the bolster is in the middle of your back and your shoulders just reach the floor. Rest your shoulders and head on the floor. Keeping your feet and heels together, stretch your legs toward the wall and put your heels on the horizontal bolster so your feet touch the wall. Your legs should be straight out in front of you. Rest your

arms in any comfortable position. Close your eyes and relax completely, softening your abdomen and breathing deeply. Stay in this position for 3 to 5 minutes.

To come out, bend your knees, slowly roll to one side, and push yourself up to a seated position.

EFFECTS This pose can strengthen your back muscles, help you build confidence, and open your chest (improving circulation and respiration). Its gentle chin lock helps balance your thyroid and parathyroid glands. Since it is a slight backbend, it can relieve depression as well.

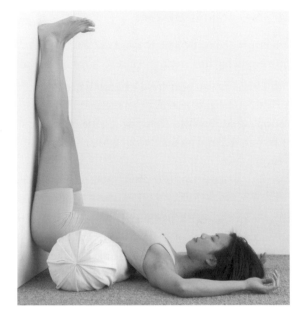

18. LEGS-UP-THE-WALL POSE† (**Viparita Karani**) Place a bolster about 3 inches from the wall. Sit on the bolster so your right hip and side are touching the wall. Using your hands to support you, lean back and swivel your body around, taking your right leg and then your left leg up the wall. Keep your buttocks close to or against the wall. (If you feel stiffness or discomfort in your legs, push your buttocks slightly away from the wall.) Lie down so your lower back and ribs are supported by the bolster, your tailbone is descending toward the floor, and your shoulders and head are on the floor. (If your neck is uncomfortable, put a folded blanket under it.) Extend through your legs and place your arms out at your sides. Rest in this position, eyes closed, for 5 minutes, or as long as you like.

To come out, gently push away from the wall until your buttocks are off the bolster and resting on the floor. Roll to one side and use your arms to help you to a seated position.

EFFECTS This pose can help calm your nerves, balance your endocrine system, and leave you feeling renewed.

†CAUTION Do not do this pose when you are menstruating.

19. CORPSE POSE (Savasana) Lie on your back with your legs stretched out in front of you. (If necessary, use a folded blanket to support your head.) Place your arms comfortably at your sides, slightly away from your torso, with your palms facing upward. Actively stretch your arms and legs away from you, then allow them to release completely. Close your eyes and let everything relax. Take a few deep breaths, inhaling into your chest without tensing your throat, neck, or diaphragm. Exhale your body into the floor, releasing your shoulders, neck, and facial muscles. Keep your abdomen soft and relaxed, and release your lower back. Remain in the pose, breathing normally, for at least 5 to 10 minutes. To come out, bend your knees, roll to one side, remain there for a few breaths, and then open your eyes and push yourself up with your arms.

EFFECTS This is a wonderful pose to develop and keep your internal focus. It helps you relax completely, reminding you that you have nowhere to go, nothing to strive for, and nothing to worry about.

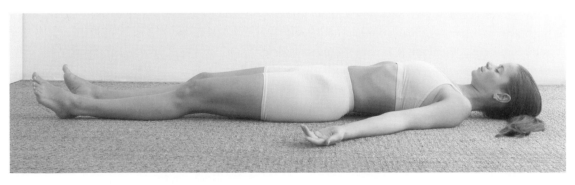

A SEQUENCE FOR EATING DISORDERS: RESTORE AND RENEW

1. Reclining Bound Angle Pose
   (Supta Baddha Konasana)
2. Bridge Pose (Setu Bandha Sarvangasana)
3. Child's Pose (Adho Mukha Virasana)
4. Head-on-Knee Pose (Janu Sirsasana)
5. Seated Forward Bend
   (Paschimottanasana)
6. Standing Forward Bend (Uttanasana)
7. Downward-Facing Dog Pose
   (Adho Mukha Svanasana)
8. Half-Moon Pose (Ardha Chandrasana)
9. Headstand (Sirsasana)
10. Inverted Staff Pose (Viparita Dandasana)
11. Camel Pose (Ustrasana)
12. Shoulderstand (Sarvangasana)
13. Plough Pose (Halasana)
14. Bridge Pose (Setu Bandha Sarvangasana)
15. Legs-Up-the-Wall Pose (Viparita Karani)
16. Corpse Pose (Savasana)

This is a wonderful sequence to do when you feel jittery, depressed, or a little out of control. If you begin by going inside yourself and taking time to breathe and relax deeply, you'll feel more centered and grounded—and have enough energy and strength to do the standing poses. (If you suffer from vomit reflux during forward bends, keep your head lifted.)

1. RECLINING BOUND ANGLE POSE (Supta Baddha Konasana) Place a bolster vertically behind you and sit just in front of it with your knees bent and your sacrum touching the bolster's edge. Put a folded blanket on the other end of the bolster to prevent any strain on your neck. Place a strap behind your back, at your sacrum; draw it forward over your hips, across your shins, and under your feet (see page xv). Put the soles of your feet together and let your knees and thighs fall to the sides. Cinch the strap securely under your feet. Lie back so your head is on the folded blanket and your torso rests comfortably on the bolster; your buttocks and legs are on the floor. (If you feel any discomfort in your lower back, add some height to your support with a folded blanket or two. If you feel any muscle tension in your legs, roll two blankets vertically and place one under the top of each thigh.) Remain in this pose for as long as you can, preferably 3 to 5 minutes or longer.

To come out, draw your knees together, slip the strap off, and slowly roll to one side. Use your hands to push yourself up to a seated position.

EFFECTS This pose opens your chest, improves respiration and circulation, helps calm jittery nerves and ease depression, and quiets an anxious mind.

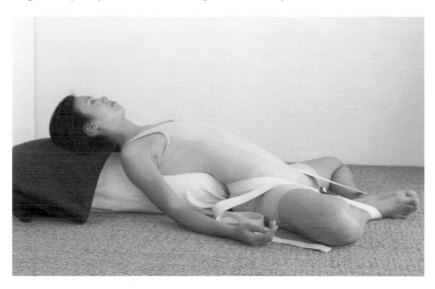

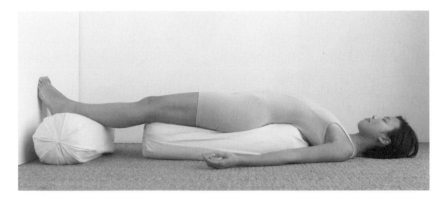

2. BRIDGE POSE (Setu Bandha Sarvangasana) Do Bridge Pose, as described on page 79. Remain in this pose for at least 3 to 5 minutes, or as long as you like.

EFFECTS This pose can help you build confidence, strengthen your back muscles, and open your chest. Its gentle chin lock helps balance your thyroid and parathyroid glands.

3. CHILD'S POSE (Adho Mukha Virasana) Kneel on the floor with a bolster placed horizontally about a foot in front of you. Place another bolster across it vertically to form a T shape. Spread your knees wide and straddle the second bolster, bringing your toes together. Bend forward and stretch your arms and trunk up and over the bolsters, pressing the vertical one into your abdomen. Rest your head on the bolsters and relax completely. Remain in this pose for several minutes, or as long as you like.

EFFECTS This is a wonderful way to help calm your nervous system and make your body, mind, and spirit feel rejuvenated.

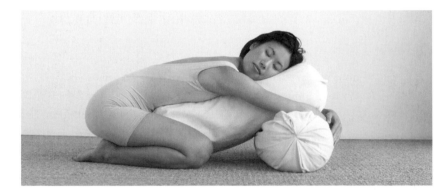

4. HEAD-ON-KNEE POSE† (Janu Sirsasana) Sit on the floor with your legs stretched out in front of you. Bend your right knee to the side so it is at a 45-degree angle to your left leg and your right heel is near your groin. Push your right knee as far back as you comfortably can; keep your left leg straight.

Place a folded blanket or a bolster on your outstretched leg, and turn your abdomen and chest so your sternum is in line with the center of your left leg. As you inhale, lift up from the base of your pelvis; as you exhale, lean your trunk forward, fold your arms on your support, and cradle your head on your arms. You should feel no pressure or strain in your back or the backs of your legs. (If you feel any strain, add more height to your support, see page 48. If you experience vomit reflux when you bend forward, keep your head up.)

Stay in this pose for as long as you like, preferably 2 to 3 minutes. Inhale while coming up, straighten your right leg, and reverse sides by bending your left knee.

EFFECTS This pose tones and strengthens your abdomen, while helping to bring a sense of calm and peace when you feel agitated or anxious. It also helps to lift and tone your uterus, and improves circulation in your pelvis.

†CAUTION Do not do this pose if you have diarrhea.

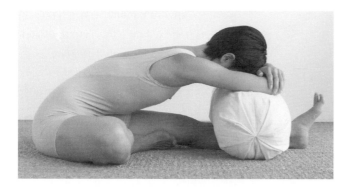

5. SEATED FORWARD BEND† (**Paschimottanasana**) Sit on your mat (or on one or two folded blankets) with your legs stretched out in front of you. Place a folded blanket or a bolster across your lower legs. Take a full, deep breath and lift your arms over your head, stretching up through your spine and lifting your sternum and head. Keep your back slightly concave. As you exhale, bend forward and extend your torso over your legs, cradling your head in your arms on your support. (If you feel strain in your back or in your legs, or if you experience vomit reflux when you bend forward, add more height to your support. See page 49.) Do not allow your buttocks to come off the floor. Remain in this pose for as long as you like, preferably 2 to 3 minutes.

EFFECTS This pose helps bring a sense of safety and peace, calming anxiety and irritability. It also works well when you need to soothe your digestive system.

†CAUTION Do not do this pose if you have diarrhea.

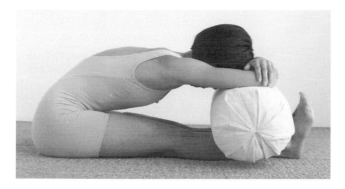

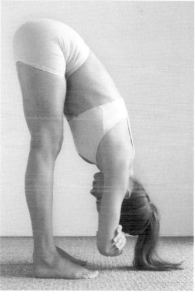

6. STANDING FORWARD BEND† (**Uttanasana**) Do Standing Forward Bend as described on page 74.

EFFECTS This pose helps calm agitation and relieve a nervous stomach.

†CAUTION If you experience vomit reflux, take your hands to the ground, lift your head, and keep your back slightly concave.

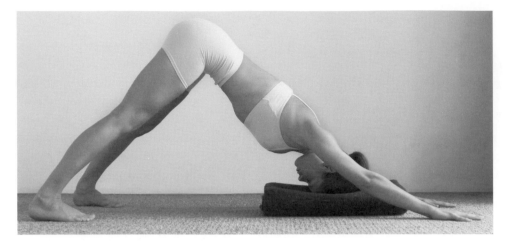

7. DOWNWARD-FACING DOG POSE (Adho Mukha Svanasana)
To find the correct distance between your hands and feet for this pose, lie facedown and place your palms by the side of your chest with your fingers well spread and pointing straight ahead. Come up on your hands and knees. That's your position. Now place folded blankets or a bolster or two vertically so your support is in line with your sternum, and resume your hands-and-knees position, turning your toes under. Exhale, press your hands firmly into the mat and extend up through your inner arms. Exhale again as you raise your buttocks high in the air and move your thighs up and back. Keep stretching through your legs and bring your heels toward the floor. Keep the legs firm and the elbows straight as you lift your buttocks upward. The action of the arms and legs serves to elongate your spine and release your head. Hold this pose for 30 seconds to 1 minute, breathing deeply. Let your head rest completely on your support, and release the base of your neck. To come out, return to your hands and knees and sit back on your heels.

EFFECTS This is a great pose to help combat depression, increase your circulation, and calm your mind.

8. HALF-MOON POSE (Ardha Chandrasana)
Do Half-Moon Pose as described on page 72.

EFFECTS This pose helps strengthen your legs, energize your body, and promote balance.

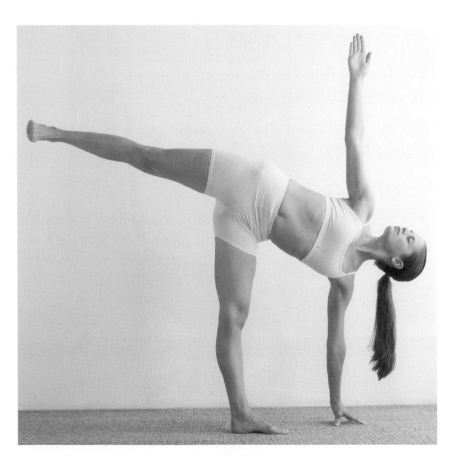

9. HEADSTAND† **(Sirsasana)** Do Headstand as described on page 76.

EFFECTS This pose is great when you want to balance your endocrine system, increase your circulation, and energize your whole body. Completing it can give you a wonderful sense of accomplishment.

†CAUTION Do this pose only if it is already part of your yoga practice. Seek the advice of an experienced teacher if you have neck problems. Do not do this pose if you have your period or suffer from back problems or migraines.

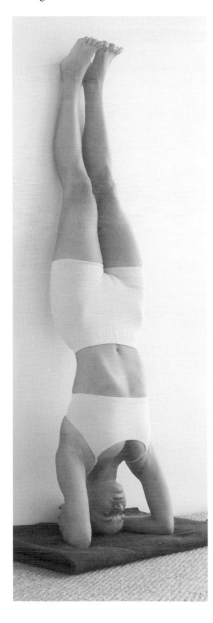

10. INVERTED STAFF POSE† **(Viparita Dandasana)** Do Inverted Staff Pose as described on page 77.

EFFECTS This exhilarating pose can promote a feeling of happiness by opening your chest, improving respiration, and increasing the circulation in and around your heart. It may also help build emotional stability and self-confidence.

†CAUTION Seek the advice of an experienced teacher if you have neck or back problems. Do not do this pose if you have a migraine or tension headache or diarrhea.

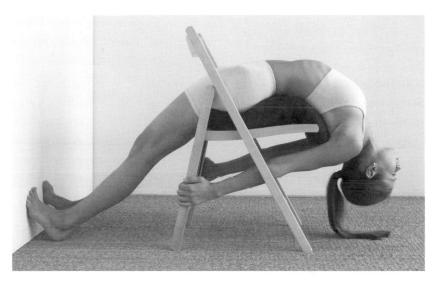

11. CAMEL POSE | **(Ustrasana)** Kneel on the floor with your knees and feet hip-width apart. Place your palms on your buttocks and as you exhale, move your thighs slightly forward and raise your side ribs. Gradually bend back as far as possible, lift your chest, and broaden your shoulders. Move your hands from your buttocks to your feet, and take hold of your heels. (If you can't reach your heels, place your hands on blocks positioned next to each ankle with your fingers pointing in the same direction as your feet.) Your thighs should be perpendicular to the floor. Take your head back, if that's comfortable, and breathe evenly for 10 to 15 seconds.

To come out, release your hands one at a time. As you exhale, slowly lift up from your sternum, using your thigh muscles. Your head should come up last.

EFFECTS This pose helps improve the circulation throughout your body, lift your spirits as it opens your chest, tone the muscles in your back, and build self-confidence.

†CAUTION Do not do this pose if you have a migraine or tension headache.

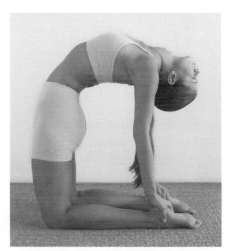

12. SHOULDERSTAND† (Sarvangasana) (Before beginning, see pages 18–19.) Lie on your back with two folded blankets supporting your shoulders and your arms stretched out beside your body. On an exhalation, bend your knees and raise your legs toward your chest. Swing your bent legs over your head; supporting your back with your hands, fingers turned in toward your spine, elbows pressed into the blankets. Raise your torso, hips, and thighs even higher, straightening your legs as they come up until your whole body is perpendicular to the floor and the top of your sternum touches your chin. Move your tailbone in to prevent your lower back from overarching. Use your hands to lift your back ribs. (If you can't keep your elbows in, come down, secure a strap around both arms, just above your elbows, and go back up.) Keep your shoulders away from your ears. Hold this pose as long as you can, preferably at least 2 minutes.

To come out, exhale as you bend your knees. Slowly roll down one vertebra at a time. Lie still for several breaths.

EFFECTS This pose is a favorite among teenagers because it helps to develop patience and emotional stability. Practice this pose when you feel irritable, anxious, or fatigued.

†CAUTION Do not do this pose if you suffer from neck or shoulder problems, if you have high blood pressure, if you are menstruating, or if you have a migraine or tension headache.

13. PLOUGH POSE† (Halasana) Lie on your back with two folded blankets supporting your neck and shoulders; your head is on the floor and your arms are down by your sides. Bend your knees and bring your thighs in to your chest. On an exhalation, swing or lift your buttocks and legs up, supporting your back with your hands, and extend your legs over your head, placing your toes on the floor behind you. (To keep your elbows in, you can use a strap around both arms, just above your elbows, before you begin.) Keep your thighs active by tightening your knees to create space between your face and your legs. Stay in this pose for at least 30 seconds and up to 2 minutes. To come out, slowly roll down. Rest with your back flat on the floor for several breaths.

EFFECTS This pose can be helpful when you need to balance your endocrine system or relax deeply. It is also good for lifting your spirits, restoring a sense of calm, taming irritability and anxiety, and building self-confidence.

†CAUTION Do not do this pose without the help of an experienced teacher, if you have neck problems, or if you are menstruating.

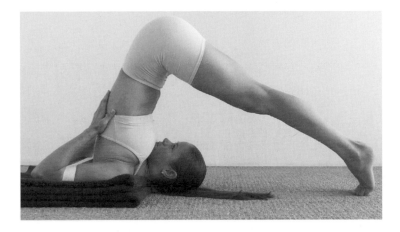

14. BRIDGE POSE (Setu Bandha Sarvangasana) Do Bridge Pose as described on page 79. Remain in this pose for as long as you like—at least 3 to 5 minutes.

EFFECTS This pose can help you build confidence, strengthen your back muscles, and open your chest (improving respiration and circulation). Its gentle chin lock helps balance your thyroid and parathyroid glands.

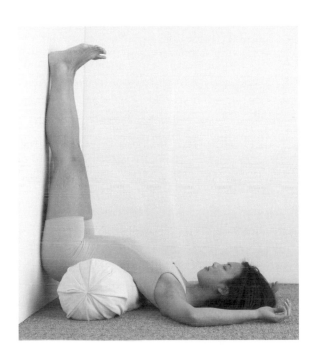

15. LEGS-UP-THE-WALL POSE† (Viparita Karani) Do Legs-Up-the-Wall Pose as described on page 80.

EFFECTS This pose can help calm your nerves, balance your endocrine system, and leave you feeling renewed.

†CAUTION Do not do this pose when you are menstruating.

16. CORPSE POSE (Savasana) Do Corpse Pose as described on page 80.

EFFECTS This is a wonderful pose to develop and keep your internal focus. It helps you relax completely, reminding you that you have nowhere to go, nothing to strive for, and nothing to worry about.

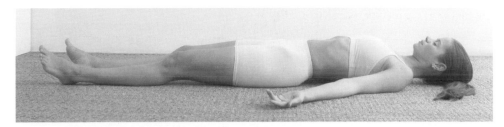

Chapter 5   *Honoring Your Menstrual Cycle*

IN THE MID-1960S, WHEN I WAS A TEENAGER, NONE OF US HAD mothers or grandmothers who taught us to celebrate our cycles, to embrace the power we received from menstruation, or to use our monthly cycles as a means of gauging our physical and emotional health. Instead, we learned that getting our periods meant only one thing: We could get pregnant if we fooled around. We were admonished if we acted sexy and coquettish; we were scolded if we got angry or felt bitchy; and we didn't get much sympathy—certainly not at school—if we complained of having cramps or premenstrual headaches.

Not much has changed over the years. If you're a teenager, you may relate to Samantha, a sixteen-year-old high school student from the Midwest, who hates having her period. It started a few years ago, when she was twelve. At first it wasn't that bad because it came so sporadically—she'd bleed one month and not the next; two months later she'd get another period and not see it again for three months. The worst part was never knowing when the Curse, as her mother called it, would show up because she rarely had any symptoms. But now that she gets her period more regularly, things have gotten more difficult. She notices that a few days before she starts bleeding, her face breaks out, she feels fat, her family (especially her little brother) annoys her even more than usual, and her friends hurt her feelings a lot. And to make matters worse, when her period does come, she gets sharp, intense cramps that just about incapacitate her for the first two days.

She hasn't talked to anyone much about these problems; it's too embarrassing. She and her friends commiserate on occasion, complaining about cramps or accusing one another of having "PMS mood swings," but none of them has ever sought advice from an adult. They simply agree that bleeding—and all the discomfort involved—is a fact of life, the scourge of being female.

Lately, however, Samantha has noticed a change. She and a couple of her friends signed up for a yoga class at school, and she still can't believe how some of the poses help her cramps. Of course, she thinks it's weird that her teacher always asks the girls if they have their "moon time," and nobody would admit it at first. But when Samantha does Half-Moon Pose (Ardha Chandrasana) and a supported forward bend, she feels so much better. Now she wonders what yoga can do to help her through PMS.

88

The answer, not surprisingly, is quite a bit. Yoga can help regulate your monthly cycle and keep you more physically and emotionally balanced. Going through puberty is not always easy, as Samantha can attest, and as you probably know firsthand. Like many teenage girls, you may sometimes feel not only that your body has betrayed you, but that you can't get a handle on your emotions, either. Yoga and even simple breathing techniques called pranayama can bring a sense of stability to those emotions, vitality to your liver, and balance to your endocrine system, a complex array of glands that produce the hormones that trigger your period in the first place. In addition, yoga puts you in tune with your body and helps you understand that menstruation is a powerful connection to other females you know, even to the earth. Samantha can't believe how many girls in her yoga class all have their period at the same time. Once she understood those connections, she didn't mind the cramps and discomfort quite as much.

To appreciate how your monthly cycle connects you to the world around you, think about your body as a microcosm of the universe. Just as the moon waxes and wanes, as the tides ebb and flow, your body moves through the stages of its cycle from ovulation to menstruation; from a feeling of lightness to a dark, moody time; from creativity to reflection. You may notice that you feel much more outgoing and energized midcycle, around ovulation time, and can't resist the need to withdraw, even push people away, just before your period starts.

A PHYSIOLOGY LESSON

Contrary to popular belief, your period doesn't begin in your uterus. The process starts in the pineal body, hidden deep within the recesses of your brain behind your eyes. This tiny, teardrop-shaped gland responds to changes in light and darkness and produces the hormone melatonin, which helps you sleep at night. According to British herbalist Amanda McQuade Crawford this gland not only registers and responds to the amount of natural and artificial light you're exposed to on a daily basis, it also signals seasonal changes and alerts the hypothalamus to begin your menstrual cycle. The hypothalamus, also a very sensitive part of your endocrine system, sits close to the emotional center of your brain and can react adversely to emotional upheaval or physical illness. The hypothalamus registers your body's most basic needs, such as hunger, thirst, sexual desire, and body temperature. When you're healthy, it provides the pituitary gland with what it needs to produce important hormones for reproduction. When your health is compromised, however, the hypothalamus may give out erroneous or incomplete information, causing the pituitary to manufacture either too many or too few female hormones, which throws your body off balance.

The hormones from the pituitary—follicle-stimulating hormone (FSH) and luteinizing hormone (LH)—stimulate the production of estrogen and progesterone, respectively, in the ovaries. This action begins on the first day of your cycle—that is, the day you start to

YOUR ENDOCRINE AND REPRODUCTIVE SYSTEMS

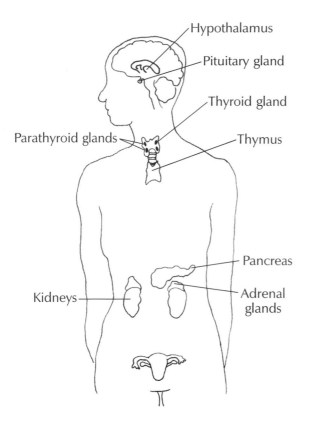

Hypothalamus
Pituitary gland
Thyroid gland
Parathyroid glands
Thymus
Pancreas
Kidneys
Adrenal glands

YOUR REPRODUCTIVE ORGANS

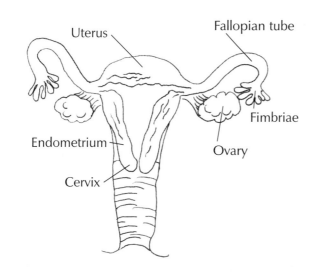

Uterus
Fallopian tube
Fimbriae
Endometrium
Ovary
Cervix

menstruate. On day one, estrogen and proges-terone are at their lowest levels. The pituitary gland responds by manufacturing FSH, which in turn stimulates the ovaries to increase production of estrogen. During this stage, which lasts until just before ovulation, an egg matures within the ovaries. At the same time, the increased estrogen allows the lining of the uterus (the endometrium) to develop and thicken, creating a safe and nour-ishing home for the egg to grow; improves circula-tion to the vagina; and lubricates the cervix as a way of inviting sperm to enter.

As your body blossoms, estrogen plays an increasingly important role. It shapes your second-ary sex characteristics, giving you rounder breasts, pubic hair, a feminine voice, and broader hips. It also governs the first half of your menstrual cycle, which prepares you for ovulation and reproduc-tion. Estrogen is at its peak during this time and affects your emotions (after all, it begins life at the insistence of the emotionally charged hypothala-mus). If your estrogen output is balanced, your emotions and your body are ripe with possibili-ties—you feel sensual, outgoing, and creative. If you experience estrogen imbalance, however, you can face debilitating menstrual cramps, infertility, fibroid tumors, and radical mood swings.

According to Christiane Northrup, M.D., author of *Women's Bodies, Women's Wisdom*, your body gives off hormonal signals during ovulation that you are fertile, sexual, and alive. Most young women find it difficult to tell when they're ovulat-ing. Generally, if you ovulate, your body signals when menstruation is about to begin. You may have cramps, mood swings, fatigue, any number of warning signs. If you don't ovulate, it's almost impossible to tell when your period is due—it just shows up, and not necessarily on a schedule. Usu-ally around the fifteenth or sixteenth day of your cycle, you will see a watery, whitish vaginal dis-charge. This "fertile flow" is an indication that you are ovulating. It may be followed by additional hormonal fluctuations—known to most women as premenstrual syndrome (PMS)—that promote bloating, swollen or tender breasts, and moodiness.

During the second half of your cycle, the luteiniz-ing phase, FSH production decreases and LH increases. The egg leaves the ovary and makes its way to the uterus, and your body prepares for the possibility of pregnancy. The hormone progesterone helps that happen. Manufactured by the corpus luteum in the ovaries, progesterone brings nourishment to the uterus through increased blood flow and forms a thick mucus plug in the cervix to keep bacteria out. If pregnancy does not occur, production of estrogen and progesterone plummets, the uterine lining dissolves, and the endometrium is shed as menstrual blood.

If progesterone production is balanced, you may feel more reflective, intuitive, and in touch with your dreams during this second stage. Too much progesterone can cause you to feel depressed, lethargic, and sexually unattractive.

To complete this monthly housecleaning, your liver and kidneys deactivate the excess estrogen and progesterone, which are eliminated from your body, along with environmental toxins, through your kidneys. If your liver is sluggish or overworked, it may not do its job efficiently, and the unneeded hormones can be reabsorbed into the bloodstream. Your body then has more hormones than it can use, which can cause such problems as heavy or irregular periods, acne, fatigue, depression, and digestive disorders.

In Ayurvedic medicine (the healing system of ancient India), physicians believe that women have a distinct advantage over men by bleeding every month. These practitioners teach that menstruation purifies the body every twenty-five to thirty-five days, gathering all the detritus and toxins that have built up over the month and moving it out of the body along with the menstrual blood. Ayurvedic physician and scholar Robert Svoboda thinks that may be why women generally live longer than men.

MENSTRUAL PROBLEMS

Amenorrhea (Delayed Menses)

Amenorrhea is the technical term for not bleeding. It's actually quite common for you to begin your period without ovulating first, like Samantha. You may have a light period one month and then no period at all for several months. This often happens because the pituitary gland, which produces the FSH and LH hormones necessary for ovulation, is underdeveloped. As we discussed earlier, when everything is normal, estrogen builds up a thick, temporary lining in the uterus, and following ovulation, progesterone stabilizes this lining. If you don't ovulate, you can't produce progesterone. And if your body produces no progesterone, estrogen gets no signal to stop thickening the uterine lining. After a while, some of this lining begins to slough off and scant bleeding will occur. Generally, the body will correct itself and there's nothing to worry about.

Unfortunately, many young women panic too soon and allow their doctors to prescribe birth control pills as a way to regulate their periods. If they don't bleed regularly because they don't ovulate, birth control pills will only prolong the problem. These pills create anovulatory cycles; they don't correct them. They will, however, encourage the body to shed the endometrium lining that has built up and provide enough progesterone to complete the process. Most holistic physicians will opt to give a girl's body time to correct itself and prescribe gentle herbal tonics like chaste tree (*Vitex agnus castus*) to balance the glandular system.

Because the hypothalamus and pituitary glands are so closely connected to the emotional center of the brain, you may stop bleeding if you're under a lot of stress. Again, missing a period on occasion because of stress doesn't usually require medical intervention, but it should cause you to reevaluate your lifestyle, and it's certainly a good reason to begin practicing yoga. Of course, prolonged amenorrhea should be discussed with a physician, because suppressed menstruation can be caused by more severe medical conditions such as diabetes, thyroid malfunction, extreme weight gain or loss, or acute emotional distress.

How Yoga Can Help Yoga works to get your period going in two very important ways. First, doing yoga consistently helps mitigate the stress that can cause your cycle to go off-kilter. Doing restful, restorative poses whenever you feel overwhelmed, overworked, and on edge will help calm your nervous system and give your reproductive system a chance to get back on track. Second, balancing your endocrine system may help the pituitary, thyroid, and hypothalamus perform correctly. Do as many of the poses in the Woman's Essential Sequence as possible, focusing on inversions, backbends, and twists. If any pose is too challenging, try the modified version or skip it entirely.

Menorrhagia (Heavy Bleeding)

Just as you can go a month or more without a period, you can also have bouts of heavy bleeding. For the most part, such bleeding is normal, as long as the blood is bright red, you don't experience clotting or heavy cramps, and you aren't wiped out every time you get your period. When the bleeding becomes excessive—that is, when you continue to soak through several pads or tampons even on the second or third day of your period—something is wrong. If menorrhagia continues month after month, it can lead to anemia and an iron deficiency, so see your doctor for an evaluation. Christiane Northrup points out that chronic stress over what she terms "second chakra issues, including creativity, relationships, money, and control of others" may be the culprit. She encourages her patients to set aside time to be creative, to mourn the loss of old relationships, and to learn to voice the joys and frustrations in new ones. When women heed the signals their bodies give them, she says, their periods often return to normal.

How Yoga Can Help If you feel weak and exhausted from excessive bleeding, Patricia recommends that you simply rest and not try to practice at all. Otherwise it's safe and helpful to practice the sequence for heavy periods that we've provided in this chapter. With the exception of Half-Moon Pose (Ardha Chandrasana), Patricia advises against doing standing poses. Standing poses require a lot of strength and energy; heavy bleeding zaps you of both. Half-Moon Pose, on the other hand, opens your pelvic region; brings space to your abdomen; and, according to Geeta Iyengar, has a drying effect on your uterus—particularly if you practice it against a wall for support. Take care not to stay in the pose too long; instead, go in and out of it a few times.

Endometriosis

Sometimes heavy bleeding can be a sign of something more serious. Endometriosis, uterine fibroids, and ovarian cysts cause severe pain and have resulted in many an untimely hysterectomy. Under normal circumstances, during the first phase of the menstrual cycle, the presence of estrogen allows the tissue within the uterine walls to thicken prior to your period. If you have endometriosis, some researchers believe that bits and pieces of this uterine lining break off and, instead of moving down and out of your body, they move upward and lodge in other areas. The most common places for this tissue to attach itself are on the pelvic organs, the pelvic side walls, and sometimes the bowel. When your period starts, these bits of tissue, stimulated by your hormones, appear to bleed as well and that's what most physicians believe produces such severe cramping. According to Mary Schatz, M.D., a physician, yoga practitioner, and author of numerous articles on therapeutic yoga, the latest theory is that endometriosis occurs when cells in the pelvic lining develop into cells like those in the uterine lining.

Whatever the cause, many holistic physicians believe stress aggravates endometriosis. Ayurvedic physicians recommend changes in diet and lifestyle, including lots of rest during the first day or so of your period, and gentle yoga asanas (poses) to relieve cramps, reduce stress, and deliver fresh blood to your pelvic region.

A number of physicians and healers agree with Christiane Northrup, who believes that endometriosis can be a wake-up call for women who compete in high-stress jobs. She writes that it is often the way a woman's body demonstrates that her "innermost emotional needs are in direct conflict with what the world is demanding of her." In other words, if you consistently and relentlessly focus your energies outward and neglect your emotional and spiritual side, you may be a prime candidate for pelvic inflammatory diseases. A consistent, supportive yoga practice can help you get in touch with—and remain aware of—your whole self.

Patricia Says

When you menstruate, and particularly during bouts of heavy bleeding, you'll want to change the focus of your yoga practice.

• Don't try to get better at or go deeper into a pose.

• Never do inversions when you are bleeding. That includes Headstand (Sirsasana), Shoulderstand (Sarvangasana), Plough Pose (Halasana), Downward-Facing Dog Pose (Adho Mukha Svanasana), and Legs-Up-the-Wall Pose (Viparita Karani) with a bolster. Inversions pull your uterus toward your head, which causes the broad ligaments to overstretch.

• Relax completely into each pose. Soften your abdomen, let your brain relax deeply, and direct your breath to any areas that feel discomfort—your abdomen, your head, your legs.

• Relax your vaginal walls completely. Now is not the time to focus on toning that area.

Cramps

Menstrual cramps—the bane of many a young woman's monthly cycle—vary widely in intensity and form. My daughter gets sharp, colicky cramps. Complete with constipation and periodic bouts of diarrhea, they bring her to a fetal position for the first twenty-four hours of her period. A friend of hers suffers from the dull, achy variety that lodges in her lower back and leaves her feeling lethargic, bloated, and nauseous. Other women complain of migraines, leg cramps, and breast pain or tenderness that herald the start of their periods.

My daughter and her friend suffer from what is called primary dysmenorrhea, the most common form of menstrual cramping. This is not associated with any other kind of pelvic disease or inflammation; it's menstrual cramps, pure and simple. Secondary dysmenorrhea is menstrual pain caused by something else going on in the body—pelvic inflammatory disease, endometriosis, or adenomyosis (a condition in which the glands in the lining of the uterus grow deeply into the uterine wall, causing the wall to bleed when you menstruate). Secondary dysmenorrhea can be quite serious, and it's important to consult your health practitioner if your cramps are unusually severe, don't respond to dietary changes or stress management, or are accompanied by heavy bleeding. Although yoga can often help relieve the pain associated with secondary dysmenorrhea, our focus here will be on the primary kind.

Western physicians believe that primary dysmenorrhea is caused by an overabundance of the hormone prostaglandin $F_2\alpha$ in the menstrual blood. When this hormone is released into the bloodstream, the smooth muscle of the uterus spasms, and you experience cramps. You can blame a diet high in animal protein and dairy products for too much prostaglandin $F_2\alpha$ in your system, as well as a lifestyle filled with unrelenting stress.

Susan Lark, M.D., author of several self-help books for women, believes that primary dysmenorrhea occurs as either spasmodic or congestive cramps. Spasmodic cramps are most commonly found in teenagers and women in their early twenties. Women sometimes find this type of cramping subsides after their first pregnancy. Congestive cramps, on the other hand, make life miserable for women in their thirties and forties and seem to worsen after childbirth. These dull, achy cramps are accompanied by bloating, breast tenderness, weight gain, irritability, and headaches.

How Yoga Can Help A favorite pose for many women suffering from heavy bleeding or menstrual cramps is Reclining Bound Angle Pose (Supta Baddha Konasana), using straps, bolsters, blankets, and eyebags. The epitome of restorative poses (Patricia calls it the "Mother of All Asanas"), it provides support for your entire body and allows you

Patricia Says

• Soft instrumental music can help you turn inward, quiet your mind, and relax more deeply.

• Sometimes when you go to class during your period, you can get caught up in the energy of the class and end up working too hard. So, practice at home; that way you can gauge how much strength you have and can adjust your practice accordingly.

• Practice with awareness. Take care to work internally, not aggressively or muscularly during times of heavy bleeding, cramping, fatigue, or agitation.

to relax completely. It's particularly beneficial for lower-back aches during menstruation, according to Judith Hanson Lasater, author of *Relax and Renew: Restful Yoga for Stressful Times*. Judith believes these backaches are often the result of overstretching in the ligaments that hold the sacrum and the pelvic bone together. She explains in her book that hormonal changes during your period create instability in those ligaments and render them susceptible to injury. This instability often causes the dull ache many women get in their lower back just before their period. By supporting your sacrum and legs with a strap and bolsters, you allow your body to remain passive. Geeta Iyengar goes a step further and recommends that your legs be supported on top of a bolster as well.

Any of the poses in the Sequence for Healthy Menstruation can help soothe cramps. Try several to determine which ones work best for you. Some women find relief in bending forward with something pressed hard against their bellies. If that works for you, try Child's Pose (Adho Mukha Virasana), hugging a bolster or two, or any of the seated forward bends. If you prefer creating space in your abdomen, allowing the breath to flow freely to release your muscles, you may benefit from any of the supported reclining poses like Bridge Pose (Setu Bandha Sarvangasana) or Inverted Staff Pose (Viparita Dandasana). If you suffer from dull, achy cramps in your back, you may prefer a gentle twist, like Simple Seated Twist Pose (Bharadvajasana) from the Woman's Essential Sequence (see page 13). Experiment until you find something that relieves your type of pain.

No matter which poses you choose, don't worry about getting better or further along in your practice. Give up trying to get your leg straighter or your back more open, and focus on caring for yourself, purifying each cell of your body and bathing it in the breath. Bri Maya Tiwari, an Ayurvedic healer, told me years ago that if I pampered myself on the first full day of my period—no work, no worries, no cooking, no writing—my reproductive health would improve enormously. And she was right. So do these poses as though you were treating yourself to an hour or so of pure indulgence.

PREMENSTRUAL SYNDROME

A catch-all phrase if there ever was one, PMS can include any of over 150 symptoms. Do you feel irritable, edgy, or "hot under the collar"? You have PMS. Anxious, moody, or ungrounded, and barely able to remember your own name? You have PMS, too. How about bloated, achy, and depressed—in fact, you could cry if someone looked at you sideways? You guessed it, PMS. You may also have periodic bouts of acne, heart fibrillations, insomnia, herpes, hives, migraines, salt or sugar cravings, or even asthma, and these would all be PMS symptoms.

According to Christiane Northrup, the type of symptom doesn't matter much; it's the way it occurs. Generally speaking, she explains that women should see a pattern of flare-ups each month. Some women feel anxious and flighty about a week before their period, and as soon as they begin to bleed, they feel better. Others may get angry and rage uncontrollably two weeks before their period, only to fall into a depression the next week and feel appreciably better the first or second day of their period. I get intense sugar cravings—particularly of the chocolate variety—about ten days before I start. If I give in to my weakness, I not only end up with a horrific headache a few days later, but my joints ache and swell until I'm through with the first or second day of my cycle.

In order to alleviate premenstrual syndrome, it's important to understand its physical and emotional causes. On a physical level, most physicians agree that an imbalance of hormones and a sluggish liver contribute to PMS symptoms. If you feel anxious, irritable, and moody, you may have an overabundance of estrogen in your body or not enough progesterone to balance it. If you are depressed and confused, can't sleep, and can't remember anything, too much progesterone may be the culprit. Regardless of which hormone predominates, it could be a sign that your endocrine system is not doing its job efficiently and has failed to produce the correct amount of the hormones you need. If you experience bloating, breast tenderness, and weight gain, your pituitary gland and adrenals may be to blame. Susan Lark says the pituitary secretes too much adrenocorticotropic hormone (ACTH), which makes its way to the adrenal glands above the kidneys. The adrenals, in response, overreact by secreting too much of their own hormones, which get sent to the kidneys, which in turn retain salt and water and produce less urine.

Ayurvedic scholar and healer Robert Svoboda calls PMS a woman's "monthly dysfunction syndrome" and believes it to be a result of the disharmony created during the early part of the menstrual cycle. In other words, if you eat junk food, drink lots of caffeinated beverages, function with very little sleep, shelve your exercise routine, and consistently fail to deal with your feelings (especially negative ones like anger and hurt), you can count on problems later in the month.

Ayurvedic medicine postulates that a woman's biological rhythms are in tune with nature's own. Nancy Lonsdorf, coauthor of *A Woman's Best Medicine: Health, Happiness, and Long Life through Ayurveda*, explains that "anything that throws off our biological rhythms can create menstrual problems. Since each cycle operates in phase with every other cycle, if we are off-rhythm in our sleep cycle, this can easily throw off our menstrual cycle." Therefore, according to ayurveda, by regulating your daily routine, you can correct monthly imbalances and hopefully lessen PMS symptoms. For some women, however, PMS symptoms have gone on for so long they need herbal support, diet revisions, and major lifestyle changes to get back on track.

My favorite definition of PMS comes from Joan Borysenko, author of *A Woman's Book of Life: The Biology, Psychology, and Spirituality of the Feminine Life Cycle*, who deems it "emotional housecleaning," the time during a woman's cycle in which she is more apt to confront what's bothering her and release it. Remember the image of your menstrual cycle linked to the lunar cycle? It's a wonderful image. As the moon comes into its fullness, so do you. Estrogen-dominant, you are alive, sexy, creative, and energized. As the moon begins to wane, you move into the luteinizing phase of your cycle. This progesterone-dominant time is when you go inward, becoming more in tune with your dreams, more in touch with your deepest, even darkest emotions. Suddenly something you've repressed all month long seems overwhelming and you just have to express it, get it out, deal with it. Women who are in touch with their emotions and needs during this time often discover many of their physical PMS complaints subside.

How Yoga Can Help

Yoga helps alleviate PMS in a number of ways. On a physical level, it relaxes your nervous system, balances your endocrine system, increases the flow of blood and oxygen to your reproductive organs, purifies your liver, and strengthens the muscles surrounding all these organs. Psychologically, yoga works to ease stress and promote relaxation so the hypothalamus can regulate your hormones more efficiently. It offers you the time—and often the permission—you may need to go inside, listen to your body, and respond to what you hear.

The sequence on page 108 is designed to alleviate symptoms you already have. In order to decrease the frequency of PMS, however, it's important to practice yoga consistently. Done regularly, the essential and energizing sequences in chapters 1 and 2 should help. If you feel irritable or angry, do the poses with some form of support (see the modifications) so you can rest your head on a bolster or chair. Resting your head cools your brain and eases any tension you may be feeling.

Inverting—turning yourself upside-down—is the best way to create balance and stability within your body's systems. If you feel irritable or anxious during PMS, Patricia recommends doing your inversions with support, as we've shown them in this chapter. You'll get the same results without having to work so hard. Headstand (Sirsasana) stimulates the pituitary gland and pineal body, both vital for good menstrual health, and increases circulation to your brain. For some women, however, Headstand can be too unsettling during PMS; they find that Shoulderstand (Sarvangasana) with full body support gives them more freedom around their throat (thereby balancing the thyroid and parathyroid glands), opens their chest, and softens their abdomen. Plough Pose (Halasana) enlivens your adrenal glands and kidneys. If you feel depressed and lethargic, any of the chest- and shoulder-opening poses will help. For many women, creating this kind of space in their body quells the agitation they feel and lifts their spirits.

RETURNING TO NORMAL

Once your period is over, you're probably eager to return to your normal routine, including your daily yoga practice. Patricia believes you shouldn't rush things. Your body needs to regain strength and stamina. We've provided several poses at the end of the chapter that you'll find beneficial for the first three to five days after you stop bleeding. In the meantime, keep the following dos and don'ts in mind:

- Don't do backbends right away—they're too aggressive. Allow your body to recover from the fatigue of your monthly cycle first.

- Do incorporate inversions immediately because they help dry up your uterus, restore your endocrine system, increase circulation to your abdominal region, and help your body regain its strength.

- Don't do a lot of standing poses the first couple of days if you still feel fatigue. Ease into them.

STAYING HEALTHY ALL MONTH LONG

The most important thing you can do to minimize menstrual problems is to take care of your body and honor yourself every day. If you know, for example, that drinking coffee or soda brings on premenstrual headaches, find a decaffeinated substitute. By avoiding greasy foods and sugary desserts, cutting down on alcohol and caffeinated beverages, and substituting home-cooked meals for processed foods, you may find much of your physical and emotional discomfort goes away. Here are some other suggestions many women have found helpful.

Patricia Says

To get the most out of these menstrual sequences, focus on creating space between your rib cage and your abdomen. Relax your abdomen, pelvic region, and vaginal walls. Pay particular attention to your breathing. Direct your breath wherever you feel constriction. If your abdomen feels tight, breathe into it to soften and comfort it. If you feel constricted in your diaphragm or around your chest and heart, direct your breathing there. If you have cramps, breathe all the way down into your uterus. Directing your breath in this way brings an internal focus to your practice and allows you to relax deeply, resting your entire body. The Sequence for Healthy Menstruation is gentle, nourishing, and designed to make you feel completely cared for.

1. *Get sufficient rest.* If you do nothing else for yourself, rest during the first day or two of your period. You'll be amazed at how much better you feel the rest of the month. This doesn't mean you should sleep during the day—that can make you feel sluggish and depressed. It does mean you should relax, read that book you've been meaning to get to, take walks with no particular place to go. If you have children, find quiet activities you can do together. If you have to go to school or work, be easy on yourself, schedule a lighter-than-usual load, and take the evening off.

2. *Be selfish.* The first day or two of your period is a time for reflection. If you meditate, now is a good time to practice loving kindness toward yourself, your family, and your friends. Do things that make you feel good about being you.

3. *Exercise in moderation.* Unless you are plagued with debilitating cramps the first day of your period, exercise is fine; just don't overdo it. Walking or gentle yoga stretches (see the healthy menstruation sequence starting on page 100) work best. During the rest of the month, a consistent yoga practice and moderate

aerobic exercise should help prevent PMS and menstrual problems from occurring in the first place.

4. *Eat pacifying foods.* During the first day or two of your cycle, eat warm foods that are easy to digest, such as rice, cooked green vegetables, and soups. Avoid cold, raw foods, as well as anything else that's hard to digest, such as red meat, cheese, and chocolate. Sip warm water throughout the day to aid digestion.

5. *Modify your routine.* Baths disrupt the natural rhythm of your menstrual flow, so shower the first few days of your period. After that, treat yourself to a warm oil massage or a facial to destress your nervous system and soothe your mind. Whenever you can, wear menstrual pads rather than tampons, especially during the first few days of your period, to encourage the downward flow of blood.

A SEQUENCE FOR HEALTHY MENSTRUATION

1. Reclining Bound Angle Pose
   (Supta Baddha Konasana)
2. Child's Pose (Adho Mukha Virasana)
3. Head-on-Knee Pose (Janu Sirsasana)
4. Three-Limb Intense Stretch (Triang
   Mukhaikapada Paschimottanasana)
5. Seated Forward Bend
   (Paschimottanasana)
6. Wide-Angle Seated Pose I
   (Upavistha Konasana I)
7. Wide-Angle Seated Pose with a Twist
   (Parsva Upavistha Konasana)
8. Wide-Angle Seated Pose II
   (Upavistha Konasana II)
9. Inverted Staff Pose (Viparita Dandasana)
10. Bridge Pose (Setu Bandha Sarvangasana)
11. Corpse Pose (Savasana)

1. RECLINING BOUND ANGLE POSE (Supta Baddha Konasana) Place a bolster vertically behind you and sit just in front of it with your knees bent and your sacrum touching the bolster's edge. Put a folded blanket on the other end of the bolster to prevent any strain on your neck. Place a strap behind your back, at your sacrum; draw it forward over your hips, across your shins, and under your feet (see page xv). Put the soles of your feet together and let your knees and thighs fall to the sides. Cinch the strap securely under your feet. Lie back so your head is on the folded blanket and your torso rests comfortably on the bolster; your buttocks and legs are on the floor. (If you feel any discomfort in your lower back, add some height to your support with a folded blanket or two. If you feel any muscle tension in your legs, roll two blankets vertically and place one under the top of each thigh.) Remain in this pose for as long as you like, breathing deeply.

To come out, draw your knees together, slip the strap off, and slowly roll to one side. Use your hands to push yourself up to a seated position.

EFFECTS This pose can help relieve menstrual cramps, spasms, and heaviness in your uterus; take pressure off your pelvic area; and open your chest, clearing your mind and calming your nerves during times of stress.

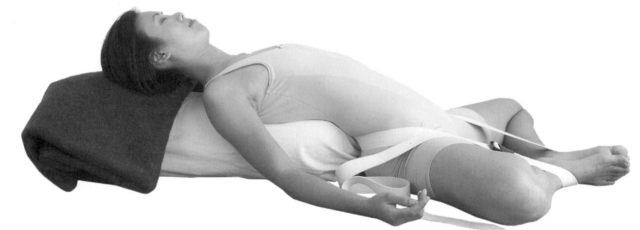

2. CHILD'S POSE (Adho Mukha Virasana) Kneel on the floor with two bolsters placed in a T shape directly in front of you, one end of the vertical bolster between your knees and the other on top of the horizontal bolster. Spread your knees wide and straddle the bolster, bringing your toes together. Bend forward and stretch your arms and trunk up and over the bolster, pressing it into your abdomen. Rest your head on both bolsters and relax completely. Close your eyes, release your vaginal muscles, soften your abdominal muscles, and breathe into your pelvic region. Remain in this pose for several minutes, or as long as you like.

EFFECTS Many women find hugging the bolster into their abdomen relieves menstrual cramps and helps them release any tension in their muscles.

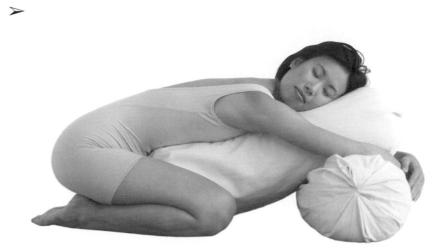

3. HEAD-ON-KNEE POSE† (**Janu Sirsasana**) Sit on the floor with your legs stretched out in front of you. Bend your right knee to the side so it is at a 45-degree angle to your left leg and your right heel is near the right side of your groin. Push your right knee as far back as you comfortably can; keep your left leg straight.

Place a folded blanket or a bolster on your outstretched leg, and turn your abdomen and chest so your sternum is in line with the center of your left leg. As you inhale, lift your trunk up from the base of your pelvis; as you exhale, reach your arms out in front of you as you lean your trunk forward. Fold your arms on your support and cradle your head on your arms. Your head should rest without straining your neck, and you should feel no pressure or strain in your back or the backs of your legs. (If you feel any strain, add more height to your support or rest your head on a padded chair seat, see page 48.)

Stay in this pose for 1 to 2 minutes, resting your head, the base of your skull, your eyes, and your mind. Inhale while coming up, and change sides.

EFFECTS This cooling pose has a toning effect on your reproductive organs and the supporting muscles. Many women also find it beneficial for cramps, PMS irritability, or anxiety.

†CAUTION Do not do this pose if you have diarrhea or feel nauseous.

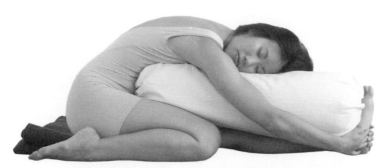

4. THREE-LIMB INTENSE STRETCH† (**Triang Mukhaikapada Paschimottanasana**) Sit on one or two folded blankets on your mat with your legs stretched out in front of you. Depending on your flexibility, place folded blankets or a bolster or two on your left leg for support. Bend your right knee and bring your right foot back by the side of your right hip, toes pointing back. Extend your trunk forward over your outstretched leg and clasp your foot with your hands, if possible. Turn your head to the side and rest completely on your support. Breathe quietly in this pose for 1 to 2 minutes, relaxing your shoulders, head, neck, and abdomen. To come out, lift up from your pelvic floor, drawing your abdomen in and up. Change sides.

EFFECTS You may find this calming, cooling pose good for relieving stress, anxiety, and mild menstrual cramps.

†CAUTION Do not do this pose if you are bleeding heavily or have severe cramps or diarrhea.

5. SEATED FORWARD BEND† (**Paschimottanasana**) Sit on your mat (or on one or two folded blankets) with your legs stretched out in front of you. Place a folded blanket or a bolster across your lower legs. Take a full, deep breath and lift your arms over your head, stretching up through your spine and lifting your sternum and head. Keep your back slightly concave. As you exhale, bend forward and extend your torso over your legs, cradling your head in your arms on your support. (If you feel strain in your back or in your legs, or if you experience vomit reflux when you bend forward, add more height to your support or rest your head on a padded chair seat, see page 49.) Do not allow your buttocks to come off the floor (or blankets). Remain in this pose for as long as you like, preferably 3 to 5 minutes, keeping your abdomen soft.

EFFECTS This is a very restful pose that helps calm anxiety and relieve irritability, cramps, and headaches.

†CAUTION Do not do this pose if you have diarrhea or feel nauseous.

6. WIDE-ANGLE SEATED POSE I (Upavistha Konasana I) Sit against the wall and spread your legs wide apart; flex your feet. Adjust the flesh of your buttocks by drawing it behind you and out to the sides. (If you find it hard to sit up straight in this position,

sit on two or more blankets or a block positioned against the wall.) Place your hands on the floor behind you, draw your abdomen and floating ribs up toward your chest, and move your shoulder blades into your back. Sit up tall, press down through your legs and extend up through your spine for 30 seconds to 1 minute. To come out, relax your arms and release your legs.

EFFECTS This pose can help the circulation in your pelvic area, regulate your menstrual flow, and stimulate your ovaries.

7. WIDE-ANGLE SEATED POSE WITH A TWIST (Parsva Upavistha Konasana) Sit up tall with your legs wide apart. Place a bolster lengthwise on your right leg. Turn your abdomen, chest, and rib cage so you are facing your right leg. As you exhale, extend your trunk forward over your leg and fold your arms on the bolster to cradle your head. Your body should rest without effort; there should be no strain on your hamstrings, shoulders, or neck. Rest comfortably in this pose for 30 seconds to 2 minutes, relaxing your head, the base of your skull, your eyes, and your mind. Inhale as you come up, and change sides.

EFFECTS The gentle twisting action of this pose may help improve circulation in your pelvis, regulate your menstrual flow, and stimulate your ovaries and kidneys.

8. WIDE-ANGLE SEATED POSE II (Upavistha Konasana II) Do Wide-Angle Seated Pose I as described above, but place a vertical bolster in front of you. As you inhale, lift your trunk up from the base of your pelvis; exhale and reach your arms out in front of you as you release your torso forward completely. Rest your head on the bolster. Fold your arms on the bolster to cradle your head. Stay in this pose for 2 to 5 minutes. To come up, place your hands on either side of the bolster and roll up to a sitting position. Release your legs.

EFFECTS This pose can help blood circulate in your pelvis, regulate your menstrual flow, and calm agitation and irritability.

9. INVERTED STAFF POSE† **(Viparita Dandasana)** (Before beginning, see pages 34–35.) Place a folded blanket on a chair about 2 feet from the wall—far enough away so your feet can press into the wall when your legs are outstretched. Pile two bolsters against the wall for your feet, and put a bolster (and a folded blanket, if necessary) in front of the chair for your head. Sit facing the wall, with your feet through the chair back. Hold onto the sides of the chair and support yourself on your elbows, as you arch back slowly. Your head, neck, and shoulders should extend past the chair seat and your shoulder blades should touch the front edge of the seat.

Still holding the sides of the chair, arch back so your shoulder blades are at the front edge of the seat and your head can rest on its support. (You may need to scoot your buttocks farther toward the back of the seat.) Put your feet on top of the bolsters and against the wall, legs slightly bent, and hold the back legs or sides of the chair. Straighten your legs, pressing your feet into the wall, and roll your thighs in toward each other. Rest your head on the bolster. Keep your hands on the chair sides or legs. Breathe quietly for 30 to 60 seconds.

To come out, bend your knees and place your feet flat on the floor. Grasp the sides of the chair back and lift up from your sternum. Lean over the chair back for a few breaths to release your back.

EFFECTS This is an excellent pose when you're suffering from depression or fatigue. It opens your chest, which can improve respiration and circulation, help lift your spirits, and invigorate your whole body.

†CAUTION Seek the advice of an experienced teacher if you have neck problems. Do not do this pose if you have a migraine or tension headache or diarrhea.

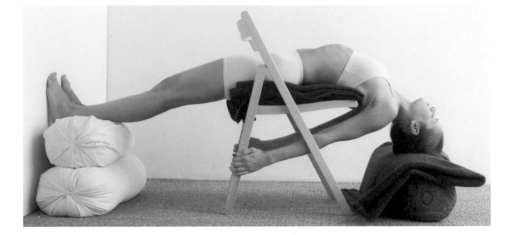

10. BRIDGE POSE (Setu Bandha Sarvangasana) Place one bolster horizontally against the wall and another vertically, forming a T shape. Sit on the end of the vertical bolster that is closest to the wall. Keeping your knees bent, lie back over the bolster. Slide down until the end of the bolster is in the middle of your back and your shoulders just reach the floor. Rest your shoulders and head on the floor. Stretch your legs toward the wall and put your heels on the horizontal bolster so your feet touch the wall. Your legs should be about hip-width apart with your feet pointing toward the ceiling. Close your eyes and relax completely, softening your abdomen, and breathing deeply. Stay in this position for at least 3 to 5 minutes.

To come out, bend your knees and slowly roll to one side. Push up to a seated position.

EFFECTS This restful pose can be beneficial for depression, as well as anxiety and irritability.

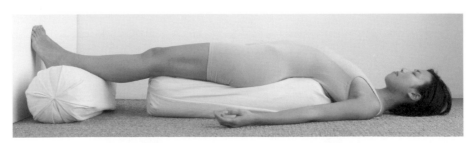

11. CORPSE POSE (Savasana) Lie on your back with your legs stretched out in front of you. (Use a folded blanket to support your head, if necessary, and an eyebag over your eyes to block out any external sensations.) Place your arms comfortably at your sides, slightly away from your torso, with your palms facing upward. Actively stretch your arms and legs away from you, then allow them to release completely. Close your eyes and let everything relax. Breathe deeply, inhaling into your chest without tensing your throat, neck, or diaphragm. Exhale your body into the floor, releasing your shoulders, neck, and facial muscles. Keep your abdomen soft and relaxed, and release your lower back. Remain in the pose, breathing normally, for 5 to 10 minutes. To come out, bend your knees, roll to one side, remain there for a few breaths, and then open your eyes and push yourself up with your hands.

EFFECTS This deeply relaxing pose allows you to release your abdominal muscles and vaginal walls. It helps relieve fatigue, as well as abdominal and lower back cramps.

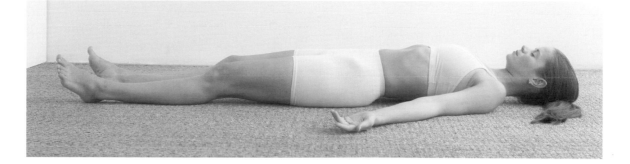

1. Bound Angle Pose (Baddha Konasana)
2. Wide-Angle Seated Pose I (Upavistha Konasana I)
3. Half-Moon Pose (Ardha Chandrasana)
4. Reclining Bound Angle Pose (Supta Baddha Konasana)
5. Bridge Pose (Setu Bandha Sarvangasana)
6. Corpse Pose (Savasana)

A SEQUENCE FOR HEAVY PERIODS

1. BOUND ANGLE POSE (Baddha Konasana) Sit against the wall with your back straight and your abdomen lifted. Bending your legs, open your knees out and bring the soles of your feet together. Hold the tops of your feet and draw your heels in toward your perineum (the pubic bone). The outer edges of your feet should remain on the floor. Lengthen your spine upward, leading with the crown of your head. Stretching your inner thighs from groin to knee, gently lower your knees as far as possible. Place your hands on the floor behind you to sit up straighter, and lift your abdomen. Stay in this position for 30 seconds or more, breathing normally. (If you are menstruating or your hips are tight and you can't lengthen your spine, sit against the wall on a block or blanket about 4 inches thick.)

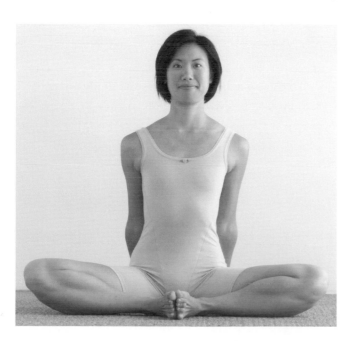

To come out, relax your arms and bring your knees up one at a time. Stretch your legs out in front of you.

EFFECTS This is a terrific pose to help alleviate cramps, heavy bleeding, and a feeling of heaviness in your abdomen.

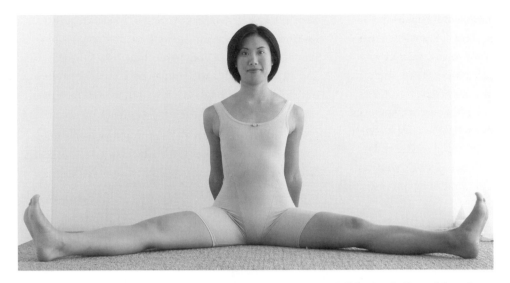

2. WIDE-ANGLE SEATED POSE I (Upavistha Konasana I) Do Wide-Angle Seated Pose I as described on page 103. Take care to completely relax your pelvic area, vaginal walls, and abdominal muscles.

EFFECTS This pose may be especially beneficial in slowing heavy bleeding associated with fibroid tumors and endometriosis. It massages your reproductive organs and gently lifts your uterus, which has a drying effect.

3. HALF-MOON POSE (Ardha Chandrasana) Do Extended Triangle Pose (Utthita Trikonasana) to the left (see page 6). Bending your left knee, place the fingertips of your left hand on a block at the wall, about a foot in front of your left leg. Come up onto the toes of your left foot. Exhale, simultaneously straightening your left leg and raising your right

up until it is parallel to the floor. Your right leg, hips, shoulders, and head should rest against the wall. Turn your pelvis and chest toward the ceiling. Stretch your right arm up in line with your shoulders and open your chest and pelvis farther. Draw your shoulder blades into your back and look up at your right hand or straight ahead. Hold for 15 seconds, breathing normally. To come down, bend your left leg, reach your right leg back, and return to Extended Triangle Pose. Inhale, come to standing and repeat on the other side. Return to Mountain Pose (Tadasana).

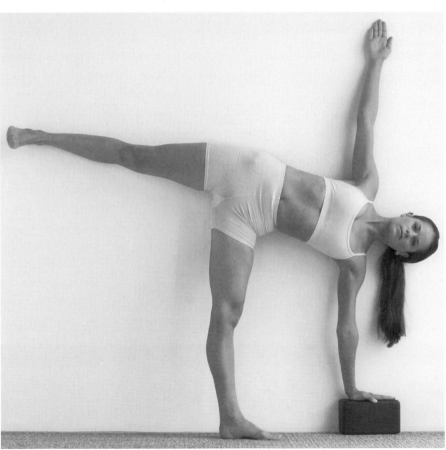

EFFECTS This is an excellent pose to help stop heavy bleeding and relieve the cramping associated with fibroid tumors and endometriosis.

4. RECLINING BOUND ANGLE POSE (Supta Baddha Konasana) Sit in the middle of a vertical bolster with a folded blanket at the end of it for your head. Place a strap behind your back, at your sacrum; draw it forward over your hips, across your shins, and under your feet. (For belt placement, see pages xv and 100.) Put the soles of your feet together and let your knees and thighs fall to the sides. Cinch the strap securely under your feet. Lie back so your head and shoulders are off the bolster (and resting on the blanket) and your feet are on the bolster.

Breathe normally, softening your belly and releasing your pelvic floor. Remain in this pose as long as you like—5 to 10 minutes at least.

To come out, draw your knees together, slip the strap off, and slowly roll to one side. Use your hands to push yourself up to a seated position.

EFFECTS This modified pose helps relieve menstrual cramps, spasms, and heaviness in your uterus by taking pressure off your pelvic area.

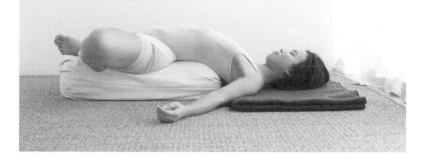

5. BRIDGE POSE (Setu Bandha Sarvangasana) Do Bridge Pose as described on page 104. Breathe calming breaths into your abdomen and chest, and remain in this pose for 5 to 10 minutes, or as long as you like.

EFFECTS Resting in this pose helps to relieve tension in your abdomen and heaviness in your uterus and eases menstrual cramping.

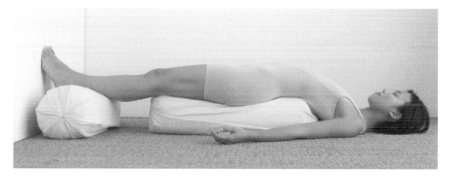

6. CORPSE POSE (Savasana) Do Corpse Pose as described on page 105. Keep your abdomen soft and release your vaginal walls. Remain in this pose for at least 5 to 10 minutes, breathing into your belly.

EFFECTS This pose helps relax and restore your entire body and quiet your mind.

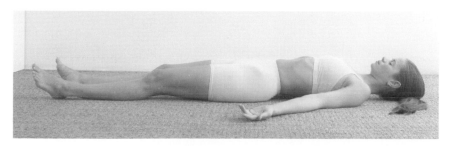

1. Reclining Bound Angle Pose
   (Supta Baddha Konasana)
2. Cross Bolsters Pose
3. Reclining Big Toe Pose II
   (Supta Padangusthasana II)
4. Downward-Facing Dog Pose
   (Adho Mukha Svanasana)
5. Headstand (Sirsasana)
6. Shoulderstand (Sarvangasana)
7. Plough Pose (Halasana)
8. Wide-Angle Seated Pose II
   (Upavistha Konasana II)
9. Bridge Pose
   (Setu Bandha Sarvangasana)
10. Corpse Pose (Savasana)

A SEQUENCE FOR PREMENSTRUAL SYNDROME

1. RECLINING BOUND ANGLE POSE (Supta Baddha Konasana) Do Reclining
Bound Angle Pose as described on page 100, taking care to soften your
abdomen and release your pelvic floor. Breathe calming breaths deep into
your abdomen. As you exhale, let your abdomen broaden and recede toward
your spine. Remain in this pose for at least 5 to 10 minutes.

EFFECTS This pose is excellent for helping you ease the anxiety, irritability,
fatigue, and depression associated with premenstrual stress.

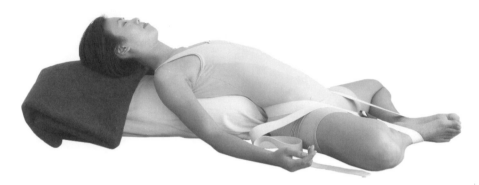

2. CROSS BOLSTERS POSE Place a bolster on your mat and lay another one
across the center of the first to form a cross. Sit on the middle of the top
bolster and carefully lie back so your spine is supported on the bolster and
the back of your head touches the floor. (If that is too much of a stretch or
puts strain on your neck, place a folded blanket underneath your head.) Place
your arms on either side of your head, palms up, elbows bent, and relax
completely. (If you feel any strain in your lower back, raise your feet on a
block.) Relax in this pose for several minutes, softening your abdominal
muscles and breathing deeply. To come out of the pose, bend your knees and
roll to one side. Help yourself up using your hands.

EFFECTS This pose opens your chest; improves respiration; and helps relieve
the fatigue, headaches, and depression associated with PMS.

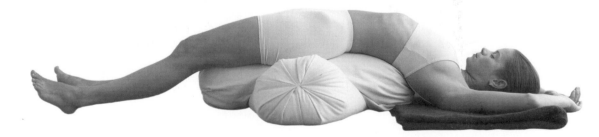

3. RECLINING BIG TOE POSE II (Supta Padangusthasana II) Place a bolster on the floor about 6 inches to your right so the bottom edge is in line with your right hip. Loop a strap around your right foot as shown in the photo, holding the long end with your left hand. Raise your leg straight up to the ceiling, run the long end of the strap behind your head, and straighten your left arm out to the side. On an exhalation, ease your right leg out to the side and down onto the bolster. Pull gently on the strap with your left hand to add a little resistance. Rest comfortably for at least 1 to 2 minutes. Repeat this pose with your left leg.

EFFECTS This pose helps relieve lower back pain and ease cramps and general pelvic discomfort.

4. DOWNWARD-FACING DOG POSE (Adho Mukha Svanasana) To find the correct distance between your hands and feet for this pose, lie facedown on your sticky mat. Place your palms on the floor by each side of your chest with your fingers well spread and pointing straight ahead. Come up on your hands and knees, and turn your toes under. (If you feel agitated, have a headache, or experience fatigue with your PMS, place a folded blanket or two or a bolster vertically on the floor so your support is in line with your sternum and will provide support for your head, see page 84.)

Exhale, press your hands firmly into the mat and extend up through your inner arms. Exhale again as you raise your buttocks high in the air and move your thighs up and back. Keep stretching through your legs and bring your heels toward the floor. Keep the legs firm and the elbows straight as you lift your buttocks upward. The action of the arms and legs serves to elongate your spine and release your head. Hold this pose for 30 seconds to 1 minute, breathing deeply. Let your head rest completely and release the base of your neck. To come out, either return to your hands and knees and sit back on your heels.

EFFECTS This pose helps tone and relax your nervous system, relieving anxiety, irritability, and depression.

5. HEADSTAND† (**Sirsasana**) (Before beginning, see pages 16–17.) Place a folded blanket against the wall. Kneel in front of it with your feet and knees together. Interlace your fingers firmly, thumbs touching and your hands cupped. Position your hands no more than 3 inches from the wall, your elbows shoulder-width apart. Your wrists, forearms, and elbows form the foundation for this pose.

Lengthen your neck and place the crown of your head on the blanket. The back of your head should be in contact with your hands. Press your forearms into the floor and lift your shoulders away from the floor. Maintain this action throughout the pose. Straighten your legs, raise your hips toward the ceiling, and walk your feet in until your spine is almost perpendicular to the floor. As you exhale, lift one leg at a time, and bring your feet to the wall.

Keep your heels and buttocks against the wall. Roll your thighs in, lift your tailbone, lengthen your legs upward, and keep your feet together. Remember to balance on the crown of your head, support yourself by pressing your forearms into the floor, and continue to lift your shoulders away from your ears. Keep your breathing even, your eyes and throat soft, and your abdomen relaxed. With regular practice, you can slowly learn to bring your buttocks and heels away from the wall. Hold the pose as long as you can, up to 5 minutes.

To come out, exhale and bring your legs down to the floor one at a time. Bend your knees, sit back on your heels, and rest for a few breaths before raising your head.

EFFECTS By counteracting the effects of gravity, this pose helps recirculate blood to your heart, so it is good for overall circulation. It also helps you feel energized and refreshed, relieving depression and confusion.

†CAUTION Do this pose only if it is already part of your yoga practice. Seek the advice of an experienced teacher if you have neck problems. Do not do this pose if you have your period or suffer from back problems or migraines.

6. SHOULDERSTAND† (**Sarvangasana**) (Before beginning see pages 18–19.) Lie on your back with two folded blankets supporting your shoulders and your arms stretched out beside your body. On an exhalation, bend your knees and raise your legs toward your chest. Pressing your hands into the floor, swing your bent legs over your head; support your back with your hands and press your elbows firmly into the blankets. Raise your torso up until it is perpendicular to the floor and your knees are close to your chest. Supporting your back, raise your legs until your thighs are parallel to the floor; raise them some more until your knees point toward the ceiling. Now raise your legs completely and extend up through your heels until your whole body is perpendicular to the floor. Move your tailbone up and in and use your hands to lift your back ribs. Feel that your whole body is long and straight. Move your shoulders away from your ears. Hold this pose as long as you can, preferably at least 2 minutes.

To come out, exhale as you bend your knees. Slowly roll down. Lie still for several breaths.

EFFECTS This pose encourages the supply of fresh, oxygenated blood to your thyroid and parathyroid glands and helps soothe your nerves, stimulate your kidneys, and calm your mind.

†CAUTION Do not do this pose if you suffer from neck or shoulder problems, if you have high blood pressure, if you are menstruating, or if you have a migraine or tension headache.

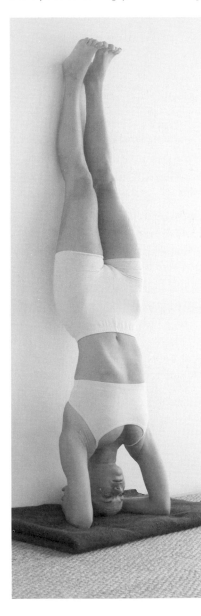

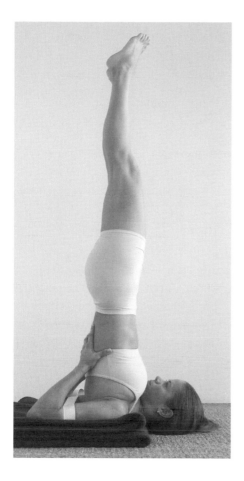

7. PLOUGH POSE† **(Halasana)** Lie on your back with two folded blankets supporting your shoulders; your head is on the sticky mat and your arms are down by your sides, palms pressed into the floor. Bend your knees and bring your thighs in to your chest. On an exhalation, swing or lift your buttocks and legs up, supporting your back with your hands, and extend your legs over your head, placing your toes on the floor behind you. Keep your thighs active by tightening your knees to create space between your face and your legs. Stay in this pose, breathing deeply and slowly, for several minutes. To come out, slowly roll down one vertebra at a time. Rest with your back flat on the floor, breathing deeply, for several breaths.

EFFECTS This pose helps balance your endocrine system and quiet your sympathetic nervous system so your mind feels uncluttered and your whole body can relax deeply. Helps relieve throat problems and congestion, and may improve thyroid and parathyroid function.

†CAUTION Do not do this pose if you suffer from neck or shoulder problems, or if you are menstruating.

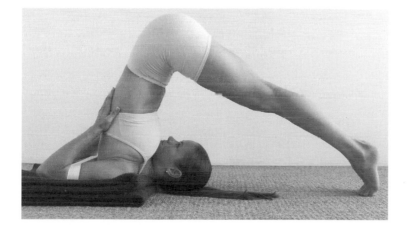

8. WIDE-ANGLE SEATED POSE II
(Upavistha Konasana II) Do Wide-Angle Seated Pose II as described on page 103.

EFFECTS This pose helps calm your endocrine system and pacify your adrenal glands. It may also be good for regulating your period.

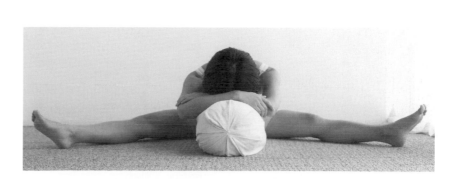

9. BRIDGE POSE (Setu Bandha Sarvangasana) Place a block vertically against the wall and have another at your side. Lie on your back with your arms at your sides and your knees bent. Raise your hips and chest as high as possible and support your back with your hands. Keeping your head and shoulders flat on the floor, lift your spine even farther, increasing the arch, and place the other vertical block under the fleshy part of your buttocks. Stretch out one leg at a time, resting each heel on the vertical block against the wall. Release your arms so that your hands reach just beyond the block under your sacrum. Hold the pose for at least 30 seconds, breathing normally.

To come out, bend your knees and place your feet on the floor. Then release the block under your sacrum and slowly roll down one vertebra at a time. Hug both knees to your chest and rest for several breaths.

EFFECTS This pose is good for toning and improving circulation to your kidneys and adrenal glands and for helping to regulate your menstrual cycle. If you feel irritable or anxious, try the supported version described on page 104.

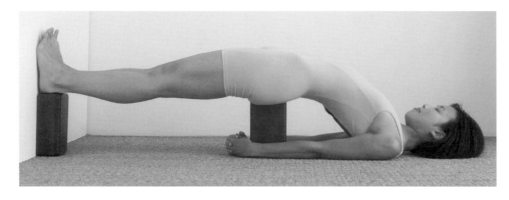

10. CORPSE POSE (Savasana) Do Corpse Pose as described on page 105, but place a bolster behind you with one end at the base of your spine and a folded blanket on the other end to support your neck and head. Keep your breathing smooth and effortless.

EFFECTS This wonderfully restorative pose helps relax your mind, quiet your nervous system, and rejuvenate your whole body.

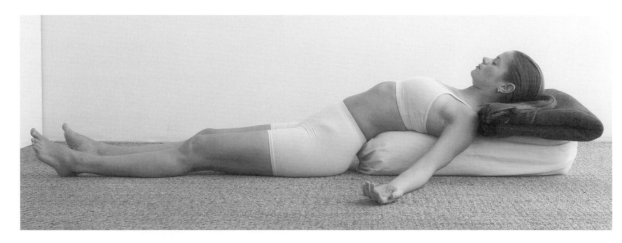

1. Downward-Facing Dog Pose
   (Adho Mukha Svanasana)
2. Standing Forward Bend (Uttanasana)
3. Wide-Angle Standing Forward Bend
   (Prasarita Padottanasana)
4. Headstand (Sirsasana)
5. Shoulderstand (Sarvangasana)
6. Plough Pose (Halasana)
7. Head-on-Knee Pose (Janu Sirsasana)
8. Corpse Pose (Savasana)

A SEQUENCE FOR POSTMENSTRUATION (3 TO 4 DAYS AFTER YOU STOP BLEEDING)

1. DOWNWARD-FACING DOG POSE (Adho Mukha Svanasana)

Do Downward-Facing Dog as described on page 109. If you feel tired or stiff, rest your head on a bolster or folded blanket.

EFFECTS This pose helps increase the blood supply to your brain and enhance circulation in your chest.

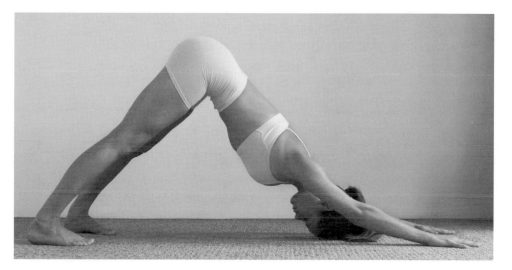

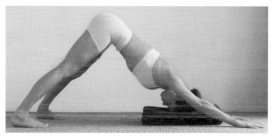

Modification

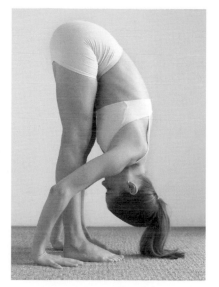

2. STANDING FORWARD BEND (Uttanasana) Stand in Mountain Pose (Tadasana). Balance the weight evenly between your feet, lengthen up through your inner thighs, and roll your thighs in. Keep your legs and knees firm as you lift your arms overhead, stretching up through your waist and ribs. As you exhale, bend forward from your hips and release your side body and head down toward your knees. Press your hands into the floor next to your feet. (If you can't touch the floor, rest your hands on blocks or on your shins.) Breathe normally for 30 to 60 seconds. To come out, keeping your legs active, put your hands on your hips and slowly lift up to standing.

EFFECTS This pose brings a sense of calm and peace when you feel agitated or anxious. It tones your liver, spleen, and kidneys and lifts and tones your uterus.

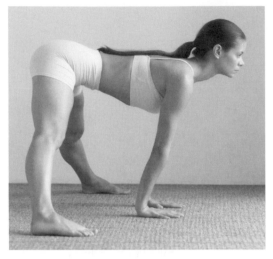

3. WIDE-ANGLE STANDING FORWARD BEND (Prasarita Padot-tanasana) Step your feet apart about 4 feet (or as wide as possible), keeping the outer edges of your feet parallel. Tighten your quadriceps to draw your kneecaps up and keep your thighs well lifted. On an exhalation, bend forward from your hips and place your hands on the floor—in line with your shoulders (A). (If you feel strain in your lower back, place your hands on blocks.) Lift your hips toward the ceiling, draw your shoulder blades into your back, and look up, keeping your entire spine concave. Remain this way for 10 to 15 seconds.

Keeping your trunk extended, exhale, bend your elbows, and release the crown of your head toward the floor—resting it on the floor, if possible (B). Keep your legs firm, but relax your shoulders and neck. Breathe deeply and let your trunk release downward. Stay in this pose for 30 to 60 seconds. To come out, return to the concave back position, bring your hands to your hips, and raise your trunk. Step your feet together.

EFFECTS This pose can be helpful when you're trying to combat fatigue, calm your mind, tone your abdominal region, and soothe jittery nerves. It also lifts your uterus, improves circulation in your pelvis, and helps restore equilibrium to your central nervous system.

B

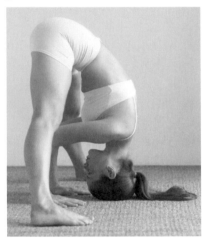

114

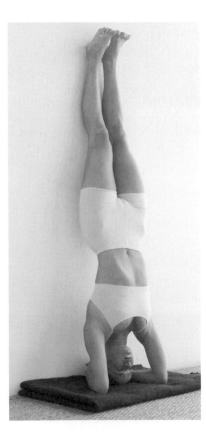

4. HEADSTAND† (Sirsasana) Do Headstand as described on page 110.

EFFECTS This rejuvenating pose is excellent for rebalancing your endocrine system and helps recirculate blood to your heart.

†CAUTION Do this pose only if it is already part of your yoga practice. Seek the advice of an experienced teacher if you have neck problems. Do not do this pose if you have your period or suffer from back problems or migraines.

Headstand for Advanced Practitioners

If you have a strong yoga practice, one that already includes Headstand (Sirsasana), you may want to add these poses to your postmenstrual sequence.

HEADSTAND WITH OUTSTRETCHED LEGS (Upavistha Konasana in Sirsasana) Do Headstand as described on page 110. Spread your legs wide, stretching from your groin through your heels. Keeping your legs straight, stretch up through your spine and broaden your chest. Remain this way for 10 to 15 seconds.

HEADSTAND WITH SOLES OF FEET TOGETHER (Baddha Konasana in Sirsasana) From the previous pose, bend your legs, spread your knees outward, and press the soles of your feet firmly together. Remain in this position for another 15 to 20 seconds, keeping your knees wide apart, and breathe normally. Straighten your legs and return to the wide-leg position, then to your original Headstand position, before coming down.

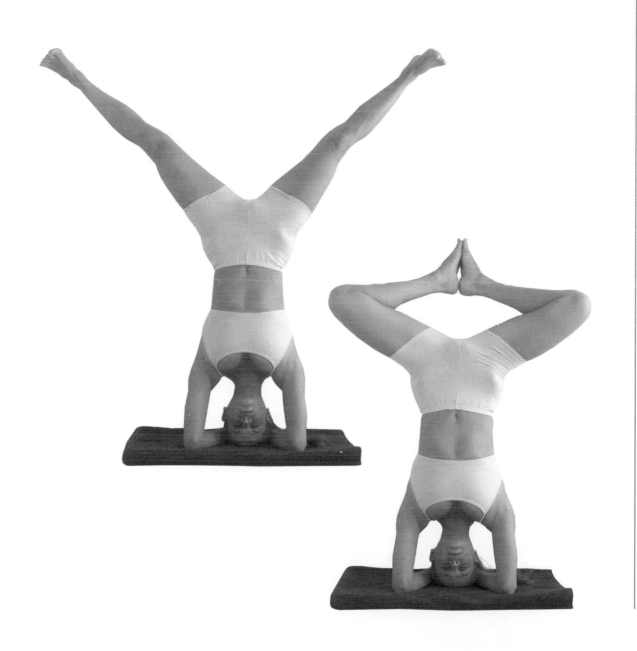

5. SHOULDERSTAND† (Sarvangasana) (Before beginning see pages 18–19.)
Lie on your back with two folded blankets supporting your shoulders and
your arms stretched out beside your body. On an exhalation, bend your knees
and raise your legs toward your chest. Pressing your hands into the floor,
swing your bent legs over your head; support your back with your hands and
press your elbows firmly into the blankets. Raise your torso up until it is
perpendicular to the floor and your knees are close to your chest. Supporting
your back, raise your legs until your thighs are parallel to the floor; raise
them some more until your knees point toward the ceiling. Now raise your
legs completely and extend up through your heels until your whole body is
perpendicular to the floor. Move your tailbone up and in and use your hands
to lift your back ribs. Feel that your whole body is long and straight. Move
your shoulders away from your ears. Hold this pose as long as you can,
preferably at least 2 minutes. To come out, exhale as you bend your knees.
Slowly roll down. Lie still for several breaths.

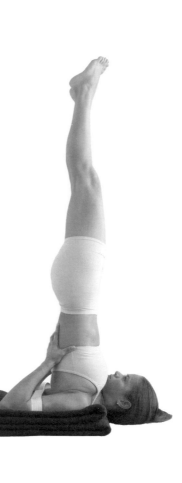

If this version of the pose is too difficult, try the modified version in the
Woman's Restorative Sequence (see page 50).

EFFECTS This pose may help improve thyroid and parathyroid function. It
soothes your nerves; stimulates your kidneys; and calms your mind, bringing
a sense of peace, strength, and new resolve when you feel tired, listless,
unstable, or nervous.

†CAUTION Do not do this pose if you suffer from neck or shoulder problems,
if you have high blood pressure, if you are menstruating, or if you have a
migraine or tension headache.

6. PLOUGH POSE† (Halasana) Lie on your back with
two folded blankets supporting your neck and shoulders;
your head is on the floor and your arms are down by
your sides, palms down. Bend your knees and bring your
thighs in to your chest. On an exhalation, swing or lift
your buttocks and legs up, supporting your back with
your hands, and extend your legs over your head, placing
your toes on the floor behind you. (To keep your elbows
in, you can use a strap around both arms, just above
your elbows, before you begin.) Keep your thighs
active by tightening your knees to create space
between your face and your legs. Stay in this
pose, breathing deeply and slowly, for at
least 30 seconds and up to 2 minutes. To
come out, slowly roll down one vertebra at a time. Rest with your back flat
on the floor, breathing deeply,
for several breaths.

If this pose is
too difficult, try

Half-Plough Pose (Ardha Halasana) as described in the
Woman's Restorative Sequence (see page 51).

EFFECTS This pose helps balance your endocrine system
and quiet your sympathetic nervous system. Resting this
way can help tame irritability and anxiety. It also tones
your abdominal organs, elongates and strengthens your
spine, and relieves fatigue.

†CAUTION Do not do this pose if you have neck problems
or if you are menstruating.

7. HEAD-ON-KNEE POSE (Janu Sirsasana) Sit with your legs stretched out in front of you. Bend your right knee to the side so it is at a 45-degree angle to your left leg and your right heel is near the right side of your groin. Push your right knee as far back as you comfortably can; loop a strap around the ball of your left foot and then straighten your left leg.

Turn your abdomen and chest to the left so your sternum is in line with the center of your left leg. With an exhalation, bend forward from your hips and pull back on the strap, straightening both arms; keep your head and back lifted. Inhale and lift your trunk up from the base of your spine. Remain like this for 15 to 20 seconds, if possible.

EFFECTS Because of the gentle twist, this pose has a toning effect on your reproductive organs and the supporting muscles.

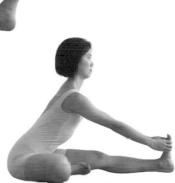

Modification

8. CORPSE POSE (Savasana) Do Corpse Pose as described on page 105, taking care to relax your facial muscles completely and drop the sides of your sacrum toward the floor to release your buttocks. If you have trouble relaxing your eyes in the beginning, drape an eyebag over them to block out any external distractions. Remain in the pose, breathing normally, for 5 to 10 minutes. To come out, bend your knees, roll to one side, and remain there for several breaths; gently push yourself up with your hands.

EFFECTS This restorative pose helps relax your mind, quiet your nervous system, and refresh and invigorate your whole body.

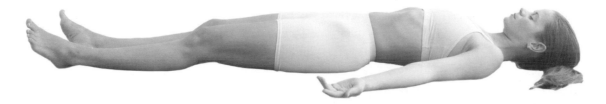

Chapter 6 *Supporting Your Immune System*

CARRIE AND HELEN HAVE BEEN ROOMMATES AND BEST FRIENDS for years. They've lived together ever since they started college, and now they're both in graduate school. They get along famously, but Carrie admits there's one thing that drives her crazy about her friend. Helen never gets sick. "I mean never. I get colds, flus, bronchitis, stuff like that, all the time; but not Helen," she explains. "I hated living in the dorm our first two years because whenever anyone came down with anything, I knew I'd get it next." And she did. Helen, on the other hand, somehow always skated by, seemingly immune to the viruses and bacteria that roamed the dormitory halls in search of stressed-out, nutritionally challenged, sleep-deprived students. Even now that the two young women rent a decent-sized apartment in the Northwest and share everything from hair products to toenail clippers, the germs find Carrie and leave Helen alone. Carrie wants to know why this happens. Aren't most viruses and bacteria equal-opportunity inhabiters?

Well, yes and no. Viruses and bacteria do take up residence in your body without much regard to whether you invite them in or attempt to keep them out. But what makes you sick or keeps you well is the combined interaction of your immune system, your emotional well-being, and your mental health. Holistic practitioners—Eastern and Western—call this the mind-body connection. Western scientists call it psychoneuroimmunology (PNI), a technical word for the study of how the mind (psyche) affects the way the body functions. PNI scientists like Candace Pert, author of *Molecules of Emotion: Why You Feel the Way You Feel* and research professor at Georgetown University Medical Center, have shown that a woman's emotions and beliefs about herself directly influence her health.

So, your emotional state has as much to do with your physical health as does the virulence of an invading virus or bacterial organism. For example, have you ever noticed that when you feel positive about your life, you have no trouble handling the day-to-day challenges that come up? But when you feel out of control, angry, and unable to express your feelings, even the smallest interruption in your schedule can cause disproportionate stress and physical symptoms such as heart palpitations, sweaty palms, and an inability to think straight?

Carrie knows this well. She acknowledges that her susceptibility to colds and flus may be the result of her state of mind. She certainly doesn't always handle stress as well as she should, and she often feels out of control. Her workload leaves her exhausted, and financial woes keep her worried most of the time. Never being one to share her feelings, she stuffs them inside and keeps going. Running to get to class on time is about the only exercise she gets. She also suffers from PMS, which manifests as a serious case of "poor me" for about a week or so before her period.

Helen, on the other hand, is generally upbeat. With a schedule that's as grueling as Carrie's, she has little time for herself, but makes it a point every night before bed to write in her journal, where she can process the day's activities and emotions. She rarely misses her early-morning yoga class and takes dance classes twice a week. Overall, she says, she feels in control of her life; in fact, she enjoys what she's doing and learning. Although she wishes she could slow down a little, she takes care (especially during exam time) to eat mindfully, acknowledge her emotions, and do things that honor her body.

Clearly, three major differences distinguish the roommates' behavior. First of all, Carrie feels out of control and Helen doesn't; second, Helen freely expresses her feelings and Carrie holds hers inside; and third, Helen exercises and practices yoga consistently and Carrie rarely finds the time. But still, why is Carrie the only one to get sick when a virus is going around—especially when they share the same food, utensils, and even cosmetics? Because the health of a woman's immune system and its ability to ward off disease depend on the health of all her bodily systems—including the nervous system, the endocrine system (ovaries, pituitary, adrenals, hypothalamus, and thyroid), and the lymphatic and circulatory systems. And all of these systems provide valuable information to assist immune function. Of course, the way she handles stress and expresses her emotions has profound effects on her immune system's ability to do its job.

Carrie and Helen have about the same amount of stress in their lives, but they view it quite differently. Carrie feels the stress she's under is beyond her control; it's determined by outside forces and she can do little about it, besides quitting school or taking medication. Helen believes stress is a natural part of her life, even a necessary part of the creative process that pushes her to change and grow. She believes that although she can't always control the amount of stress she comes into contact with, she can control how she responds to it.

THE IMMUNE RESPONSE

So, what is happening inside Carrie and Helen? How does feeling stuck and out of control cause Carrie's immune system to malfunction? How does expressing her emotions help Helen's immune system do a better job? And why does yoga make a difference? Mary Schatz,

Patricia Says

Cultivating the following habits can help you promote a healthy immune system:

• Get a good night's sleep. Ayurvedic physicians say the best time for a restful sleep is between 10:00 p.m. and 6:00 a.m. That's when your body restores and rejuvenates.

• Eat foods that are high in antioxidants and fiber but low in fat.

• Get in touch with and learn to express your emotions on a regular basis. If you need outside help to begin the process, by all means, seek out holistic practitioners who specialize in mind-body modalities.

M.D., author of *Back Care Basics: A Doctor's Gentle Program for Back and Neck Pain Relief* and a longtime yoga practitioner, believes that everyone operates from either an external locus of control or an internal one. Carrie has an external locus. She believes that outside forces control her stress levels and that, no matter what she does, she can't change what's happening to her. Helen, on the other hand, lives with an internal locus of control. She knows she can directly influence her body's responses to outside stresses in her life. Carrie subconsciously gives her body two distinct messages—first, that it's in danger, and second, that it's too weak and worthless to counteract that danger. Helen also sends her body subconscious messages, but they say everything is under control and she's confident her body and mind can handle anything that comes their way. Using PNI scientific hypotheses and research on how the immune system protects the body from invading organisms, it's easy to see why a positive attitude and a daily yoga practice can be powerful immune-system allies.

The immune system performs a complex job. It must distinguish everything that is you from everything that is not you. Generally you can coexist happily with the air you breathe, the food you eat, the clothes you wear, even the friendly bacteria that live in your intestines. But sometimes a harmful organism sneaks in and invades your cells. That's when your immune system—the spleen, bone marrow, lymph nodes, and different kinds of white blood cells—goes to work.

It's somehow reassuring to have your own built-in, internal security force, ever diligent and on the lookout for harmful invaders. Even your skin, the first line of defense, acts to ward off unwelcome germs. Your sweat and sebaceous glands give off substances that prevent bacteria from entering your system. Mucus membranes filter out most organisms that threaten the respiratory tract, and your stomach increases its gastric juices to render food bacteria harmless. Your respiratory organs, intestines, and reproductive organs also contain powerful enzymes that destroy the protein coverings of invading bacteria. If a virus or bacterium succeeds in getting past this first line of defense, it has an entire army of white blood cells awaiting it. These cells

Kim's Story

After the birth of her second child (by cesarean section), Kim's immune system went on strike. She was sick at least once a month, sometimes every two weeks. "My ailments weren't life-threatening," she remembers. "Just a string of head colds, stomach flu, and respiratory gunk. I tried vitamins, herbs, antibiotics, naturopathic remedies, massage, longer yoga practices, and taking more time off from work. Nothing seemed to help. After losing 70 percent of my hearing from a double ear infection (my hearing eventually came back) and having a staph infection take hold on my face, I was desperate.

"I turned to yoga. My teacher, Claudia Kuhns, teaches classes for people with immunosuppressive diseases. I explained my problems, and Claudia recommended a series of daily inversions. Ugh! After eight years of yoga, inversions rated right up there with backbends as my least favorite poses. But I was determined to cure myself, so I started doing a series of short inversions (10 to 30 seconds) every day. At first, I was exhausted after just a few poses, but after several weeks the poses started to get a little easier. We discussed that the exhaustion was probably due to my body going through a major reset.

"The first benefit of the inversions was that my too-frequent periods began to go back to a twenty-eight-day cycle. This happened the first month of my inversion practice. By the third month, as the length of my poses began to increase, I realized I hadn't been sick at all since I started this new practice! After one year, I've only been sick two days. Occasionally, I feel as if I'm fighting off some ailment, so I do an extra headstand, load up on vitamins, and go on my way."

For Kim's situation, her teacher's recommendation included more advanced poses like Handstand (Adho Mukha Vrksasana) and Elbow Balance (Pincha Mayurasana), as well as Downward-Facing Dog (Adho Mukha Svanasana) and Headstand (Sirsasana) for at least thirty seconds each and Inverted Staff Pose (Viparita Dandasana) on a chair, Bridge Pose (Setu Bandha Sarvangasana) on blocks, supported Shoulderstand (Sarvangasana), and Legs-Up-the-Wall Pose (Viparita Karani) for between two and five minutes each.

search out and destroy offending organisms, then clean up and repair the damage done.

In order to do a good job, the immune system must communicate effectively with the nervous and endocrine systems so it destroys only the invaders and repairs only your own tissues. Immune cells not only live in the lining of your lungs and intestines, on your skin, and in all mucous membranes, but they travel throughout your body responding to whatever it needs.

This seems like a pretty automatic response. How would feeling out of control or emotionally stuck change how your immune system works? First of all, as Candace Pert explains in her book, the neuro-peptides that transport thoughts and emotions throughout your body also control the routing and migration of the white blood cells that destroy disease-bearing organisms. These same neuropeptides also bind to receptors in your cells just the way viruses do. For example, reovirus (the one that causes colds) binds to the same receptors as norepinephrine, which your body manufactures when you feel happy and energetic. So it's possible that Helen's upbeat, positive feelings are literally taking up the space in her cells where reovirus would normally reside. If the virus can't find a host cell in which to reproduce, it can't do any harm.

Second, immune cells not only appear to respond to the neuro-peptides from the brain, but they also produce some of their own. As Edward Blalock, an immunologist from University of Texas, comments, "No state of mind exists that is not reflected by a state of the immune system."

FIGHT OR FLIGHT

Everybody's familiar with what scientists call the fight-or-flight response. If you've ever stepped off the curb and barely missed being hit by a car, you know what this response feels like: As your adrenaline soars, your blood pressure rises, your heart pounds wildly, you sweat like crazy, your mind goes on hyperalert, and your breath becomes shallow and quick. To bring as much power as possible to your sympathetic nervous system (which controls this response) so you can react quickly and efficiently, your body diverts energy from your digestive, reproductive, and immune systems, slowing them down to a bare maintenance level.

Once you realize you're out of danger, you begin to calm down and your nervous system returns to normal. People like Carrie, however, who constantly feel the threat of external stressors, don't give their systems a chance to calm down and return to a balanced state. They stay on hyperalert. Their adrenal glands become exhausted from constantly pumping adrenaline into the body; their digestive and immune systems remain sluggish; and the neurotransmitters that deliver messages of well-being are seriously lacking. If everything continues in this vein, immune surveillance can shut down, creating an opening for opportunistic viruses and bacteria to enter the body.

These days, unprecedented challenges from the outside world—pesticides, pollution, radiation, processed foods, prescription or recreational drugs—bombard your body and may prove too much for your immune system to handle.

Some evidence suggests that lack of sleep is just as detrimental to the immune system as unrelenting stress. According to research by the National Sleep Foundation, deep (non-REM) sleep allows your immune system to replenish and in particular to increase production of prolactin and interleukin-1, two hormones responsible for enhanced immune function. Further evidence suggests lack of sleep retards phagocytosis (destruction of invading organisms) and prevents lymphocyte production.

In essence, your physical body gets signals from your emotional self that say either "All is well, happy, and healthy," or "I can't cope; I'm in danger of losing it." These signals can be as subtle as taking a slow, deep breath (all is well) or clenching your jaw (danger signal), or as overt as being head-over-heels in love or grief-stricken by a loved one's death. Signals of well-being allow your immune cells to circulate freely; indications of stress or danger shift your body's resources away from the immune system to the sympathetic nervous system, which sounds the fight-or-flight alarm.

SO WHAT'S A BODY TO DO?

This is probably a good time to reevaluate your lifestyle and determine the best way to enhance and support your immune system. Dietary choices, a daily yoga practice, and herbal and vitamin supplements are all important steps. However, researchers are discovering that it's not so much what you do—that is, which therapy you turn to or which diet you embark on—that helps you heal, but your belief that such action will work. As Patricia reminds her students, learning to express emotions, honoring the wisdom of your body, and taking time for reflection and relaxation give a powerful signal to your body and spirit that they are loved. There are many ways a yoga practice can help you do that and bring your mind and body back to a state of balance and well-being.

HOW YOGA CAN HELP

Improve Your Circulation

Good surveillance—the seek-and-destroy mission of the immune cells—depends on good circulation. Remember that immune cells not only live in specific sites in your body, but also roam freely throughout the bloodstream and lymphatic fluids looking for foreign organisms.

Foods for a Healthy Immune System

• Fruits and vegetables high in vitamins C and A, which are antioxidants that stimulate immunity and counteract the effects of free radicals in the body.

• Essential fatty acids—particularly omega-3—found in freshwater fish; ground-up flax seeds; and oils from borage, evening primrose, and flaxseed, which have been found to regulate immune function in the body.

• Whole grains, which are high in vitamins and fiber and improve digestion so the body can more easily rid itself of toxins and waste.

• Sea vegetables—such as kelp, hizake, or dulse—which are high in trace minerals and vitamins. Seaweed provides nourishment to all the endocrine glands, particularly the thyroid and parathyroid. Include the milder tasting sea vegetables in soups or stews. Hizake and dulse are flavorful, but kelp is an acquired taste. Seaweed is also available in capsule form.

Certain products should be avoided, because they can undo all the good done by the healthy foods listed. Such products include refined sugar and anything containing caffeine.

Patricia Says

• Spend some time with nature as often as possible. Go to the park, a local forest preserve, or even your own backyard. Smelling the flowers, listening to the birds, or watching a beautiful sunset is calming and nurturing and helps restore your sense of connection to the world around you.

• Walk, ride your bike, or jog—exercise increases immune function and produces endorphins that signal the body that you feel happy and worthwhile.

• Do a consistent daily yoga practice that focuses not only on postures, but on conscious breathing. Yoga, meditation, and journal writing can help you reconnect with your higher self.

• Practice loving kindness on a daily basis—not only toward other people, but toward yourself. Count your blessings, each and every one of them, every day.

• Laugh a lot. Laughter stimulates immunity, while prolonged grief suppresses it.

And, because your immune system relies on information from the central nervous and endocrine systems, good circulation allows immune cells to communicate freely with the pituitary gland, pineal body, hypothalamus, lymphatic tissues, and other immune cell sites like the gastrointestinal tract, respiratory tract, and skin.

Inversions are yoga's gift to your circulation system. Headstand (Sirsasana), Shoulderstand (Sarvangasana), and Plough Pose (Halasana) all improve blood flow to the endocrine glands. When you are in a pose, Patricia says it helps to visualize what yoga masters call the squeezing, soaking, and massaging action of the posture. In Shoulderstand, for example, you can feel how a chin lock exerts gentle massage pressure on the throat, "squeezing" out the stale blood. As you release the pose, visualize the area being soaked with new, healthy immune cells and flooded with blood to regulate their function. By turning everything upside down, inversions energize and stabilize the whole system. According to yoga researcher, Krishna Raman, author of *A Matter of Health*, yoga's squeeze-and-soak action pushes out cellular toxins more efficiently than other forms of exercise.

He also writes that the massage action in general brings freshly oxygenated blood to your skin, which promotes "healthy output of antibacterial secretions," enhances blood flow to your respiratory tract, and pushes blood into your bone marrow, increasing your body's ability to produce immune cells. What most women know is that Shoulderstand (Sarvangasana) makes them feel joyful and balanced, energized and peaceful at the same time.

Balance Your Central Nervous System

B. K. S. Iyengar, a master of yoga's therapeutic applications, believes that certain yoga poses quiet your sympathetic nervous system (the fight-or-flight instigator), replenish your adrenal glands when they have been working overtime, and promote a general feeling of well-being. He says that forward bends calm the sympathetic response and stop the adrenals from firing. Patricia notes that supported forward bends (using a bolster or chair so your back muscles do less work) give a feeling of being supported literally, of being safe from outside stressors.

Once the adrenals are calm, twisting poses can replenish and backbends can energize them. Krishna Raman explains it similarly: "Forward bends recuperate, backbends stimulate, passive poses energize, and inverted poses refresh."

Fill Your Heart, Clear Your Mind, and Enliven Your Spirit

Nothing works quite like yoga in bringing you back to your essential nature, your true self. In *A Woman's Best Medicine: Health, Happiness, and Long Life through Ayurveda,* coauthor Nancy Lonsdorf explains how loving yourself (and others) keeps you healthy. She says that a feeling of love in your heart creates a life-sustaining environment, "a collective emotional desire among all your cells" to be truly alive. Patricia teaches over and over again that yoga can help you find that love from inside. She says standing poses offer the strength you need to stand on your own two feet; backbends help you stay open to and flexible in challenging situations; inversions teach you to stay centered even when your life turns upside-down; balancing poses remind you that you can stay focused and balanced in the midst of stress; forward bends and restorative poses offer you a safe haven, an opportunity to return to your core and replenish yourself.

Patricia believes your yoga class can serve as your "personal growth lab" in which the lessons you learn through your practice can be applied to daily life. Ellen, a sixteen-year-old from Massachusetts, says forward bends have been a good teaching tool for her. She finds she shies away from them because she can't do them as well—or as gracefully—as she can do backbends. Knowing that about herself helps her look at what else she avoids.

Let Your Breath Make a Difference

Scientists have studied the effects of relaxation and deep breathing on the body and have found that a person can consciously alter functions once thought to be autonomic (unconscious), including heart rate, digestion, and even cellular functions. Many women have been able to control the amount of pain they feel during natural childbirth. And everyone's heard of yogis and swamis who can significantly reduce their heart rate through meditation. Other studies suggest that deep breathing, biofeedback, and self-hypnosis can render white blood cells more effective in immune surveillance. Common sense will tell you it's impossible to clench your fist, jaw, or stomach muscles when you take slow, deep breaths and concentrate on exhaling.

Relaxed, conscious breathing gives your body the signal that life is good, that you feel safe. Fast, shallow breathing indicates danger and pushes your body into the fight-or-flight response, suppressing immune function and activating your sympathetic nervous system. Breathing exercises (pranayama) and resting postures such as Corpse Pose (Savasana) and Reclining Bound Angle Pose (Supta Baddha Konasana) help balance your sympathetic and parasympathetic nervous systems, initiating the relaxation response, and help improve blood oxygenation, which is necessary for good health. Patricia says that breathing up into your chest brings more oxygenated blood to the area and gives your body and mind a sense of well-being and openness. These techniques can further focus your attention on a single point and prevent you from reacting to onslaughts of outside stimuli.

Patricia Says

Patañjali, second-century sage and author of the *Yoga Sutra,* wrote that chanting the syllable OM removes all obstacles to practice, helps turn your mind inward, and brings you right to the source of wisdom, of true self (Sutras I:27/28). Choose a word or phrase for yourself, one that can help you get through a hard time. Choose another one that will serve as a guiding principle for your life. Let it ride on the waves of your breathing; let it be the vehicle to calm and nourish you.

The postures Patricia provides in this chapter are designed to balance your immune system in general, and to calm and restore your sympathetic nervous system in particular. It's beyond the scope of this book to tailor sequences to specific immune dysfunctions, such as rheumatoid arthritis, multiple sclerosis, Crohn's disease, or cancer. However, practicing many of the restorative poses in this book will offer support and balance to your entire system and thus counteract the feelings of despair and anxiety that often come with these conditions. (Further suggestions for rheumatoid arthritis can be found in chapter 8; Crohn's disease sufferers will find helpful advice in chapter 12.)

1. Reclining Bound Angle Pose
   (Supta Baddha Konasana)
2. Head-on-Knee Pose (Janu Sirsasana)
3. Downward-Facing Dog Pose
   (Adho Mukha Svanasana)
4. Headstand (Sirsasana)
5. Shoulderstand (Sarvangasana)
6. Plough Pose (Halasana)
7. Simple Seated Twist Pose
   (Bharadvajasana)
8. Legs-Up-the-Wall Pose (Viparita Karani)
   and Cycle
9. Corpse Pose (Savasana)

A SEQUENCE FOR ENHANCED IMMUNITY

1. RECLINING BOUND ANGLE POSE (Supta Baddha Konasana) Place a bolster vertically behind you and sit just in front of it with your knees bent and your sacrum touching the bolster's edge. Put a folded blanket on the other end of the bolster to prevent any strain on your neck. Place a strap behind your back, at your sacrum; draw it forward over your hips, across your shins, and under your feet (see page xv). Put the soles of your feet together and let your knees and thighs fall to the sides. Cinch the strap securely under your feet. Lie back so your head is on the folded blanket and your torso rests comfortably on the bolster; your buttocks and legs are on the floor. (If you feel any discomfort in your lower back, add some height to your support with a folded blanket or two. If you feel any muscle tension in your legs, roll two blankets vertically and place one under the top of each thigh.) Remain in this pose for as long as you like, breathing deeply.

To come out, draw your knees together, slip the strap off, and slowly roll to one side. Use your hands to push yourself up to a seated position.

EFFECTS This pose helps quiet your mind, calm your nerves, and relieve anxiety during times of stress.

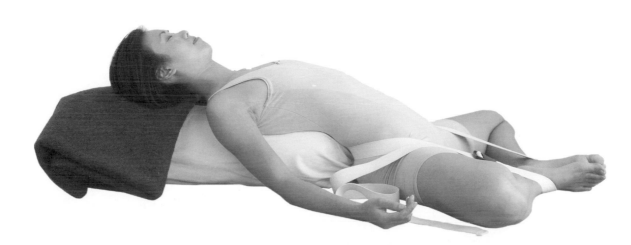

2. HEAD-ON-KNEE POSE† (Janu Sirsasana) Sit on the floor with your legs stretched out in front of you. Bend your right knee to the side so it is at a 45-degree angle to your left leg and your right heel is near the right side of your groin. Keep your left leg straight.

Place a folded blanket or a bolster on your outstretched leg, and turn your abdomen and chest so your sternum is in line with the center of your left leg. As you inhale, lift your trunk up from the base of your pelvis; as you exhale, reach your arms out in front of you as you lean your trunk forward. Fold your arms on your support and cradle your head on your arms. Your head should rest without straining your neck, and you should feel no pressure or strain in your back or the backs of your legs. (If you feel any strain, add more height to your support or rest your head on a padded chair.)

Stay in this pose for as long as you like, preferably 2 to 3 minutes, resting your head, the base of your skull, your eyes, and your mind. Inhale while coming up, and change sides.

EFFECTS This pose can bring a sense of calm and peace to your whole body.

†CAUTION Do not do this pose if you have diarrhea.

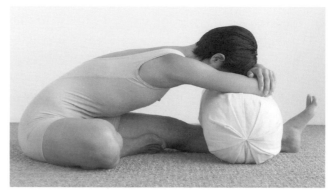

3. DOWNWARD-FACING DOG POSE (Adho Mukha Svanasana) Begin on your hands and knees; curl your toes under. (If you don't feel well, place a bolster or a folded blanket or two vertically on the floor so it's in line with your sternum and will provide support for your head.)

Exhale, press your hands firmly into the mat and extend up through your inner arms. Exhale again as you raise your buttocks high in the air and move your thighs up and back. Keep stretching through your legs and bring your heels toward the floor. Keep the legs firm and

the elbows straight as you lift your buttocks upward. The opposing action of the arms and legs serves to elongate your spine and release your head. Hold this pose for 30 seconds to 1 minute, breathing deeply. Let your head rest completely and release the base of your neck. To come out, return to your hands and knees and sit back on your heels.

EFFECTS This pose helps increase circulation to your heart and lungs, calm and soothe your mind, and it gently energizes your whole body.

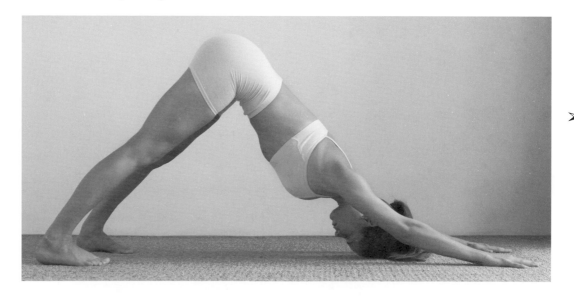

4. HEADSTAND† **(Sirsasana)** (Before beginning, see pages 16–17.) Place a folded blanket against the wall. Kneel in front of it with your feet and knees together. Interlace your fingers firmly, thumbs touching and your hands cupped. Position your hands no more than 3 inches from the wall, your elbows shoulder-width apart. Your wrists, forearms, and elbows form the foundation for this pose.

Lengthen your neck and place the crown of your head on the blanket. The back of your head should be in contact with your hands. Press your forearms into the floor and lift your shoulders away from the floor. Maintain this action throughout the pose. Straighten your legs, raise your hips toward the ceiling, and walk your feet in until your spine is almost perpendicular to the floor. As you exhale, lift one leg at a time and bring your feet to the wall.

Keep your heels and buttocks against the wall. Roll your thighs in, lift your tailbone, lengthen your legs upward, and keep your feet together. Remember to balance on the crown of your head, support yourself by pressing your forearms into the floor, and continue to lift your shoulders away from your ears. Keep your breathing even, your eyes and throat soft, and your abdomen relaxed. With regular practice, you can slowly learn to bring your buttocks and heels away from the wall. Hold the pose as long as you can, up to 5 minutes.

To come out, exhale and bring your legs down to the floor one at a time. Bend your knees, sit back on your heels, and rest for a few breaths before raising your head.

EFFECTS This is a good pose for overall circulation and respiratory health; it makes your whole body feel energized and refreshed.

†CAUTION Do this pose only if it is already part of your yoga practice. Seek the advice of an experienced teacher if you have neck problems. Do not do this pose if you have your period or suffer from back problems or migraines.

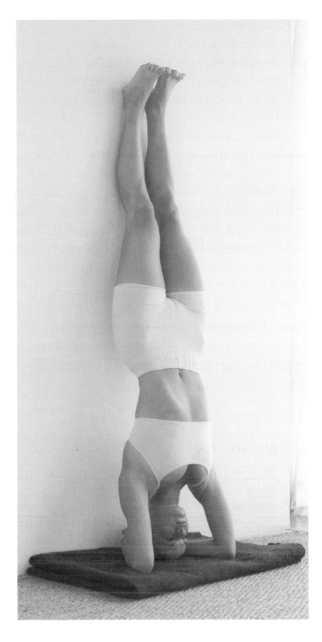

Modification

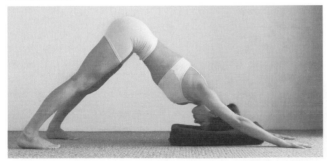

5. SHOULDERSTAND† (**Sarvangasana**) (Before beginning see pages 18–19.) Lie on your back with two folded blankets supporting your shoulders and your arms stretched out beside your body. On an exhalation, bend your knees and raise your legs toward your chest. Pressing your hands into the floor, swing your bent legs over your head; support your back with your hands and press your elbows firmly into the blankets. Raise your torso up until it is perpendicular to the floor and your knees are close to your chest. Supporting your back, raise your legs until your thighs are parallel to the floor; raise them some more until your knees point toward the ceiling. Now raise your legs completely and extend up through your heels until your whole body is perpendicular to the floor. Move your tailbone up and in and use your hands to lift your back ribs. Feel that your whole body is long and straight. Move your shoulders away from your ears. Hold this pose as long as you can, preferably at least 2 minutes.

To come out, exhale as you bend your knees. Slowly roll down. Lie still for several breaths.

EFFECTS This pose helps supply fresh, oxygenated blood to your thyroid and parathyroid glands, soothe your nerves, stimulate your kidneys, and calm your mind.

†CAUTION Do not do this pose if you suffer from neck or shoulder problems, if you have high blood pressure, if you are menstruating, or if you have a migraine or tension headache.

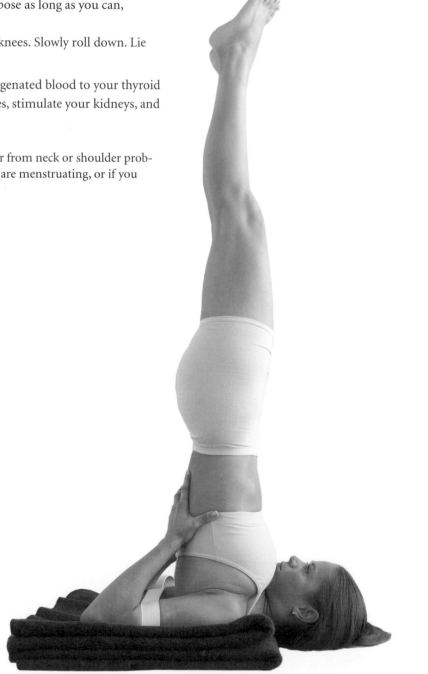

6. PLOUGH POSE† **(Halasana)** Lie on your back with two folded blankets supporting your neck and shoulders; your head is on the floor and your arms are down by your sides. Bend your knees and bring your thighs in to your chest. On an exhalation, swing or lift your buttocks and legs up, supporting your back with your hands, and extend your legs over your head, placing your toes on the floor behind you. (To keep your elbows in, you can use a strap around both arms, just above your elbows, before you begin.) Keep your thighs active by tightening your knees to create space between your face and your legs. Stay in this pose for at least 30 seconds and up to 2 minutes. To come out, slowly roll down one vertebra at a time. Rest with your back flat on the floor for several breaths.

EFFECTS This pose is good for balancing your endocrine system and calming your sympathetic nervous system so your mind feels empty and you can relax deeply. Helps relieve throat problems and congestion.

†CAUTION Do not do this pose if you suffer from neck or shoulder problems, or if you have your period.

7. SIMPLE SEATED TWIST POSE† **(Bharadvajasana)** Sit up straight with your legs stretched out in front of you and your left hip elevated on a folded blanket or two. Bend both legs to the right so your feet are next to your right hip. Keeping your thighs and knees facing forward, make sure your right ankle rests on the arch of your left foot and that you are not sitting on top of your foot.
Draw your shoulder blades into your back, broaden your chest, and extend your spine upward. On an exhalation, turn your abdomen, ribs, chest, and shoulders (in that order) to the left; place your right hand on the outside of your left thigh and your left hand on the floor behind you (or on a block). Take several breaths, holding the posture for 20 to 30 seconds. Relax your face, neck, and throat. Come back to the center position, straighten your legs, and change sides.

EFFECTS This pose can help improve circulation in and around your abdomen, kidneys, liver, and spleen. It is beneficial if your digestive system has been compromised due to stress.

†CAUTION Do not practice twists if you have diarrhea.

8. LEGS-UP-THE-WALL POSE† (Viparita Karani) AND CYCLE Place a bolster about 3 inches from the wall. Sit on the bolster so your right hip and side are touching the wall. Using your hands to support you, lean back and swivel your body around, taking your right leg and then your left leg up the wall. Keep your buttocks close to or against the wall. (If you feel stiffness or discomfort in your legs, push your buttocks slightly away from the wall.) Lie down so your lower back and ribs are supported by the bolster. Your tailbone should descend toward the floor. Your shoulders and head are resting on the floor (A). (If your neck is uncomfortable, put a folded towel or blanket under it.) Extend through your legs and place your arms out at your sides, elbows bent and palms up. Rest in this position, eyes closed, for 5 minutes.

CYCLE Without moving your torso, allow your legs to open out to the sides (B). Remain in this position, breathing normally, for 3 to 5 minutes.

Then bend your knees, cross your legs at the ankles, and continue in the pose for another 3 to 5 minutes (C).

Gently push away from the wall until your buttocks are just off the bolster and resting on the floor; the backs of your thighs and legs are on the bolster (D). Rest in this position for 5 minutes, or as long as you like.

To come out of the pose, uncross your legs, push gently away from the bolster, and roll to one side. Breathe quietly for a few breaths, then use your arms to help you to a seated position.

EFFECTS This deeply relaxing pose calms your sympathetic nervous system and helps stop the fight-or-flight response.

†CAUTION Do not do this pose when you are menstruating.

A

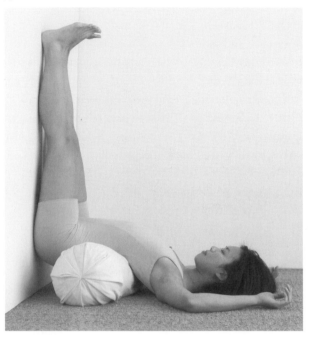

B

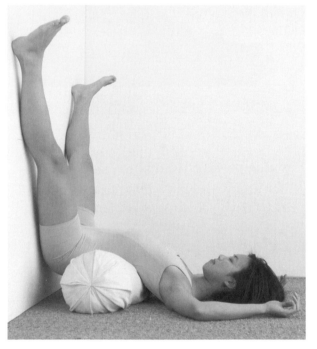

C

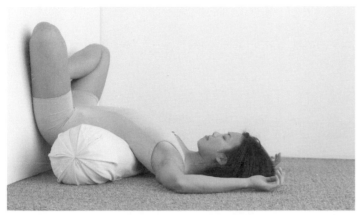

D

9. CORPSE POSE (Savasana) Lie on your back with your legs stretched out in front of you. (Use a folded blanket to support your head, if necessary, and an eyebag over your eyes to block out any external sensations.) Place your arms comfortably at your sides, slightly away from your torso, with your palms facing upward. Actively stretch your arms and legs away from you, then allow them to release completely. Close your eyes and let everything relax. Breathe deeply, inhaling into your chest without tensing your throat, neck, or diaphragm. Exhale your body into the floor, releasing your shoulders, neck, and facial muscles. Keep your abdomen soft and relaxed, and release your lower back. Remain in the pose, breathing normally with a slight emphasis on the exhale, for 5 to 10 minutes. To come out, bend your knees, roll to one side, remain there for a few breaths, and then open your eyes and push yourself up with your arms.

EFFECTS This pose helps soothe your sympathetic nervous system, rejuvenate your whole body, and refresh your mind.

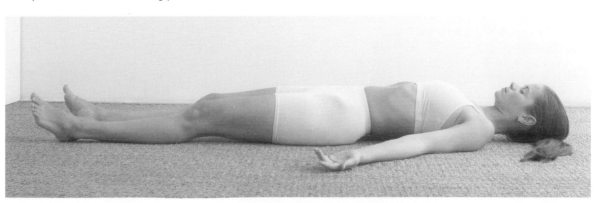

PART THREE

Coming into Fullness

Introduction

Several years ago I went to see an ayurvedic healer, a doctor trained in the medical art and science of ancient India, because I was falling apart, but I couldn't explain the symptoms in a way that made sense to my family physician. I didn't feel like myself—I was scattered, anxious, and weepy; I couldn't sleep; pains radiated down my back into my legs; and I had lost ten pounds I didn't need to lose. After reading my pulses for a long time, the doctor looked up at me and said, "My dear, you appear to have a heart problem." Seeing my look of alarm, she quickly explained that the problem didn't stem from any malfunction in the muscle; indeed, my arteries were clear and open. My difficulty came from taking into my own heart the suffering of those around me. "Do you mean I absorb other people's pain?" I asked. "No," she sighed, "You inhale it. And you don't do anyone any good, especially yourself, if you lose yourself in the process of taking care of others."

Someone once described a woman's health as the barometer of her environment, created and molded out of her relationships and the collective joys, fears, and tragedies of those around her. When all is right with the world, she is calm; when those she loves are in turmoil, she internalizes the stress and gets sick. On the surface, nothing is inherently wrong with wanting to make everything better. But it took getting sick for me to realize that I had bought into the myth of woman as ultimate caregiver, the "don't worry, I'll take care of everything" mentality that for years defined the perfect wife and mother, and later the myth of Superwoman. And it took falling apart for me to realize what was missing from that equation—I had neglected, as so many women had, to become a caregiver for myself as well.

As you enter your thirties, you straddle a fine line between being present in the world and being swallowed up by that world. If you've entered this stage in balance (and with your inner voice intact), you come ready to explore what the world has to offer and ready to share your gifts with that world. If you have lost touch with your inner voice, this stage of life brings lots of challenges, both physical and emotional. Not surprisingly, the most common physical complaints from women in this age group are stress-related. Tension headaches and migraines make you feel like you're literally bursting at the seams. Back pain comes from tension, stress, doing the wrong kind of exercise (or not taking the time to do any at all), and working too much. And even joyful occasions such as pregnancy stress your body and emotions.

A consistent, mindful yoga practice offers you a respite from the world, a break from all the responsibilities you shoulder, and a way of coming home to yourself. Yoga gives you a chance to focus on your core, refuel, fill up your tank of compassion, and put things back in perspective.

Yoga has long-range benefits as well. If you begin perimenopause with adrenal glands depleted from stress, for example, you increase

135

your chances of experiencing the hot flashes, fatigue, and anxiety characteristic of that transition time. If, on the other hand, you get to that life stage balanced and healthy, you're more likely to ease into it relatively unscathed.

Even if you're a beginning student, you can reap the benefits of yoga. First of all, yoga can immediately put you in direct communication with your body and your breathing. Stephen Cope, author of *Yoga: The Quest for the True Self,* points out that the only way to return to the self is to get out of your head and into your body; to physically, kinesthetically experience your physical being. And more often than not, what you experience physically will often mirror what you feel emotionally and what you need spiritually.

A commitment to yoga practice is the ultimate form of self-care; practice is a time to do something just for yourself. And that alone, Patricia says, can change your relationship with others. Physically it may open the chest and bring flexibility to the hips. Spiritually and emotionally, it opens the mind and the heart, and you're left with more love to give and a bigger capacity to receive it.

Chapter 7 *Preparing for Labor, Birth, and Postpartum*

PREGNANCY

When I got pregnant with my second child, I knew almost immediately. Within a week, my breasts felt sore. And a few days later, a sharp, familiar pain shot across the side of my belly when I jumped out of bed to turn off my alarm. The doctor at the clinic told me I was crazy, that there was no way for me to know that soon. But, sure enough, the blood test confirmed what I already felt deep inside. By that point in my life, I had been meditating and doing yoga for a long time, and it wasn't unusual for me to notice changes in my body and fluctuations in my emotional state. Although some of the symptoms I felt mimicked typical premenstrual problems, I knew the timing of these new feelings ruled out PMS.

Intuition such as this is not unusual, especially for someone who practices yoga. Although no signs of pregnancy are visible for weeks or sometimes even a couple of months after conception, a lot of activity takes place deep within your body. In fact, well before the fertilized egg makes its way down the fallopian tube and into the uterus, your body has begun to get ready for this monumental occasion. As soon as the sperm and egg successfully connect, armies of hormones kick into high gear, not only to create a hospitable environment in which the fetus can thrive, but to prepare your uterus for labor and delivery and your breasts for milk production. Your brain, adrenals, lungs, and heart join your endocrine system in supporting your uterus and providing the space and nourishment the fetus needs to grow.

There was no need for me to discontinue my yoga practice; in fact, yoga was the best thing I could do for myself and my baby—physically, emotionally, and spiritually. Physically, I needed yoga to keep my body strong and flexible at a time when it had to contend with additional weight and hyperactive hormones. I knew the asanas could give me tools to combat the fatigue, backache, digestive disorders, and headaches that were sure to come at some time during my pregnancy; the breathing exercises would be powerful allies during labor and delivery. A daily practice would strengthen my endocrine and nervous systems, both of which are vital for a healthy pregnancy and birth. By squatting, bending, and stretching, my muscles could release and

137

lengthen, allowing the breath to flow with my movements and calm any fears and anxieties I had about the months—and years—ahead of me.

Emotionally, yoga releases deeply stored feelings of anger, fear, anxiety, and sadness through its gentle attention to the body and breath. These strong, negative emotions can affect you on a physical level as well. As yoga teacher Janet Balaskas explains in her book *Preparing for Birth with Yoga: Exercises for Pregnancy and Childbirth*, when a woman feels angry or sad, her body moves to shield her from the pain by tensing her muscles, rounding her shoulders, or constricting her breath. According to Balaskas, the "physical tightness deadens the feelings . . . which become deeply buried." Most meditation teachers will agree that as these emotions come to the surface through yogic postures and breathing, the muscles themselves release and your body feels freer, lighter.

Releasing pent-up emotions can put you in touch with your intuition and your inner power. As your muscles relax and your breathing deepens, you can tune in to your body and begin to understand what's going on inside. One of my yoga teachers, Jill Minye, always tells her students that yoga is about waking up the body, feeling the spirit within. She says yoga brings awareness of sensation, of the breath, and of the self. As you ground yourself in your practice, you feel and trust the power of your body, you learn to listen to your instincts and to connect with the life growing inside you. A daily yoga practice provides at least an hour a day when you can communicate with your baby in utero and surrender to the process.

The Inside Story

Even before you know you're pregnant, your body is preparing to support and nourish the tiny life growing inside of you. Although most of the changes take place in your reproductive organs, your digestive, circulatory, cardiovascular, and respiratory systems also change pretty dramatically, responding to the powerful increase in hormone production.

By the time the tiny embryonic cell travels down the fallopian tube to your uterus—about twenty-one days—it has multiplied several times, forming a cluster of cells. Some of these cells will develop into a fetus; others will form the amniotic membrane that protects the fetus; and still others will create a yolk sac. Between the yolk sac and the amniotic membrane, cells come together to create the umbilical cord.

Once the placenta forms (by the third month), it manufactures enormous amounts of estrogen—more than a nonpregnant woman would produce in one hundred years—using both your adrenal glands and those of the baby. Progesterone also comes from the placenta at this point at a rate many times higher than prepregnancy levels. The increased estrogen causes your uterus to grow and produces changes in your cervix, vagina, and breasts. Progesterone supports and nourishes

Patricia Says

• Don't practice yoga during the first trimester if you have a history of miscarriage; after the first trimester, do only supported, restorative poses.

• Do poses that help create space between your rib cage and your abdomen, which will increase your comfort level and create more room for the baby.

the fetus, keeps your uterus from contracting, and maintains the health of your blood vessels and uterine lining. Together the two hormones relax your body's smooth muscle tissue, making it easier for your uterus to expand and for your body to accommodate the increased demand for fluids and blood.

Another hormone from the placenta, aptly called relaxin, softens the ligaments and connective tissues surrounding your pelvis and spine so they too can accommodate your uterus as it grows and expands. The hypothalamus contributes additional endorphins to bring about a sense of well-being and pleasure while you're pregnant and even help mitigate the pain of labor and delivery. And your adrenals work closely with the hypothalamus to contribute adrenaline and noradrenalin to make sure the involuntary functions of your body—digestion, circulation, breathing and, when the time is right, uterine contractions—are carried out properly.

The pituitary gland also helps ensure that the baby is born efficiently. It manufactures oxytocin to make your uterus contract during the birth process and your milk glands produce milk afterward. Because the hypothalamus and pituitary gland sit so close to the emotional center of your brain, stress can prevent oxytocin from doing its job effectively, thereby inhibiting labor and, later on, stopping the flow of milk into the milk ducts. Oxytocin also triggers a slight feeling of sexual arousal that Joan Borysenko calls a little "trick of nature to ensure that we will enjoy nursing our babies." This increase in oxytocin brings about the feeling of contentment and nurturance, and it helps you bond to your baby in a deeply profound way.

The First Trimester

Even though I was lucky and never had morning sickness, I did feel pretty seasick the first couple months. My sore breasts and crampy belly made me feel as though I had permanent PMS, and although I've never been one to take afternoon naps, by 4:00 PM I could barely keep my eyes open. Sometimes I experienced pure joy; other times, I would burst into tears at the slightest provocation.

My friend Angie, on the other hand, had it bad. The only thing that helped her most days was warm ginger tea, saltine crackers (when she could keep them down), and a bolster tucked under her as she lay in Child's Pose (Adho Mukha Virasana). Because I felt as though I had vertigo, bending forward made me feel dizzy and faint, but breathing deeply in Half-Moon Pose (Ardha Chandrasana) with my head and body against the wall helped tremendously. Amy Cooper, a yoga teacher from northern California, says many of her students prefer standing poses when they feel nauseous. These poses can help ground you, bring stability to your body, and increase circulation.

No one knows for sure what causes morning sickness, a fairly common occurrence for the first three months of pregnancy. Most doctors hold the hormone human chorionic gonadotropin (HCG) partially responsible. The placenta manufactures this hormone in the very early stages of pregnancy to prevent your body from dissolving the corpus luteum too early and rejecting the fetus. When HCG tapers off after about twelve weeks, once the placenta is firmly established, the nausea or vomiting should subside. Anxiety and a sluggish digestive system can also contribute to morning sickness. Supported forward bends and other restorative poses often help alleviate symptoms.

During this time, the increase in hormones will cause your smooth muscle tissue to relax and soften so your uterus has the ability—and the room—to expand. This softening benefits the uterus but causes your digestive tract, made up almost solely of smooth muscle tissue, to slow down. As a result, constipation, gas, and indigestion occur early on and can last throughout the pregnancy. Frequent urination, also caused by excess hormones and the increase in bodily fluids, starts well before the fetus is large enough to press against your bladder. In fact, for some women, having to go more often is a sure sign that they're pregnant.

With so much activity taking place in your body, it's no wonder you feel exhausted, especially at the beginning. Since I had been taking yoga before I got pregnant, I continued to practice my usual routine the first few months. But I immediately added more restorative, meditative poses that allowed me to visualize what was going on inside me. It somehow helped to know that my breasts were sore because they were expanding and preparing to nourish my baby; the stitch in my side wasn't nearly as painful once I realized that it came from my uterus getting bigger and changing position; and I didn't even mind urinating so much when I remembered that all the excess fluid made it easier to transport food to the baby.

The Baby During the first two weeks of pregnancy, the egg travels down the fallopian tube and implants itself in the uterine lining. Before the ninth week, the cells undergo rapid changes, creating new organs and systems almost daily. From the ninth week on, the fetus concentrates on perfecting and fine-tuning the organs and systems already developed. By the end of the first trimester, the baby is completely formed, but very tiny. Because so much emphasis is placed on the fetus's development, it's vitally important during these first few months to take good care of yourself—abstaining from alcohol, drugs, and environmental chemicals and supplementing your diet with a good prenatal vitamin.

Your Yoga Practice My friend Carole, pregnant with her first child, didn't feel the need to alter her yoga practice at all the first three months. Although she found herself incredibly sleepy by midafternoon, she revved up her energy with backbends; if she felt unfocused and anxious, doing inversions kept her sane; and forward bends helped stave off the morning queasiness she experienced, especially if she forgot to eat right away.

Donna Fone, a well-known yoga teacher with three children, agrees that her practice didn't need to change too much at first. But she still recommends enrolling in a prenatal yoga class, whether you're new to yoga or have a longtime routine. "It's nice to be in a class of all pregnant women doing yoga," Donna explains. "I think the focus is different; it teaches you things you could never learn in a regular class, like how to adjust for pregnancy, how to change the pose for yourself as you get bigger." While yoga in general creates space for the baby inside your body, prenatal yoga classes begin to make space for the baby in your mind. Plus, they build a sense of community among women going through similar experiences. Donna does recommend giving up twisting poses as early as the first trimester. She explains that a twisting action cleanses and flushes your system. You don't want to do anything that gives your body the signal to flush or expel. The Simple Seated Twist Pose (Bharadvajasana) is fine, however. The emphasis in this twist is on lifting and extending your spine, making room for the baby. Its action comes from your back, not from your pelvis.

Donna encourages women to include chest and shoulder openers in their daily practice as soon as possible. She says these will help keep your chest open and your joints flexible; you'll definitely notice the difference after a few months of nursing (which can cause your chest to cave in) and carrying your baby (which rounds your shoulders and tightens your muscles and joints).

Jen, a new mother at thirty-two, chose to wait until after the first trimester to resume her yoga practice. Although she knew intellectually that yoga was gentle enough not to cause any danger, she still worried about miscarriage—it had taken her so long to get pregnant in the first place, she didn't want to take any chances. Certainly, if you experience any first-trimester bleeding or have had a previous miscarriage, wait until your pregnancy is firmly established before doing yoga.

The Second Trimester

During this time, most women feel fabulous—full of energy and downright sexy. I certainly did; in fact, I've never felt healthier. My hair thickened, my complexion looked rosy, and the whole world made me happy. Even my appetite came back, as the HCG hormone levels dropped off.

By the fourth month, if you sit very still and pay close attention, you should be able to feel the baby move. Some women say it feels like butterfly flutters or gentle air currents. In the next month or so, you most likely will experience kicks, jabs, pokes, and thrusts from side to side. Your baby can now hear the sound of your voice.

During the second trimester, your uterus continues to expand, reaching past your belly button by the sixth month. You'll continue to gain weight, about half of which comes from the increased fluid your body produces. This fluid circulates through your bloodstream and

Poses to Avoid after the First Trimester

- Any positions in which you lie on your belly
- Any poses in which you lie flat on your back without support
- Any posture that contracts your abdominal muscles
- Twists that compress your abdominal muscles
- Any pose that doesn't feel good

into your soft tissues, muscles, and organs. It softens the ligaments, makes your body more receptive to the baby, prepares you for the ardors of labor and delivery, and provides the placenta with adequate blood flow and nourishment. You begin to store fat more efficiently, which your baby will need at the end of your pregnancy. Your body needs more blood now (for you and the baby), and by the end of this trimester, your blood volume will have increased about 40 percent. The walls of your blood vessels relax enough to speed up the delivery of oxygen and nutrients to the baby. Unfortunately, as many women discover, the valves of the large veins in your legs or anus also relax, resulting in varicose veins and hemorrhoids. You may also notice that your gums bleed more easily and that you feel more sexually aroused.

The Baby By now the baby's sex organs have formed and the ribs and spine have hardened. Her skin is red and wrinkly, and she has tiny eyelashes and faint outlines of eyebrows. She has hair on her head, and she can hear outside sounds. She's definitely moving around and responding to what she hears. The focus during these three months is on growth more than development. The baby's head is no longer as large as the rest of the body combined; her neck and shoulders are more able to hold the head upright, and she even has her own set of finger- and toeprints.

Your Yoga Practice As their bellies grew, both Carole and Donna saw their practice shift away from anything that would compress their abdomen. They both continued doing inversions, however, because it gave them relief to have the baby lift up in their pelvis. Carole says the baby's comfort became the focus of her yoga. Patricia wholeheartedly agrees. Yoga during pregnancy, she says, is all about making more room for the baby. If you do Mountain Pose (Tadasana), for example, don't stand with your feet together; that closes off your pelvic area. Place them hip-width apart to create more space. A traditional Downward-Facing Dog Pose (Adho Mukha Svanasana) may be fine during the first few months, but as your belly gets bigger, you may be more comfortable placing your hands on blocks or even on the back of a chair. Choose poses from this point on for their ability to open up the front of your body, create space for your belly, and extend your spine.

Patricia suggests modifying the poses so they're more comfortable for you and your baby. Do Extended Triangle Pose (Utthita Trikonasana) or Half-Moon Pose (Ardha Chandrasana), for example, with your hand on a block and your body pressed against the wall. Have the security of a wall behind you when you practice inversions, just in case—and remember to spread your legs to create space. The only twists recommended now are Simple Seated Twist Pose (Bharad-vajasana) and/or Standing Spinal Twist Pose (Utthita Marichyasana) (see chapter 8). These twists lift and extend your spine and open your shoulders without compressing your abdomen. Use a wall for support in both poses.

The Third Trimester

By the time you've reached your third trimester, the whole world can tell you're pregnant! Your uterus—by now about five hundred times its normal size—has expanded all the way to your rib cage, which is where you'll often find your baby's feet. That can make breathing a bit of a challenge sometimes. Your breasts may get bigger and more sensitive. The biggest complaints woman have during this time include heartburn and indigestion, breathlessness, constipation, an inability to sleep, and—by the ninth month—frequent trips to the bathroom.

Patricia Says

The most important criterion for your yoga practice these last few months is comfort. Find poses that feel good, help you get in touch with your body, communicate with your baby, and alleviate any anxiety you feel about the upcoming labor and delivery. Your focus should turn inward. Use these months to rest and replenish and to embrace what is happening to you.

Softening tissues can again cause discomfort by slowing your body's ability to digest food, which may cause constipation and indigestion and can lead to swelling in your hands and feet. None of these conditions should cause alarm, but if swelling is accompanied by a sudden rise in blood pressure or the presence of protein in your urine, you should seek medical advice.

At the beginning of the ninth month, the baby usually drops into position, although this can happen earlier or later. If you've felt a lot of pressure in your rib cage and upper abdomen during most of your pregnancy, you may feel a sense of relief—more room to breathe. On the other hand, you may feel that the baby is sitting directly on your bladder, and you'll be running to the bathroom a lot more.

Many women experience Braxton-Hicks contractions in the last three months. These "silent," painless contractions help prepare your uterus for delivery by softening and dilating your cervix. Many women welcome such prelabor contractions as a clear sign that the end is in sight.

The Baby All five senses have awakened by now. Your baby can see, smell, hear, taste, and respond to touch. She's preparing for her world debut and has mastered the sucking and swallowing skills she'll need. By the seventh month, her brain has fully developed, her nervous system is advancing, and some researchers suggest that she now possesses the ability to remember. You won't feel her moving quite as much; she'll be sleeping much of the time. You may feel her hiccuping, however. The baby fattens up during the last two months; her fingernails and toenails grow, and she receives the antibodies from you that she'll need to survive in the world.

Your Yoga Practice Carole stopped doing inversions after the seventh month. Headstand (Sirsasana) no longer felt comfortable, and by the beginning of the ninth month, she certainly didn't want to confuse her baby or discourage her from heading down into the birth canal. Patricia feels that all inversions should stop as soon as a woman experiences heaviness in her pelvis, abdomen, and chest area and breathing becomes more difficult. For both Carole and Donna, extreme backbends gave way to more passive variations that helped keep their chest and shoulders open. After about the fourth month, neither of them did Corpse Pose (Savasana) lying flat or any other supine position that would put undue compression on the vena cava (the largest vein in the body responsible for pumping deoxygenated blood to the heart). Instead, they enjoyed lying on their side, comforted and bolstered by lots of pillows. They did this pose several times a day, in fact. Most midwives will encourage you to get all the rest you can now. You'll need to be prepared not only for the birthing process, but for the sleepless nights of early motherhood that lie ahead.

How Yoga Can Help

The pregnancy sequence we provide in this chapter works for most women at all stages of pregnancy. It includes a wide variety of poses—standing, seated, bending forward, opening backward, and gently twisting side to side. Practice these poses as often as you like, but discontinue any that no longer feel comfortable. One caveat, however: Before you begin any exercise program—especially if it's new to you—talk to your physician or midwife.

Standing Poses These poses energize and strengthen your body, open your chest and abdominal area, and extend your spine. They help realign your posture and serve to ground your energy and strengthen your spirit. Because your spine must bear the load of your uterus and the extra weight, it has to stay strong and flexible; standing poses can help. They generally strengthen your abdominals without putting pressure on the fetus. Some women in the later months have trouble standing for long. If that's the case, use a wall for support; don't stay in the pose past what's comfortable (10 to 20 seconds is fine); and come out of the pose slowly and deliberately so you don't get dizzy. In all standing poses, make sure your legs are at least hip-width apart.

Learning to squat is invaluable for labor and delivery. Begin early on so you get the hang of it. All standing poses are good preparations for childbirth as well, since they require stamina and determination. Twisting standing poses are generally not recommended after the first trimester.

Standing Forward Bends Done with a concave back (with your head up), these postures extend your spine, take pressure off your lower back, and lengthen your hamstrings. Forward bends also improve circulation to your legs, kidneys, and pelvis as they relax your pelvic floor muscles, increase your energy, and realign your spine. They can help give space and elasticity to the back of the vaginal and cervical wall and can relieve the heaviness of your uterus. Do Wide-Angle Standing Forward Bend (Prasarita Padottanasana), resting your hands on a chair so you keep as much space as possible for the baby and still derive maximum benefit from the pose.

Backbends Supported backbends offer many benefits during pregnancy. They tone your anterior spinal muscles and stretch the muscles of your anterior abdominal wall and diaphragm to accommodate your uterus as it grows. They strengthen your spine; increase flexibility; improve circulation to your kidneys, uterus, and pelvis; reduce water retention; and lift your spirits by opening your chest. If you already do backbends in your practice, Patricia says you can continue them safely through the first trimester, as long as you feel comfortable. After that, most women find supported, passive backbends like Reclining Bound Angle Pose (Supta Baddha Konasana) or Reclining Hero Pose (Supta Virasana) to be more comfortable. Even supported backbends can relieve the pressure of your uterus on your kidneys and bladder, and they can sometimes help calm nausea and relieve the feeling of fullness in your abdomen.

Patricia Says

- Don't overstretch your abdominals; they're vulnerable and you can strain the smooth muscles of your uterus.

- Support your hips and groin as you release your inner thighs. Many women have trouble with their hips being either too tight or too loose.

- Don't overstretch or try to go deeper just because your ligaments are loose. For example, if you do Bound Angle Pose (Baddha Konasana), place a bolster under each knee.

Seated Poses Seated poses can relieve pain in your lower back and heaviness around your pubic bone. They tone and stretch your pelvic floor, soften and stretch your vaginal opening, and strengthen your spine for sitting meditation. These poses also relieve stiffness in your hips, groin, and knees. Be gentle with yourself and don't force your body to do what doesn't feel comfortable. Patricia reminds her students that pregnancy is no time to try to get better at a pose; it's the time to reap the benefits of what you've already learned. If you have trouble sitting tall without straining, place your hands against the wall in front of you for support and stability.

Seated Forward Extensions Done with a concave back, these poses can stimulate blood flow to your kidneys; reduce stiffness in your lower back, hips, and groin; lift and tone your uterus; relax your pelvic floor; and improve circulation to your lower body. Seated extensions can be grounding. And some women swear by Child's Pose (Adho Mukha Virasana) to combat nausea, relieve anxiety, and quiet the mind.

Twists Pregnant women should avoid twisting poses that compress the abdomen or create a squeezing action in the belly or pelvis. Remember, prenatal yoga is all about creating space for the baby to move and grow. Some gentle twists, like a Simple Seated Twist Pose (Bharadvajasana), however, can relieve lower back pain, especially in the first trimester, and increase the flow of fresh blood to your adrenal glands, uterus, and ovaries.

Inversions You can practice inversions until turning upside down is no longer comfortable for you or the baby. That usually happens around the seventh or eighth month; but some women need to forswear inversions after the fifth or sixth month. Inversions release tension in your neck, shoulders, and spine; stimulate your endocrine system (the pituitary, hypothalamus, and thyroid gland), which is vital for pregnancy, labor, and delivery; provide much-needed energy; lift your uterus off your pelvic floor to relieve the heaviness you often feel; and help regulate salt and water retention by increasing the blood supply to your kidneys and hypothalamus. The easiest, gentlest inversion for pregnant women is Legs-Up-the-Wall Pose (Viparita Karani) with a bolster under your sacrum.

Breathing Exercises Don't wait until your first labor pains are imminent to start learning proper breathing techniques. To be truly effective during labor and delivery, deep breathing exercises must be almost automatic, so it's best to begin early in your pregnancy. By learning and practicing yogic breathing (pranayama) in the first few months, you can communicate healing, loving breath (prana) to your baby as he or she is growing inside of you. Geeta Iyengar recommends Interval Breathing (Viloma) with an emphasis on exhalations, and Expanding Life Force Energy Breathing (Ujjayi Pranayama), both of which we've included in this chapter. My friend Carole used these techniques with good results, but she preferred adding sounds to her exhalations. Sometimes she would let out a moan, a groan, or a loud sigh; other times, she'd utter a special sound she had chosen to help her through pain.

LABOR AND DELIVERY

In preparation for giving birth to her first child, Carole learned a method of natural delivery that taught her to focus on an object outside her body to distract her from the pain of labor. During the final stage, she began to pant, using the shallow breathing technique she had learned. All of a sudden, she remembers, "My entire body went rigid with pain, and I began to thrash around uncontrollably. The nurse told me that she would have to tie me down to prevent me from injuring myself and the baby, and then she left to get some restraints." While the nurse was out of the room, Carole realized the shallow panting had triggered her sympathetic nervous system and that her body had gone into a fight-or-flight response to the pain. She began a simple yoga breathing technique she used in her daily practice, called alternate nostril breathing (without holding her breath at the end). By the time the nurse returned with the restraints, Carole's entire body had relaxed and her daughter was born twenty minutes later.

While yoga offers a number of postures that support you during labor and delivery, its greatest gift is the power of proper breathing. Janet Balaskas writes that when you are pregnant, you not only eat for two, you breathe for two as well, providing your baby with the oxygen and healing prana (life force) she needs to grow. Your inhalation brings nourishment and vitality to her as well as to yourself, and your exhalation allows you "to release tension, to cleanse and purify" your body. It is your breath, Balaskas explains, that grounds your energy to the earth and allows your spirit to lift toward the sky.

If you've been doing yoga throughout your pregnancy (or well before), you know what a difference breathing makes to your practice.

How many times have you felt you couldn't do a pose, only to find that once you began breathing slowly and calmly, the pose came more easily? When you feel tense, agitated, or distracted, not only does the breath move up into your chest, but your movements become shallow, mechanical, and stiff. By bathing your movements in breath, you allow your body to dance the movement, to take it deeper inside, to let go and luxuriate in the feelings the movement brings. Your muscles respond by elongating, softening, and relaxing. Suddenly you feel more supple, flexible, and relaxed.

All through your pregnancy, you've allowed the yoga poses and your mindful breathing to help your muscles relax and open, your ligaments to soften and stretch, and your body to feel stronger and better aligned. Now as you go into labor, you'll want to continue moving and breathing in much the same way.

What Happens in Labor?

For the last nine months, your body has adjusted to accommodate the growing life within you. Your endocrine system and adrenals have provided the right amount of hormones, your blood and fluids have increased to transport nourishment to your baby, and the ligaments and muscles have softened—and in several instances, gotten out of the way—to allow your uterus to expand as the baby grows. Now it's time for your uterus to contract. The lower part of the uterus must stretch and the cervix must open wide enough to allow the baby to come out. The average baby weighs between seven and eight pounds, which is a lot of baby to push through that opening.

The hypothalamus and pituitary glands, so active in your menstrual cycle and during pregnancy, also play a role in the birth of your child. Because your emotions affect the way these glands work, feeling tense, afraid, nervous, or stressed directly impacts your endocrine and autonomic nervous systems (as well as the baby's) and inhibits the release of uterine-contracting hormones and the endorphins that help you bear the pain.

Improper breathing caused Carole's body to become rigid with pain, which made her contractions ineffective. Luckily, slow, deliberate deep breathing got her back on track and allowed her body to complete the birthing process without incident.

In other words, when you become frightened or tense during labor, your sympathetic nervous system goes into overdrive, triggering the fight-or-flight response. When you feel calm and relaxed, your parasympathetic nervous system kicks in, allowing your cervix to dilate and your vaginal walls to stretch.

Preparing for Labor

Prelabor contractions called Braxton-Hicks, mentioned earlier, are generally your first sign that the baby is getting ready to be born. These painless contractions feel like someone is gripping your belly from the inside and then releasing it. Once the bottom of your uterus stretches out and the baby can comfortably drop into your pelvis, these contractions can come more frequently. This generally marks the beginning of the birthing process, even though it can happen several weeks before actual labor starts. Many women are fortunate to experience a fairly active prelabor. Other women feel nothing at all. My Braxton-Hicks contractions, which felt like strong pulls on my belly, were quite effective the last three or four weeks. In fact, by the time I went into active labor, I was already dilated three centimeters and my cervix was completely effaced (thinned out).

Now is the time to get as much rest as possible. Use yoga to soothe your tired body and your spent emotions, to connect with your breathing, and to communicate with the baby inside you. Allow your partner to pamper you with massages and calming foods. Restorative poses like Reclining Bound Angle Pose (Supta Baddha Konasana) will relax and energize you; and Garland Pose (Malasana) is a squat that will prepare you for the birthing process.

A lot of women find it hard to distinguish between false and true labor. I was told that real labor pains continue even after you change positions; false labor usually stops. Walking can increase the intensity of real labor pains but will often halt false labor.

The First Stage of Labor (The Latent Phase)

Most doctors and midwives will tell you there's no need to do anything special when your labor begins, unless you have a history of fast births. For most women, this stage (called the latent phase) can last several hours, or even a day or more. The contractions are far apart at first, and the pain varies in intensity. Some women even sleep through most of it, which is precisely what you should do as much as possible. Janet Balaskas suggests keeping a collection of pillows on your bed to hug close to your body when the contractions awaken you in the night.

Even when your contractions get stronger and more rhythmic, you still needn't do a lot. This is a good time to remember your yogic breathing and to practice slowing down your exhalations. If you practiced yoga before you got pregnant, you know slow, steady, rhythmic breathing helps you get through difficult poses. That kind of breathing can help you now. Relax your pelvic floor muscles and rest as much as you can between contractions. I created a very simple mantra for myself during my labor. I inhaled the words *I am* and breathed out the word *relaxed*. The slight aspirant quality to *relaxed* helped me send my breath all the way down into my belly where it was needed. Both Expanding Life Force Energy Breathing (Ujjayi Pranayama) and Interval Breathing (Viloma) can help during this time.

The latent phase of labor takes the longest. Some women complete it in three or four hours; others are still here after twenty hours. Don't get discouraged if, after all this time and pain, your cervix has only

Patricia Says

• Don't practice inversions the last two months without guidance from an experienced yoga teacher. You can, however, do a modified Downward-Facing Dog Pose (Adho Mukha Svanasana) against a wall. Do inversions during the first two trimesters only if they are already part of your practice or you are under the guidance of an experienced teacher.

dilated one or two centimeters. That's normal. According to Emanuel Friedman, the Harvard University professor who named this phase, latency prepares your body for the more rapid, active stages of labor; the smooth muscles of your uterus use this time to get better at working together. Meanwhile, your cervix is busy preparing biochemically for the intense dilation that will soon take place. It's sort of like the early stages of a marathon run.

Many women find remaining vertical for as long as possible helps them weather these contractions. Others find sitting with their legs apart and leaning forward helps them breathe into their bellies more effectively. Just don't lie flat; that works against gravity and puts pressure on the back of your pelvis. Kneeling in a vertical position or squatting works well during this time, too. Between contractions, rest, rest, rest. If you feel like a massage, let your partner know. Some women need to go deep inside during this time and find touching too distracting; others find comfort in breathing along with the gentle strokes their partner provides. When the pain got too intense, I had trouble focusing on my breathing; it helped a lot when my husband practiced pranayama breathing with me, making his inhalations and exhalations audible enough for me to follow along.

The Active Phase

Once your cervix has dilated three or four centimeters, your labor pains should accelerate and the rate at which your cervix dilates and thins out increases rapidly. For some women, this phase can last for a short time—about forty-five minutes—or as long as five hours. The cervix has to dilate enough to allow the baby to enter through the birth canal and then pull back over his head. Some midwives call this the Transition Phase, when the labor pains can come fast and furious—every two minutes or so, lasting about sixty seconds each. You don't have a lot of resting time at this point!

Many women find it harder and harder to walk during the active stage of labor, because the pains are coming closer and closer together. Squatting, which widens the pelvis, works for some, but for others, it intensifies the contractions too much. Janet Balaskas suggests squatting between contractions and standing up while holding on to your partner during contractions.

Pushing the Baby Out

When your cervix has fully dilated (10 cm) and completely effaced, you can begin pushing. Most women know instinctively when to push; I didn't. I think if my midwife hadn't suggested pushing, I'd still be lying on the table! All midwives will explain that pushing works most effectively when it coincides with a contraction. Whatever you do, don't hold your breath and strain. In fact, focus on exhaling completely and releasing your pelvic floor as you visualize your baby moving through the birth canal and into the world.

Your yoga practice will serve you well during this intense time. The standing, squatting, and seated poses you've been doing will allow you to maintain the birthing position you choose—whether you squat, kneel on all fours, or lie semisupine on your side. You need the help of gravity to push your baby out, so avoid lying flat on your back or in any position where your weight is on your sacrum or coccyx.

LIFE AFTER THE BIRTHING PROCESS

Now that you've given birth, what you do in the first few weeks will greatly influence your ability to care for your baby and yourself in the upcoming months. Carrying a baby to term requires tremendous physical and mental energy, but the real demands start after the midwife goes home and you're left to feed, rock, carry, change, and love your baby and then feed, rock, carry, change, and love her some more, with what feels like only a few minutes of sleep in between. Even if you have a loving partner who can share the new responsibilities and joys, the baby really needs you—physically and emotionally. The problem is that your baby needs a mother who is rested, calm, and healthy, but you feel exhausted, stressed, undernourished, and emotionally fraught. But it doesn't have to be this way.

When I gave birth to my oldest daughter, Sarah, I prided myself on getting right back to business. My labor was blessedly short; I healed physically rather quickly; and I resumed my normal life, with a tiny baby in her little pack snuggled up against my chest. After three weeks of the Supermom mentality, I burned out and ended up with quite a case of the "baby blues."

A friend of mine had a much different experience. Raised by her Chinese mother and Russian grandmother, Anna gave birth at home to a baby boy. Her grandmother and mother immediately took care of everything. Her grandmother bathed Anna and her baby together, cooked for her, massaged her feet, and made sure Anna slept uninterrupted whenever her son fell asleep. Anna was not allowed to even come downstairs the first ten days after delivery! Her sole duties were to feed, love, and care for her son and herself. Her mother, who tended to the household tasks of cleaning, washing diapers, and changing the baby, also rocked and sang to her new grandson and took him outside for his daily ration of fresh air.

Of course, in retrospect, it's not hard for me to see who had the better deal, but back then I thought how odd it was not to do it all yourself. Anna's mother and grandmother, however, knew instinctively that a woman's body and emotions need time to recuperate and strengthen. A lot goes on physiologically during the first six weeks after giving birth, and you need time to adjust. First of all, don't expect to lose all the weight you gained during pregnancy as soon as you deliver. You'll probably shed ten to twelve pounds right away and

Patricia Says

Now that your baby has come, you'll be eager to resume your yoga practice. Here are a few tips that should help you practice with awareness.

• When you were pregnant, you concentrated on poses that created space between your rib cage and pelvis, made room for your growing uterus, and opened your hip joints. Now your focus should be on toning and strengthening, and bringing your uterus back into place. Focus on drawing in and up. Avoid poses that stretch your groin like Reclining Bound Angle Pose (Supta Baddha Konasana), Bound Angle Pose (Baddha Konasana), Wide-Angle Seated Pose I or II (Upavistha Konasana I or II), or Reclining Big Toe Pose II (Supta Padangusthasana II).

another five or six after the first week or two by urinating all that excess body water you've been carrying around (about three quarts). Most new mothers discover that they perspire profusely the first week or so, which expels still more fluid. Of course, once your uterus shrinks back to its prepregnancy size and shape, you'll lose even more weight.

Restoring Your Uterus

In the first weeks after childbirth, your body must concentrate on repairing itself, particularly in restoring and restructuring the uterus. During that process, your uterus sloughs off blood, clots, and cells from its top layer. This lochia acts like a heavy period and can last about ten days. The color of the discharge will gradually change from dark red to pale pink and finally to a milky color, and the odor will start out strong and gradually diminish. By the end of three weeks, the lochia should vanish.

Your uterus also needs to return to its normal size. As it softens, you will feel contractions, much like you did when you were in labor (though not as painful). Nursing will help your uterus contract faster, and many women feel these contractions the first couple of weeks they feed their babies. These "after-pains" are caused by oxytocin, the powerful hormone that also regulates your milk flow. You can lessen the pain by massaging your uterus often. Reclining Hero Pose (Supta Virasana), well supported, or Corpse Pose (Savasana) can help. Drink lots of fluids, but urinate often—a full bladder adds to the discomfort. Not surprisingly, stress intensifies the pain, so practice restorative poses like Corpse Pose or Seated Forward Bend (Paschimottanasana) with a pillow pressing against your belly.

Getting Your Figure Back

While many women find themselves too tired or busy to even think about exercising, the desire to look thin and fit drives some to start back too soon. Resist the urge. Wait until your uterus has healed and returned to its normal size and your hormone levels have stabilized— most specialists recommend six weeks. Geeta Iyengar suggests waiting two to three weeks before resuming any yoga. Then, start slowly with some pranayama breathing and Corpse Pose (Savasana), both of which will tone your abdominals, help your uterus diminish in size, and increase your flow of milk. Gentle restorative chest openers like Reclining Hero Pose (Supta Virasana) are fine right away, as are old-fashioned Kegel exercises. Donna Fone recommends supported forward bends. She found them helpful in drying and "closing up" her uterus.

After six weeks, if you're not too exhausted, you can begin the postpartum sequence in this chapter, which includes some abdominal strengtheners and poses to lift and tone your uterus. Six to seven weeks after giving birth, you can add inversions if you've stopped bleeding; and you can do twists by the eighth week. Generally, three

• As you do poses that strengthen and tone your abdominal muscles and bring your reproductive organs into place, visualize your muscles moving toward one another, knitting themselves back together. Think of your uterus lifting up and into place, as you move your abdomen up and back toward your spine. Downward-Facing Dog Pose (Adho Mukha Svanasana) and Great Seal Pose (Maha Mudra) actively tone your pelvic organs and floor.

• Concentrate on poses that open your chest, lengthen your upper back, and bring your shoulder blades into your back ribs. This helps relax the muscles you tense while nursing and will lift your spirits if you feel blue.

• What you do with your body has a profound impact on your emotions—stand up straight, walk with dignity, open your chest, and periodically raise your arms over your head. Focus on the inhalation to bring healing prana (energy) into your body and fill your spirit with joy.

months after delivery (depending on your energy level), you can resume your usual yoga routine. You can even include your little one in your practice; you'll both have a great time doing the poses together at various times throughout the day. Then when she goes down for a nap, or later in the evening when your husband's at home, you can practice by yourself.

If you've had a cesarean section or any labor or delivery complications, Patricia cautions you not to do any yoga until the wound heals, with the exception of Corpse Pose (Savasana), Reclining Hero Pose (Supta Virasana), and gentle pranayama exercises. After the wound heals completely (usually at least two months), you may add a supported Shoulderstand (Sarvangasana), supported Bridge Pose (Setu Bandha Sarvangasana), Legs-Up-the-Wall Pose (Viparita Karani), and Great Seal Pose (Maha Mudra) to balance your hormones, tone your uterus, and strengthen your abdominals. Wait a full six months before resuming your usual yoga routine.

Amy Cooper, a California yoga teacher specializing in pre- and postnatal yoga, recommends stretching and strengthening the iliopsoas muscle (commonly referred to as the psoas, it runs from your spine to your groin), which tightens, shortens, and weakens during pregnancy. Try a Reclining Hero Pose (Supta Virasana), which appears in this chapter, and a supported Upward-Facing Dog Pose (Urdhva Mukha Svanasana), as shown in chapter 8.

Improving Digestion

Unfortunately, many women suffer from constipation following the birth of their child—a normal but annoying side effect. This is usually caused by the enormous amount of estrogen produced during labor and delivery, exacerbated by the fact that they haven't eaten or drunk much since labor began, they may have hemorrhoids, or (if they've had an episiotomy) they could be afraid their stitches will tear.

Yoga can help ease the digestive disorders associated with postpartum recuperation. (Refer to chapter 12 for helpful yoga poses.)

Nursing Your Baby

Lots of books and advice exist for new mothers who nurse their babies, so I won't duplicate all that. However, I do want to say that although nursing is one of the most incredible activities I've ever done, it's not so easy at the beginning. Don't get discouraged and give up too soon. Like so many physiological responses in your body, hormones control the amount of milk you produce and the timing of that production. Any stress you feel can effect how those hormones do their job. When the baby sucks at your breast, the autonomic nerves there send a signal to the hypothalamus that it's time to let down some milk. If you're calm and relaxed, the hypothalamus (remember it's near the emotional center of your brain) then triggers the pituitary gland to release oxytocin, which causes the muscles in your breast to contract. If you're stressed, exhausted, or worried your milk won't release easily and both you and your baby will end up frustrated.

It all goes back to the fight-or-flight response (discussed in detail in chapter 6). If a mother perceives danger, her autonomic nervous system reacts, arresting the let-down reflex and preparing her to either run or protect her baby. In more primitive times, such threats came on suddenly and infrequently. These days, unrelenting stress from overwork, lack of sleep, anxiety, or myriad other stimuli can trigger the fight-or-flight response and inhibit your flow of milk.

Especially if you're a new mother, it's important to create a calm environment that is free of distractions, so you can relax and allow the milk to flow to your baby. Any of the restorative poses given in this book, especially Reclining Hero Pose (Supta Virasana), Easy Seated Forward Bend (Adho Mukha Sukhasana), and Half-Plough Pose (Ardha Halasana), will help put you in the right frame of mind for nursing. See the Woman's Restorative Sequence (chapter 3) for instructions. Also, give your body (and your emotions) a few weeks to adjust to the new demands. In other words, be patient.

Postpartum Depression

After Sarah was about three weeks old, I fell apart. I wasn't prepared for the demands of a new baby (especially one who cried all the time). I had always been self-sufficient and now I had to rely on my husband for support; I craved adult companionship; and my body wasn't as strong and lean as it had been before (and I expected it to be, even after only three weeks). The baby blues hit me hard, and it took almost three months of yoga, meditation, and an understanding husband to lift me out of the doldrums. My friend Kathryn thinks all women should be warned about postpartum depression. She said hers manifested as sheer terror. She was frightened at the thought of being responsible for such a tiny being—a responsibility she knew would last a lifetime. She was terrified that her life would never again be solely her own and wasn't quite sure she could live up to the awesome task of providing for, nurturing, and guiding her daughter through life.

Both of us took solace in knowing our feelings weren't unusual. Many doctors attribute a new mother's incredible highs and attendant lows to the rise and fall of pre- and postnatal hormones. But I think the depression most of us feel has other causes as well. Typically, the baby blues come on about the same time as your milk pours into your breasts, engorging them and making them hurt like crazy; the same time the baby begins fussing more; and the same time the novelty of the situation has worn off—everyone else is back to their daily routine and Mom is all alone with her newborn. Life suddenly seems overwhelming and the responsibility of caring for a new and very tiny human being is sometimes more than you can bear.

Concentrate on poses that open your chest, expand your breathing, and reenergize your spirit, like Reclining Hero Pose (Supta Virasana), Shoulderstand (Sarvangasana), Bridge Pose (Setu Bandha Sarvangasana), and others from chapter 10. I also felt better if I just took a little time to do something for myself—taking a walk, meditating, visiting a friend, going to a postnatal class—anything that would clear my head and recharge my batteries. Don't be afraid to ask for help; no one ever said this was going to be easy, nor did anyone mean for you to do it all by yourself. Postnatal yoga classes offer a wonderful opportunity—whether you go by yourself or with your baby—to practice and, equally important, to connect with other moms. If your depression lasts longer than a couple of weeks, seek outside help.

1. Hero Pose (Virasana) Cycle
2. Reclining Hero Pose (Supta Virasana)
3. Child's Pose (Adho Mukha Virasana)
4. Reclining Bound Angle Pose (Supta Baddha Konasana)
5. Garland Pose (Malasana)
6. Simple Seated Twist Pose (Bharadvajasana)
7. Mountain Pose (Tadasana)
8. Extended Triangle Pose (Utthita Trikonasana)
9. Half-Moon Pose (Ardha Chandrasana)
10. Wide-Angle Standing Forward Bend (Prasarita Padottanasana)
11. Wide-Angle Seated Pose I (Upavistha Konasana I)
12. Bound Angle Pose (Baddha Konasana)
13. Legs-Up-the-Wall Pose (Viparita Karani)
14. Corpse Pose (Savasana)

A SEQUENCE FOR PREGNANCY

1. HERO POSE† (Virasana) **CYCLE** Kneel on a folded blanket with your knees together and your feet pointing straight back, slightly wider than your hips. (If you feel any pressure in your knees, legs, or lower back, spread your knees farther apart.) You will move from this pose directly into the next, so place a bolster vertically behind you and another one underneath it to form a T shape—for a slanted surface. You will not use the bolsters in this pose. Sit between your feet on a block or a bolster.

ARMS OVERHEAD (Parvatasana) Stretch your arms out in front of you with the palms facing you; interlock your fingers (A). Turn your palms out and stretch your arms over your head. Press your palms toward the ceiling and straighten your elbows. Draw your shoulder blades into your back, lift your sternum (breastbone), and stretch your trunk up from the bones in your buttocks. Hold this pose for 10 to 20 seconds. Sitting up tall and stretching from your waist, bring your arms down, reverse the interlock of your hands, and repeat.

COW-FACE (Gomukhasana) ARMS Take your left arm behind you and stretch the forearm up your back as far as you can; the back of your hand is against your back. Reach your right arm over your head and, bending at the elbow, reach down your back toward your left hand. Interlace your fingers (or hold a strap if you can't catch your hands). Keep your right elbow pointing toward the ceiling and your head up (B). Roll your shoulders back and open your chest. Breathe normally in this pose for 30 seconds to a minute. Repeat with your arms reversed.

PRAYER (Namaste) HANDS Bring your palms together behind your back with your fingers pointing down toward your waist. Turn your hands so your fingers go in toward your waist and then up your back so they point toward the ceiling. Move your hands up the middle of your back, pressing your palms together. Roll your shoulders back while you spread and lift your chest. Push your elbows back (C). (If this is too difficult, fold your arms behind your back and cup an elbow in each hand to work on broadening your chest.)

Hold this arm position for 60 seconds before releasing and stretching your arms to the side with your palms up. Do not shake your wrists; instead, stretch through your elbows, wrists, and fingers.

EFFECTS This pose is recommended to help ease swelling in your legs and prevent varicose veins. The different arm positions are excellent for keeping your chest open and your shoulders flexible. They are also very useful post-partum if you plan to breast-feed your baby, because they counteract the forward-shoulder, closed-chest position that is an inevitable part of nursing.

†CAUTION If you feel any strain in your knees, separate them slightly and sit on a bolster or block. If you are a beginner, don't stay in this pose longer than 1 minute.

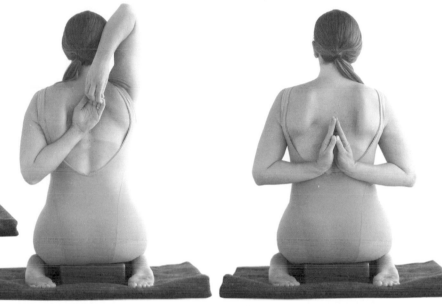

A

B

C

2. RECLINING HERO POSE (Supta Virasana) From Hero Pose (Virasana), lean back onto your forearms and gently let your trunk rest on the bolsters behind you, with your head on the bolster. Rest your arms in a relaxed position at your sides. Close your eyes, and concentrate on giving your baby deep, nurturing breaths. Initially, stay in this pose for 1 or 2 minutes. If it's comfortable, you can increase your time to 5 minutes.

EFFECTS This pose helps ease swelling in your legs and prevent varicose veins. It may also relieve heartburn and morning sickness by lifting your diaphragm off your stomach, and ease digestive disorders and constipation. It also stretches the hip flexors, which tend to tighten during pregnancy because of postural changes.

3. CHILD'S POSE (Adho Mukha Virasana) From Reclining Hero Pose (Supta Virasana), use your arms to push yourself up, leading with your sternum. Keep your head back until you come all the way back up to sitting. Spread your knees so they are wider than your hips (giving enough room for your belly) and bring your big toes as close together as possible. Position your two bolsters in front of you, stacking one on top of the other. Bend forward from your hips and stretch out your arms, elongating your spine. As you move your torso forward, toward the bolsters, keep your pelvis close to your heels. Release and lengthen the back of your neck and relax your shoulders. Rest your head on the bolsters in front of you. Hold this pose for several minutes, or as long as you feel comfortable. Come up very slowly and sit comfortably for a few breaths.

EFFECTS This pose relaxes your back and lengthens your spine. It releases tension in your hip joints and groin area and encourages the pelvic canal to widen.

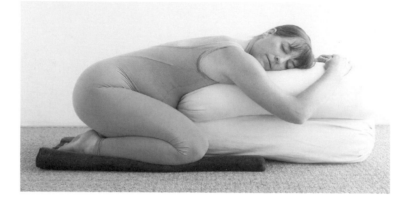

4. RECLINING BOUND ANGLE POSE (Supta Baddha Konasana) Place your bolsters behind you again, forming a T-shaped, slanted surface with the vertical bolster on top. Sit just in front of them with your knees bent and your sacrum touching the vertical bolster's edge. Secure the strap as shown on page xv. Lie back so your head and torso rest comfortably on the bolster and your buttocks and legs are on the floor. You shouldn't feel any discomfort in your lower back. (If you feel any strain in your neck, place a folded blanket under your head and neck. If you feel any muscle tension in your legs, roll two blankets vertically and place one under the top of each thigh.) Rest in this pose for as long as you like, breathing deeply. In the last two or three months, place a block between your feet to broaden your pelvis in preparation for childbirth.

To come out, bend your knees to release the strap and push the block away with your feet. Roll to one side, rest for a couple of breaths, and come up.

EFFECTS This is an excellent way to open your pelvis both vertically and horizontally and make more space for the baby. It relieves nausea and promotes easy breathing. Because it is a gentle backbend, it will open your shoulders and relieve tension in your upper back.

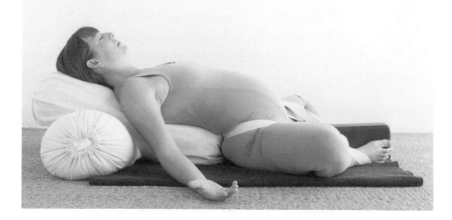

5. GARLAND POSE† **(Malasana)** Stand with your back against a wall, your feet about 18 inches apart. Slowly drop your weight into your heels, as though you were going to sit down in a chair. If you wish, you can lean forward slightly from your hip joints, so your back is free but your sacrum and buttocks are still supported by the wall. Put your hands together in prayer position at your breastbone. Press your elbows against your knees slightly to keep them apart and remain in this position, with your inner arches raised and your heels pressed into the floor, for 30 seconds or more. Work up to 3 minutes. Alternatively, you can come in and out of the pose several times until it gets easier. (If you have trouble keeping your heels down, place a rolled mat or towel under them. Some women prefer using a bolster or two, or even a low stool, to squat on.) Breathe as normally as possible, with the emphasis on your exhalation, releasing the muscles in your pelvic floor and elongating your spine.

EFFECTS During pregnancy, this pose helps keep your hip joints and pelvis mobile. Practicing this pose in your ninth month may encourage the baby to drop down into the birthing canal. It's an ideal pose for labor and delivery.

†CAUTION Do not practice this pose if you have hemorrhoids, painful varicose veins, or a cervical stitch.

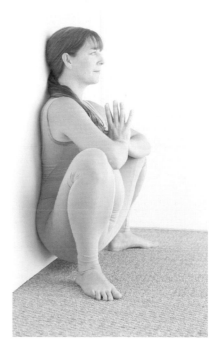

6. SIMPLE SEATED TWIST POSE† **(Bharadvajasana)** Sit up on two folded blankets with your legs stretched out in front of you and the wall on your right. Bend both legs and bring them sideways next to (or near) your left hip. Keeping both buttocks on the blankets, draw your shoulder blades into your back, broaden your chest, and extend your spine upward. On an exhalation, turn your abdomen, ribs, chest, and shoulders to the right, and place both hands on the wall at shoulder height. Take several breaths, holding the posture for 60 seconds, and be aware of turning the baby as you turn your abdomen. Relax your face, neck, and throat. Come back to the center position, straighten your legs, and change sides.

EFFECTS This pose keeps your spine flexible and relieves back strain. It also helps strengthen your oblique muscles without putting any pressure on the fetus.

†CAUTION Do not practice twists if you have diarrhea.

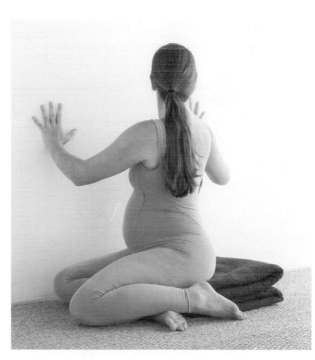

7. MOUNTAIN POSE (Tadasana) Stand up straight with your back resting against the wall. Place your feet hip-width apart and parallel to each other. Distribute your weight evenly between the front of your feet and your heels. Tighten your knees by pulling your quadriceps (front thigh muscles) up. Raise your sternum and broaden your chest by rolling your shoulders back to the wall and drawing your shoulder blades into your body. Lift your abdomen up and draw your tailbone in and down without pushing your thighs forward. Extend your arms downward with your palms facing your thighs and your fingers together. Keep your shoulders moving away from your ears. It is normal to have some space between your lower back and the wall, but only just enough to slip your hand through. Stand in this posture for 30 seconds or longer, breathing normally.

EFFECTS With your constantly changing weight distribution, it is essential to maintain good posture to prevent back problems, and this pose helps correct alignment problems. Good posture will also help you feel physically lighter and psychologically optimistic.

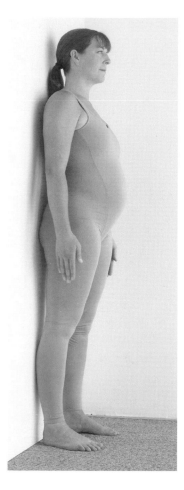

8. EXTENDED TRIANGLE POSE (Utthita Trikonasana)
Stand up straight with your back against the wall. Step your feet about 3 feet apart; turn your left foot out 90 degrees so the side of your foot is parallel to the wall, and turn your right foot slightly inward. The heel of your left foot should line up with the arch of your right. Place a block between the outside edge of your left foot and the wall. Stretch your arms out to the sides, draw up through your quadriceps, and lift your abdomen and chest. On an exhalation, keeping your back and the backs of your arms against the wall, extend your trunk to the left and bring your left hand down on the block. Press your hand into the block; stretch across your chest and up through your right arm. Draw your shoulder blades in, turn your chest toward the ceiling, and look straight ahead or up at your right hand. Turn your abdomen to the right. Breathe normally in this pose for 20 to 30 seconds. On an inhalation, lift up. Repeat the pose on your right side. Turn your toes in and step your feet back together.

EFFECTS The purposes of this strengthening pose are to energize your whole body, strengthen your legs, open your chest, improve respiration and circulation, and broaden your shoulders. It also helps your spine stay flexible.

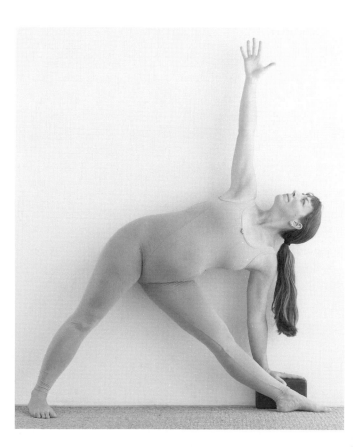

9. HALF-MOON POSE (Ardha Chandrasana)

Begin by doing Extended Triangle Pose (Utthita Trikonasana) to the left with your back against the wall. Place your left hand on a block that is between your left foot and the wall. On an exhalation, bend your left knee and take the block about 12 inches along the wall past your foot. Draw your right foot in toward the left to bring more weight onto your left leg. Come up to the toes of your right foot with your heel off the floor. On an exhalation, simultaneously straighten your left leg and raise your right leg up until it is parallel to the floor. Keep your back and right leg against the wall and turn your pelvis and chest toward the ceiling. Stretch your right arm up in line with your shoulders and open your chest and pelvis farther. Turn your abdomen toward the ceiling, away from your right thigh. Draw your shoulder blades into your back and expand your chest as much as possible. Hold this position for 30 to 60 seconds, breathing deeply and easily.

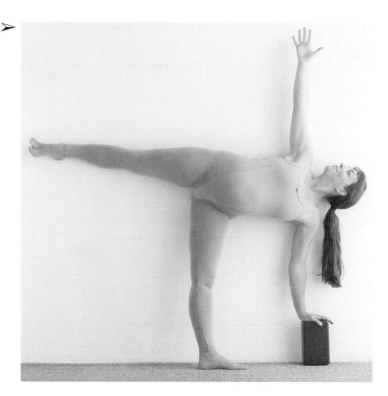

To come down, use the wall as support and bend your left leg while lowering your right leg. Come back to Extended Triangle Pose (Utthita Trikonasana). Inhale and slowly lift your torso up to standing. Do the pose on the other side.

EFFECTS This pose helps relieve morning sickness and open your pelvis and chest. It keeps your legs strong and engages your abdominals without putting pressure on the fetus.

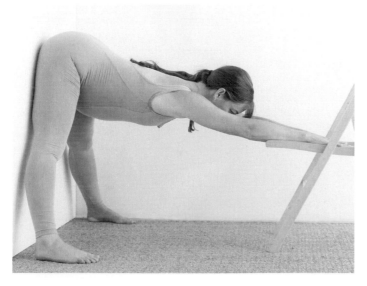

10. WIDE-ANGLE STANDING FORWARD BEND†

(Prasarita Padottanasana) Stand in a wide stance, feet parallel, with your back to the wall and a chair 3 to 4 feet in front of you. Put your hands on your hips, ground yourself through your heels, and lengthen up through the crown of your head. Bend forward from your hip joints, moving your shoulders away from your ears, and supporting your buttocks at the wall. Extend your arms straight out in front and place your forearms on the chair seat. Your torso should now be parallel and your legs perpendicular to the floor. Your spine should feel long, your belly open, and your shoulders relaxed. You should feel a nice stretch in your hamstrings. Look toward your hands and breathe normally, slightly emphasizing the exhalation, for 30 to 60 seconds.

To come out of the pose, release your arms, place your hands on your hips, and slowly come back to a standing position, resting against the wall for a few breaths.

EFFECTS This pose helps improve circulation in your legs, relax your pelvic floor muscles, and energize your whole body.

†CAUTION Do not practice this pose if it makes you dizzy or if you suffer from low blood pressure during pregnancy.

11. WIDE-ANGLE SEATED POSE I (Upavistha Konasana I)
Sit on two folded blankets with your back against the wall, spread your legs wide apart, and sit up straight. Place your hands on the edge of the blankets, just behind your thighs. Press your thighs and arms down and lift up through the sides of your trunk. Keep lifting the baby by drawing up through your abdomen from your pelvic floor. Sit like this as long as possible, from 1 to 3 minutes, without straining. Breathe normally, as you visualize creating more space in your womb for the baby to grow. To come out of this pose, bend your knees one at a time.

EFFECTS This pose helps broaden and tone your pelvic area to give the baby room to move. It also strengthens your spine, pelvic floor, and inner thighs and increases mobility in your hips. It is said to ease labor pains and promote an easy delivery if practiced regularly throughout pregnancy.

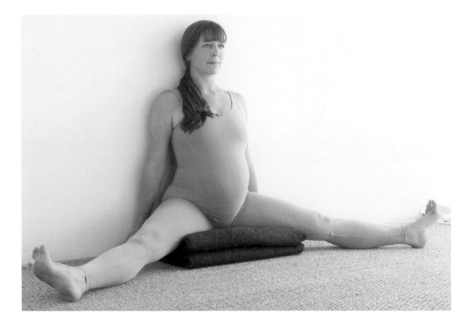

12. BOUND ANGLE POSE (Baddha Konasana) Sit on two folded blankets against the wall, with your back straight and your abdomen lifted. Bending your legs, open your knees out and bring the soles of your feet together. (After the fifth month, place a block between the soles of your feet to further broaden your pelvis.) Keep the outer edges of your feet on the floor. Lengthen your spine upward, leading with the crown of your head. Visualize moving the baby up as you lift up through your abdomen from your pelvic floor. Stretching your inner thighs from the groin to the knee, gently lower your knees as far as possible. Place your hands on the floor behind you to sit up straighter, and lift your abdomen. Stay in this position for 30 seconds or more, breathing normally. To come out, place your feet on the floor and straighten your legs out in front.

EFFECTS This pose helps broaden your pelvis, strengthen your spine, improve your posture, relax your pelvic floor muscles, and tone your abdominal region. It can also help position your pelvis for the birthing process.

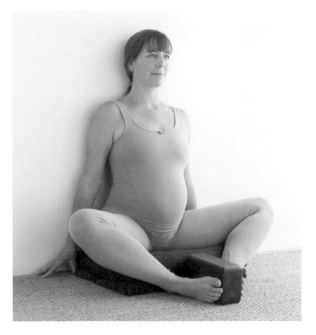

13. LEGS-UP-THE-WALL POSE (Viparita Karani) Place a bolster about 3 inches from the wall with a folded blanket in front of it for your head and shoulders. Sit on the bolster so your right hip and side are touching the wall. Using your hands to support you, lean back and swivel your body around as you take first your right leg and then your left leg up the wall. Keep your buttocks close to or against the wall; if they moved away from the wall as you lifted your legs, place your feet on the wall and use your hands for support to lift your hips and move your buttocks back into position. (If you feel stiffness or discomfort in your legs, push your buttocks slightly away from the wall.) Recline so that your lower back and ribs are supported by the bolster, your tailbone reclines toward the floor, your legs are at least hip-width apart, and your shoulders and head are on the blanket. Extend through your legs and place your hands on your belly so you can communicate with your baby. Rest in this position, eyes closed, for 5 minutes.

EFFECTS This calming pose can help ease fatigue in general, but especially in your legs; relieve nausea; and reduce swelling in your legs. It can be used in place of Corpse Pose (Savasana), if you prefer.

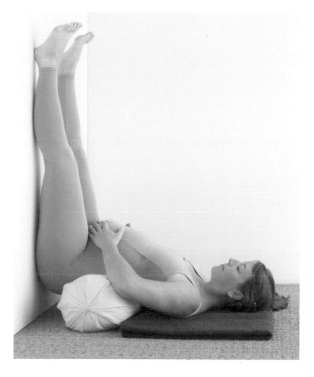

14. CORPSE POSE (Savasana) For the first trimester of pregnancy, you may practice this pose as described in the Woman's Essential Sequence (page 23). From the fourth month on, practice this pose on your side. Sit on one hip, knees bent to one side. Place a bolster between your knees and one in front of you. Using your arms for support, carefully lie down on your side and then hug the bolster with both arms. Rest your head comfortably to the side and remain in the pose for as long as you like. Optimal comfort is key here, so use as many bolsters as you wish, as long as your whole body—including your

neck and head—is in a straight line. Practice this deep relaxation pose as often as you like, switching sides for comfort. Focus on your breathing, allowing it to bathe your belly and your baby with loving kindness. To come out of the pose, use both hands to gently push yourself up to a seated position. Remain there for a few breaths before standing.

EFFECTS This deeply relaxing pose soothes your sympathetic nervous system, relieves fatigue and anxiety, and restores emotional balance.

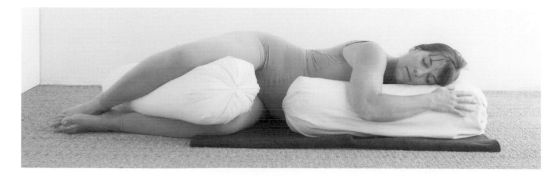

Breathing Exercises for Labor and Delivery

Practice these breathing exercises during your pregnancy, in preparation for the birthing process.

Expanding Life Force Energy Breathing (Ujjayi Pranayama) Begin in a comfortable position, like Reclining Bound Angle Pose (Supta Baddha Konasana). Close your eyes and relax completely, with your hands resting by your sides, palms up toward the ceiling. Breathe with your mouth closed. As you inhale, feel your lungs expanding and your chest broadening to receive the breath. Every inhalation lengthens your spine, creating space for your baby. You will feel the breath on your palate as it produces a slight hissing sound. As you exhale, surrender your femurs (thighbones) to the ground. Every exhalation roots you to the earth, offering you support and strength. The breath also makes a sound coming from the back of your throat as you exhale. Some practitioners say it reminds them of Darth Vader in *Star Wars.*

Breathe steadily for several breaths. Once you're completely relaxed, inhale normally. Pause for a second and then exhale slowly, releasing all the air from your lungs. Your breathing should be steady, with your exhalations longer than your inhalations. Repeat this cycle 12 to 15 times.

Now reverse it: Inhale long deep breaths, pause for a second, and then exhale normally, making your inhalation longer than your exhalation. Keep your chest lifted and allow your breath to expand the sides of your torso. Repeat this cycle 12 to 15 times.

In the last phase, inhale slowly and deeply; exhale slowly and silently until your lungs empty completely. Your inhalation and exhalation should be the same. Repeat this cycle 12 to 15 times, ending on an exhalation.

Interval Breathing (Viloma) Begin by inhaling deeply. Exhale from the top of the breath downward, emptying your lungs in three parts. Exhale a little bit and pause for 2 seconds. Exhale a little more and pause again. Continue to exhale until your lungs are empty; pause for 3 seconds. Breathe normally for several breaths, then begin again. Continue the practice for 5 or 6 cycles.

After your last exhalation, take your next inhalation in three parts: pull air into the bottom of your lungs, pause for 1 second, draw more air into the middle part of your lungs, pause again, and then breathe all the way in up to the top part of your chest and pause. Exhale completely, releasing your lower body into the floor and allowing your upper body to rise up. Breathe normally for several breaths, then begin again. Practice this exercise for 5 or 6 cycles.

Always end your pranayama practice with 5 to 10 minutes of Corpse Pose (Savasana), supported with pillows or bolsters.

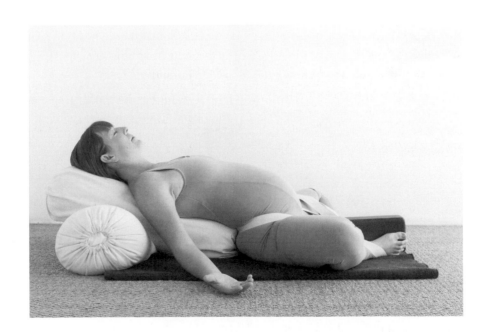

A SEQUENCE FOR POSTPARTUM RECOVERY (AFTER 6 WEEKS)

1. Tree Pose (Vrksasana)
2. Downward-Facing Dog Pose (Adho Mukha Svanasana)
3. Great Seal Pose (Maha Mudra)
4. Upward-Facing Leg Stretch (Urdhva Prasarita Padasana)
5. Shoulderstand (Sarvangasana)
6. Half-Plough Pose (Ardha Halasana)
7. Bridge Pose (Setu Bandha Sarvangasana)
8. Legs-Up-the-Wall Pose (Viparita Karani)
9. Corpse Pose (Savasana)

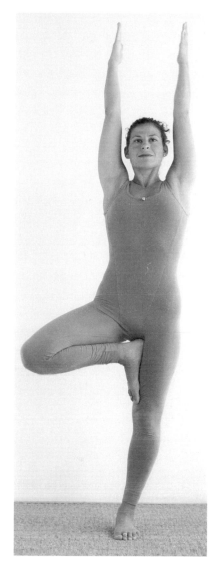

1. TREE POSE (Vrksasana) Stand with your feet hip-width apart. Bend your right knee and place the heel of your right foot at the top of your left thigh. Press your foot into your thigh and hold it there, toes pointing downward. Balance on your left leg and either raise both arms over your head, put your palms together in front of your chest in prayer position, or hold your baby in one arm. Stay in this pose for 10 to 15 seconds, if possible.

EFFECTS This pose can help strengthen your spinal column, improve your posture, and energize your whole body.

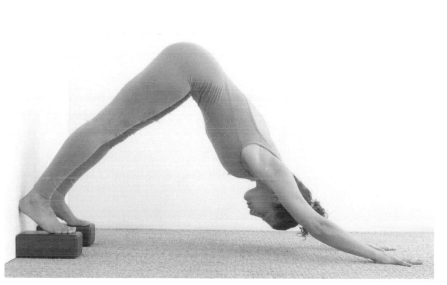

2. DOWNWARD-FACING DOG POSE (Adho Mukha Svanasana) Put two blocks against the wall to rest your feet on during this pose. Lie facedown with your feet just in front of the blocks. Place your palms on the floor by each side of your chest with your fingers well spread and pointing straight ahead. Come up on your hands and knees and step your feet onto the blocks.

Exhale and actively press your hands into the floor and your toes onto the blocks. Inhale and then on an exhalation raise your buttocks high into the air. Move your thighs up and back, keep stretching through your legs, and bring your heels toward the blocks as you lift your buttocks higher. The action of the arms and legs serves to elongate the spine and release your head. Stay in this pose for 30 seconds to 1 minute, breathing deeply. Let your head rest completely and release the base of your neck.

To come out, step off the blocks and return to your hands and knees, bringing your feet together. Keep your knees spread slightly and sit back on your heels.

EFFECTS Placing your feet on the blocks helps lift your uterus, tone your pelvic floor, and strengthen your spinal column.

3. GREAT SEAL POSE (Maha Mudra)
Sit up tall with your legs stretched
out in front of you. Bend your right
leg and place your right heel close to
your groin so your right leg is
perpendicular to your left. Extend
your arms and clasp the big toe on
your left foot with both hands. (If
you can't reach comfortably, wrap a
strap around the ball of your foot.)
Pressing your thighs into the floor,
raise your torso, and straighten your
arms. Your back should be slightly
concave and your sternum lifted.
Lower your chin toward your chest
and exhale completely. Inhale fully
and tighten your abdomen, pulling
in from the tip of your pubic bone
all the way up into your diaphragm
as you stretch your spine upward.

Hold the breath for 3 to 5 seconds;
exhale and begin the cycle one more
time. Relax, straighten your right leg
and repeat on your other side.

EFFECTS Similar to Kegel exercises,
this pose can help realign your
uterus and tone your pelvic floor
and abdominals.

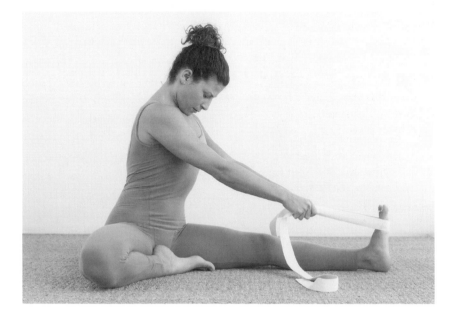

**4. UPWARD-FACING LEG STRETCH (Urdhva Prasarita
Padasana)** Lie on your back with your legs together and
your heels touching the wall at about a 60-degree angle.
Stretch your arms over your head, palms facing up, and
feel your body extending as well (A). Press your thighs,
knees, ankles, and toes together and breathe normally in
this position for a few breaths. On an exhalation, raise
both legs up so they are perpendicular to the floor (B);
remain like this for 5 to 10 seconds, breathing normally.
Exhale as you bring your legs down to the wall again.

Breathe normally for 5 to 10 seconds, then raise your legs
back to 90 degrees. Repeat 3 or 4 times. As your abdominal muscles get stronger, you can do 15 to 20 repetitions.
Make sure your hips and back are positioned firmly on
your sticky mat so you are using your abdominal muscles and not your lower back.

EFFECTS This pose stretches your spine and tones your
abdominal region, waist, thighs, and buttocks.

A

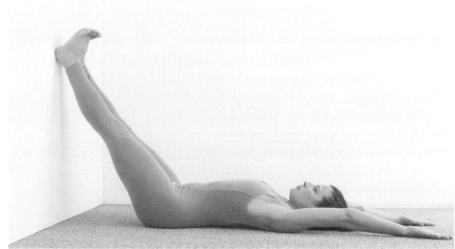

5. SHOULDERSTAND† (**Sarvangasana**) (Before beginning, see page 50.) Place a chair with its back about 8 to 10 inches away from the wall. Put a folded blanket on the chair seat, and two or three folded blankets in front of the chair. Sit backward on the chair with your legs bent over the top of the back; move your buttocks into the center of the chair seat.

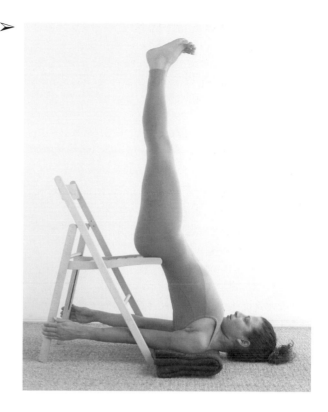

Holding the sides and then the front legs of the chair, slowly lower your torso so your neck and shoulders are on the blankets and your head is on the floor. You must extend your spine and open your chest while doing this to get the proper position. Move your hands, one at a time, to hold the back legs of the chair; your arms should be between the front legs. Rotating your thighs in, stretch your legs straight up. Keep your legs together and extended from your groin to your heels. Close your eyes, breathe normally, and bring your chest toward your chin. Hold this pose for 5 minutes.

To release from the pose, bend your knees, place your feet on the chair back, release your hands, and slide down until your sacrum rests on the blankets and your calves are on the chair seat. Rest here a moment, then roll to your side and sit up slowly.

EFFECTS This is an especially nice inversion if you feel fatigued or anxious. It may help alleviate varicose veins because it increases circulation. It can help develop patience, emotional stability, and willpower—all good qualities for new mothers.

†CAUTION Do not do this pose if you are still bleeding, have high blood pressure, or have a tension or migraine headache.

B

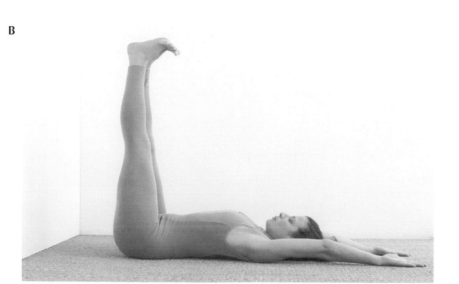

6. HALF-PLOUGH POSE† (Ardha Halasana) Place a folded blanket on top of your sticky mat with the rounded edge near the legs of a chair. Lie on your back with your legs outstretched, your shoulders on the blanket, and your head beneath the chair seat. As you exhale, bend your knees and swing or lift your buttocks and legs, so your thighs rest completely on the chair seat. (Pad the seat with blankets if you need more height for your legs to be parallel to the floor.) Move your chest in toward your chin. Bend your elbows at right angles to

your body and relax with your palms up and your eyes closed. Rest here for at least 3 to 5 minutes, if possible, breathing deeply to quiet your mind. To come out, place your hands on your back and slowly roll down, one vertebra at a time. Roll to one side and sit up.

EFFECTS This pose can help soothe your nerves, relieve fatigue, and alleviate stiffness in your shoulders and arms.

†CAUTION Do not do this pose if you suffer from neck or shoulder problems, or if you are still bleeding.

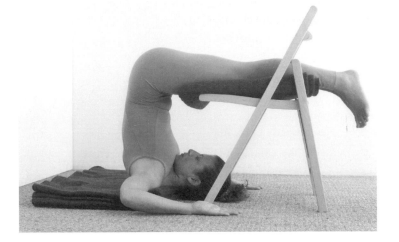

7. BRIDGE POSE (Setu Bandha Sarvangasana) Have two bolsters and a blanket on hand. Place one bolster horizontally against the wall and the other vertically, forming a T shape. Sit on the end of the vertical bolster that is closest to the wall. Keeping your knees bent, lie back over the bolster. Slide down until the end of the bolster is in the middle of your back and your shoulders just reach the floor. Rest your shoulders and head on the floor. Keeping your feet and heels together, stretch your legs toward the wall and put your heels on the horizontal bolster so your feet touch the wall. Your legs should be straight out in front of you. Rest your arms in any

comfortable position. Close your eyes and relax completely, softening your abdomen, releasing your vaginal walls, and breathing deeply. Stay in this position as long as you like.

To come out, bend your knees and slowly roll to one side. Using your hands, push yourself up to a seated position.

EFFECTS This restorative pose helps calm your mind, soothe your nerves, and open your chest (improving respiration and circulation). Some women find it beneficial to prevent varicose veins.

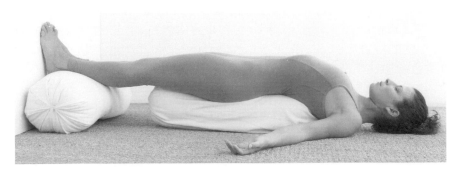

8. LEGS-UP-THE-WALL POSE† (**Viparita Karani**) Place a bolster about 3 inches from the wall. Sit on the bolster so your right hip and side are touching the wall. Using your hands to support you, lean back and swivel your body around, taking your right leg and then your left leg up the wall. Keep your buttocks close to or against the wall; if they moved away from the wall as you lifted your legs, place your feet on the wall and use your hands for support to lift your hips and move your buttocks back into position. (If you feel stiffness or discomfort in your legs, push your buttocks slightly away from the wall.) Lie down so your lower back and ribs are supported by the bolster, your tailbone is moving toward the floor, and your shoulders and head are on the floor. (If your neck is uncomfortable, put a blanket under it.) Extend through your legs and place your arms out at your sides, elbows bent and palms up. Rest in this position, eyes closed, as long as you like.

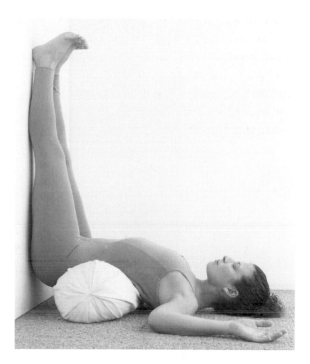

EFFECTS This supported inversion helps balance your endocrine system, soothe your nerves, open your chest, and improve respiration and circulation. Some women find it beneficial for alleviating postpartum depression.

CAUTION Do not do this pose if you are still bleeding.

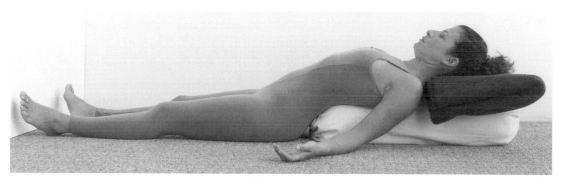

9. CORPSE POSE (Savasana) Place a vertical bolster behind you on your mat with a folded blanket at the far end of the bolster for your head. Sit with the end of the bolster touching your buttocks. Lower yourself onto the bolster and rest your head on the blanket. Relax your arms out to the sides, palms up, and let your feet relax away from each other. Focusing on your breathing, completely relax your shoulders, neck, and facial muscles. Keep your abdomen soft and relaxed. As you inhale,

allow your breath to move into your chest, but keep your throat, neck, and diaphragm free of tension. Let your eyes rest and breathe normally for at least 5 to 10 minutes.

EFFECTS This restorative pose relieves physical and mental fatigue; soothes your sympathetic nervous system, which helps relieve anxiety; and promotes a healthy milk supply.

Chapter 8 *Caring for Your Back*

IF YOU SUFFER FROM BACK PAIN, YOU MAY TAKE COMFORT IN knowing you're not alone. Back problems lead the list of physical complaints among American adults; rank as the number-one reason for lost job time; and keep thousands of orthopedic specialists, chiropractors, body workers, acupuncturists, and yoga therapists in business.

Back pain, like almost everything else in your body, has as much to do with how you feel emotionally, what you think, and the way you move through the world as it does with the muscles and bones in your back. Patricia often reminds her students that thinking affects feelings, feelings affect physiology, and the reverse is true as well. In other words, if you think you're a loser, you'll begin to feel like one, and your body language will reflect your loss of self-esteem. Ultimately your feelings will translate into rounded shoulders, lower back pain, and even compromised lung capacity. But if you walk with a purposeful stride and good posture, your emotions may rise to the occasion, and you'll actually feel confident and powerful.

For most women, back problems start in the teen years. If you're typical, you physically abused your back years ago by hauling big, heavy book bags, usually slung over one shoulder, and by bending over a desk for hours. Now you talk on the phone nonstop—for business or pleasure—with the receiver cradled between your neck and shoulder. Psychologically, you're probably no easier on yourself now than you were when you were a teen. Thirty-five-year-old Marjorie still remembers her mother constantly telling her when she was a teenager to stand up straight, walk proudly, hold her head up high. "As if I were going to walk around like I was some big shot," she told me. "I didn't want people staring at my chest. I hated my chest; I still do. And anyway, who wants to call attention to herself when she doesn't feel that great?" Sound familiar?

Marjorie says she always preferred to take up as little space as possible, and her posture still reflects that attitude. Her shoulders round forward; she often walks with her eyes cast down; and she sits or stands with her arms folded tightly across her chest. By creating a physical and emotional fortress against the world when she was still a teenager, Marjorie has spent years protecting herself from the judgments of her peers; at the same time, unfortunately, she has created problems in her neck and upper back from chronic overuse of those muscles. She suffers from what chiropractor and yoga teacher Thomas Alden, D.C., calls "overholding." It doesn't take a physical therapist or psychotherapist to figure out that Marjorie's past has affected her posture, which in turn, has reinforced her feelings of inadequacy.

Your feelings can affect your posture and the health of your back at any age. When my friend Joyce began practicing yoga in her thirties, she was having a lot of problems with her sacrum; she could barely touch her toes. Even though she knew she hated the way her body had changed after giving birth—her belly was no longer flat, her thighs had started to dimple—she had no idea that those feelings had actually messed up her posture and were causing her physical as well as emotional pain. The natural curve in her lumbar spine had flattened out and her thoracic curve had become exaggerated, all because she was trying to suck in her belly and look thinner.

Other women have problems stemming from job- and sports-related pursuits. As Dr. Alden explained to me, they tend to "over-hang" in their joints. Suzanne, a former ballet dancer and yoga teacher, is a prime example of this. Her hyperextended knees and pronated (inward-turning) feet have caused undue wear and tear on her joints. The joints, which are much more fragile than bones, must bear the body's weight and keep it in alignment.

If you have a high-stress job, you may suffer from what Tom Alden calls "performance-pattern holding." Under extreme pressure to do well, often in a male-dominated environment, you may cut yourself off from your feelings and your body. This "me-against-the-world" stance appears strong, self-reliant, and unbending to outsiders; inwardly, it is characterized by shallow breathing, tense muscles (especially in your upper back), and a clenched jaw. The shallow breathing and poor circulation this stance creates trigger the fight-or-flight response in your immune system (see chapter 6) and translate to a lot of pain in your muscles and joints.

The overholding syndrome Marjorie described can also affect women who take care of infants and young children. Any woman who has nursed a baby knows how painful your upper back and neck can feel. Lifting young children and carrying them on one hip can have disastrous effects on the alignment of your spine. If you work at home (especially at a computer) and take care of your children, you'll really need to be careful. I never thought much about my own back until recently, when my daily three or four hours at the computer turned into eight or nine. I'd forget to take breaks and by the end of the day, my neck ached, my shoulders were tight, and my lower back felt stiff. Even my left rotator cuff bothered me. It never dawned on me until I was talking to my yoga teacher that all these problems were connected and related to the way I was sitting.

By the time a woman has reached her forties and fifties, the stiffness and pain she's carried with her all her life join with fluctuating hormones to cause even more problems. The physical twinges in her hip joints, shoulders, and back turn to arthritis, and osteoporosis rears its ugly head (see chapter 14). Many aging women literally shrink at the thought of looking old and, like Marjorie, try to take up as little space as possible (maybe no one will notice the sags, bags, and rounding that age inevitably brings).

Back pain comes in many guises—from upper back and neck tightness to sciatica in the sacrum; from the swayback signature of lordosis to the humpback look of kyphosis; from the structural challenges of scoliosis to the crippling effects of osteoarthritis, osteoporosis, and spinal stenosis. While a number of back problems can be attributed to injuries, congenital defects, or even immune disorders, the majority have to do with posture and muscle tone. And most problems are aggravated by stress, pregnancy, poor nutrition, grief, work, and genetic disposition. Even serious degenerative disorders can be helped by improving your posture, reducing abnormal demand on your joints, getting adequate rest, eating right, and managing your stress level. Of course, it's important to have your back problems evaluated by a health care professional before you begin a yoga program.

CHECK YOUR POSTURE

Exactly what is healthy posture? How do you know whether everything's aligned the way it's supposed to be? Stand with your heels against a wall. If your calves, buttocks, shoulders, and the back of your head also touch the wall—and you can fit your hand between the wall and the small of your back—you have good alignment. Basically, your head should rest squarely over your shoulders, which rest over your hips, which in turn are centered over your knees. Your knees stack over your ankles with your weight distributed evenly on all four corners of your feet. Sitting in good posture (with your knees bent) means that you could draw an imaginary straight line from the center of your earlobe through your shoulder to the middle of your hip.

In order to maintain good posture, your spine must be both flexible and stable, but never rigid. Its stability supports the weight of your head and shoulder girdle and holds your body upright. Its flexibility allows your torso to bend and twist, move forward and back, and stretch side to side. The late Vanda Scaravelli, a renowned yoga teacher and author of *Awakening the Spine,* likened the spine to a tree. Its roots run down into your sacrum and legs, bringing support, stability, and balance to your body. Its trunk rises up to the base of your skull, supporting your head; its branches reach out to hold your shoulders in place.

A consistent, daily yoga practice is an ideal way to maintain good posture. Yoga helps keep your spine stable yet flexible because it offers a well-rounded routine of moving naturally in all directions.

THE MAP OF YOUR BACK

What's the prognosis if you didn't pass the posture test? It certainly doesn't mean the effects of bad posture are irreversible and that you're destined to a life of pain and suffering. Of course, it's not easy to alter the effects of bad habits cultivated over a lifetime—but it can be done, and a daily yoga practice can provide invaluable benefits. Before you can truly understand how the flexion and extension, contraction and expansion of yoga can help, however, you need to have a rudimentary knowledge of how your spine works and what's connected to what.

The spine, a complex interconnection of bones, nerves, muscles, and ligaments, begins at the top of your neck, where it supports your head, and ends at your coccyx (tailbone) at the very end of your sacrum. Attached to the spine are your arms (via the shoulder girdle), your chest (through the ribs), and your legs (by way of the pelvis). The prominent bones in the spine are called vertebrae, which you can feel as you bend forward. These interlocking spool-shaped bones are held in place by the surrounding muscles and ligaments and have bony arches that link together to form the spinal canal, which houses the nerves in the spinal cord.

Your spine isn't designed to be perfectly straight when you're standing still. Instead, three natural curves give it the strength and resilience it needs to bend, stretch, and absorb the normal daily pressures of supporting the rest of your body. Look at your back in the mirror (or observe a friend's). You can see that the cervical spine slopes inward (a concave curve) at the back of the neck. The next curve—in the upper back—moves outward (a convex curve) at the thoracic spine. A third curve finishes the movement with a concave slope at the lumbar spine (lower back), then a slightly convex turn at the tip of the coccyx. If any one of these curves is either exaggerated or flatter than it's designed to be, other parts of your spine must compensate, and pain in your back, shoulders, and even legs often results. For example, you may notice, like I did, that when the curve in your cervical spine is exaggerated, you feel pain not only in your neck but in your sacrum, the backs of your legs, your clavicle (collarbone), and your shoulder joints. Conversely, when your lumbar curve is exaggerated, it affects your hip flexors and abdominal muscles in the front of your body, sometimes your knees, and certainly the muscles alongside your spine and the intervertebral disks in your lower back (see pages xviii and xix).

Many chiropractors and body workers have a three-dimensional model of the spine in their offices to demonstrate exactly how it works. You can see the natural curves of the spine, as well as the size and shape of its vertebrae, which go from smaller in the cervical spine to progressively larger in the thoracic area and quite large in the lumbar spine, where they bear the most weight. Each vertebra stacks neatly on top of the next, separated and cushioned by intervertebral disks.

The health of your spine depends on the health of its disks. Designed to act as shock absorbers, these intervertebral cushions are made up of cartilage and fibrous tissue; they give your spine its mobility and keep the vertebrae from rubbing against one another. Each disk has a strong outer layer of interwoven fibrocartilage that houses and protects a soft, pulpy interior. If the outer layer tears, the gel-like substance inside will poke through, pressing against the spinal nerves and causing a lot of pain. This is called a herniated disk.

Like so many other parts of your body, the intervertebral disks need proper nourishment to stay strong, flexible, and functional. Since

HOW YOUR SPINE FITS TOGETHER

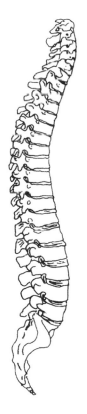

the soft interior of the disk has no blood supply of its own, it must soak up nutrients, like a sponge, from surrounding tissues. Mary Schatz, M.D., author of *Back Care Basics: A Doctor's Gentle Program for Back and Neck Pain Relief,* explains that when your body is at rest, the disks expand with nutrients (that's why you're taller when you get up in the morning); when you're active, the fluid squeezes back out to the tissues and vertebrae. As soon as you rest again, the process starts over. The action is a bit reminiscent of a bellows. If the disks are compromised in any way—through poor posture, stiffness in the spine, or injury—their spongelike action is also compromised and the disks starve. Dr. Schatz says the problems that result from these brittle, thin disks create a syndrome called degenerative disk disease.

DISKS AND VERTEBRAE

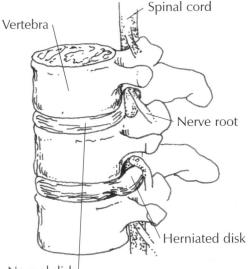

Vertebra

Spinal cord

Nerve root

Herniated disk

Normal disk

The Supporting Cast

Obviously your spine can't maintain proper alignment without help from the surrounding muscles, including the paraspinals, abdominals, hip flexors, and hamstrings. The paraspinals, as the name implies, run parallel to your spinal column. They are the muscles that feel so good when someone massages up the length of your back. They support your spine, keeping it upright and maintaining its curvature as it rotates, extends, and bends every which way. If these muscles are too tight, your spinal curves become exaggerated and you'll have a swayback. If the paraspinals are overly stretched, you won't have enough of a curve in your lower back. If one side is tighter than the other, you may have functional scoliosis (explained later in this chapter).

Upper back muscles control the flexibility and stability of your shoulders and neck. The muscles in the backs of your legs (hamstrings), the hip flexors in the front (the ones you engage when you lift up your leg), and the abdominals all affect the lumbar curve of your spine by tilting your pelvis forward or backward. If your hamstrings are too tight, they pull on your lower back and cause the lumbar curve to flatten out and the thoracic spine to round. If the hip flexors lose their flexibility, your pelvis will tilt forward and create too much of a lumbar curve. Underdeveloped abdominals don't offer enough support to your lumbar spine, causing it to press forward and create an exaggerated and potentially painful curve.

Equally important are the flexor, extensor, and rotator muscles that control movement in your joints. Flexor muscles bend the joints, extensors straighten them, and rotators twist or turn the bones in their sockets. The health and balance of these muscles affect your posture and ultimately the health of your back. According to Mary Schatz, an imbalance caused by uneven flexors, extensors, and rotators weakens joints and makes them more vulnerable to injury. The imbalance further prohibits the bones from bearing weight evenly. If this goes on long enough, it can result in arthritis.

COMMON BACK PROBLEMS

As I mentioned, most back pain responds quite well to postural realignment—particularly through yoga. And although yoga does much more than simply relieve immediate pain, most often that's what needs to happen first, before you can even start thinking about long-term solutions. Patricia and Chris Saudek, another Iyengar yoga teacher, created the back care sequence at the end of this chapter, which is beneficial for most back complaints. However, if you suffer from sacroiliac pain or sciatica, please work with a therapeutic yoga specialist to find the poses that work best for you.

Lordosis Often called a swayback because of the abnormal curvature in the lumbar spine, lordosis usually develops in response to weak abdominal muscles, tight hip flexors, or both. Pregnant women often suffer from this condition because their lower back muscles aren't strong enough to counter the forward pull of their pelvis. Women with pronounced lordosis will often stand with their weight over their toes, instead of centered over their whole foot.

If this is your underlying problem, include poses in your daily practice that strengthen your abdominals, lengthen your lower back, and stretch your hip flexors. Standing poses such as Extended Triangle Pose (Utthita Trikonasana) and Half-Moon Pose (Ardha Chandrasana) at the wall and backbends such as Bridge Pose (Setu Bandha Sarvangasana) work to stretch your hip flexors. Do Child's Pose (Adho Mukha Virasana) to lengthen your lower back.

Kyphosis An exaggerated curvature in your upper or thoracic spine, the telltale sign of kyphosis, is often called a dowager's hump. This condition appears most often in women who have tight hamstrings or shoulder muscles, walk with their heads jutting forward, or have extreme thoracic scoliosis or osteoporosis. Common among computer operators, women who are self-conscious about their chests or bellies, and elderly women, kyphosis can interfere with breathing and restrict movement of the rib cage.

Yoga poses that emphasize broadening your chest and rolling your shoulders back, as well as lengthening your hamstrings and strengthening your back muscles, can help. Standing poses like Extended Triangle Pose (Utthita Trikonasana), Revolved Triangle Pose (Parivrtta Trikonasana), and Upward-Facing Dog Pose (Urdhva Mukha Svanasana)—as either full poses or modifications using a chair—work to open your chest and strengthen your upper back. Seated poses such as Hero Pose with Cow-Face Arms (Virasana with Gomukhasana Arms) also relieve stiffness in your back and shoulders.

Sciatica Sciatic pain occurs when something presses on the sciatic nerve, which runs from your deep buttock muscles down into the muscles at the backs of your legs. That something could be a bulging intervertebral disk in your lumbar spine that's putting pressure on the

KYPHOSIS

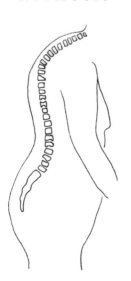

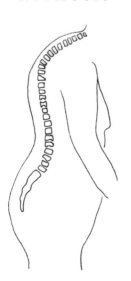

CARING FOR YOUR BACK

nerve root or the piriformis muscle (the large muscle on the side of your sacrum that rotates your leg outward), according to Mary Schatz. Lots of women experience intense sciatic pain during the late stages of pregnancy, when the weight of the fetus bears down on the nerve. Of course, if you suspect that a herniated or bulging disk is your problem, consult a specialist.

Because sciatica is so individualized, poses that may help one woman could aggravate another's pain. Although some of the poses we've offered in this chapter may alleviate the pressure, Patricia recommends working with a therapeutic yoga teacher if your pain persists.

Sacroiliac Pain A common complaint among women, sacroiliac (SI) pain is often caused by a torque or rotation in your pelvis, but it can also result from an injury to a hip joint or your lumbar spine. Ballet dancers are prime candidates for rotational stress injuries on the SI joint. Pregnant women also complain of SI problems from loose ligaments caused by the hormone relaxin. The SI joints—where the sacrum meets the ileum bones of the pelvis—are two bony protrusions just below your waist, on either side of your spine. If you suffer from a dull, persistent ache on one side above your buttocks, you probably have SI problems. You can tell which way your pelvis is rotated because one joint will protrude more—and hurt more, too. The pain, which is rarely sharp, can also show up in your groin, hamstrings, or even lower abdominals, making it hard to diagnose. Unfortunately, creating a particular yoga sequence that works for every woman's SI pain is impossible because the pain is so individualized.

Kathryn Arnold, editor of *Yoga Journal*, blames some of her sacroiliac problems on her sedentary job. She believes sitting so much causes her to overcontract her buttocks (the gluteus maximus) and overuse her lower back muscles. At the same time, she doesn't use her abdominals or adductors (inner thigh muscles) as much as she should, causing them to weaken. Like most women, Kathryn finds that standing poses make her SI pain much worse, primarily because these poses challenge her and cause her to tighten and grip the very muscles she needs to relax. She gets a certain amount of relief (and a lot of benefit) by practicing standing poses against a wall, where she feels safe enough to release the muscles in her legs and back.

Contrary to conventional therapeutic wisdom, seated twists and forward bends alleviate Kathryn's pain, possibly because, as she explains, "I get much more mobility when I'm on the ground, and I can focus on releasing my back and using my abdominals." She also believes that anyone with SI pain should work with a yoga specialist individually because what works for other people hasn't always worked for her, and what gives her more mobility could end up making someone else's problems worse.

Forward Head Position The forward head position is a classic indication of poor self-image and depression, as well as a symptom of dedicated couch potatoes and computer operators. Nursing moms also suffer from the effects of this posture, as do young moms who carry their baby in a backpack. You may think that this condition just impacts your upper back and neck muscles, but jutting your head forward has consequences throughout your entire body. Remember that in order to bend, twist, and rotate properly, your spine must be properly aligned. The vertebrae must stack correctly; the cervical, thoracic, and lumbar spines must maintain their curves; and the supporting muscles must be allowed to relax completely. When you sit, stand, or walk with your head forward on your neck, lots of things happen. Your upper back and neck muscles tighten immediately in an attempt to hold your head up. Chronically strained upper back and neck muscles can bring on tension headaches or even arthritis in that area. After a while, these same muscles become overstretched and tired from having to do all that work, which can lead to intervertebral disk problems in your neck. As your head moves out of alignment, your cervical curve decreases, your thoracic curve exaggerates, and your lumbar curve flattens. When your thoracic spine rounds, your ability to twist and rotate your upper back is compromised, which puts greater pressure on your lumbar spine to perform those functions.

As if that weren't enough, forward head position prevents other parts of your body from performing their functions, too. Your shoulder blades move out of alignment, causing rotator cuff problems and inflammation in the surrounding tissues. Your collarbones also move forward; your chest collapses inward; and your lungs—lacking adequate space to function—press against your diaphragm, moving it downward against the abdominal wall. Your abdominal muscles weaken, which in turn causes more problems in your lumbar spine. All this because you sit and walk with your head forward!

Many yoga poses address this condition, including standing poses to correct posture, shoulder and neck openers, backbends, and inversions. The back sequence at the end of this chapter is excellent for addressing the problems associated with forward head position, especially if you're in pain already. Any of the poses that address kyphosis will also help forward head problems. Of course, a daily practice of poses (such as the Woman's Essential Sequence or the Woman's Energizing Sequence) that flex, extend, and rotate your spine is ideal to prevent this syndrome.

Menstrual Back Pain

Back pain can also be caused by hormones. Some women suffer from lower back pain as part of PMS. Although no one knows for sure, most doctors think this kind of pain is somehow related to prostaglandin $F_2\alpha$, a hormone released shortly after you ovulate.

Other women experience a dull backache the first day or two of their period, which could be caused by hormonal changes as they start to bleed. According to Judith Hanson Lasater, author of *Relax and Renew: Restful Yoga for Stressful Times*, the ligaments that hold the sacrum and ileum bones of your pelvis together get overstretched and unstable during this time and become susceptible to pain and injury. Endometriosis (when bits of the uterine lining slough off and lodge outside the uterus) can create back pain, too, if the uterine lining attaches itself to the back of the pelvic wall. See the sequences provided in chapter 5 for poses that alleviate backaches and cramping.

Pregnant women and nursing moms often complain of chronic back pain, too. Hormones that create instability in the joints and ligaments may be part of the problem, but the weight of the baby in the womb can also press uncomfortably against the sciatic nerve or pelvic floor. Most of the poses shown in this chapter work well for pregnant women; however, do not do supine poses (lying on your back) after the first two months. The sequences in chapter 7 may also provide helpful suggestions. New mothers may find the sequence for postpartum in chapter 7 useful as well.

Scoliosis

Women are diagnosed with scoliosis seven times more often than men are. Researchers have found that there are three times in a woman's life that scoliosis can worsen: puberty, pregnancy, and perimenopause (times when our hormones fluctuate wildly). These fluctuations often cause looseness in the joints and less stability in the bones.

Remember that your spine must maintain its natural curves for proper alignment. These curves all slope in the same plane, which begins at the top of your neck and ends at the coccyx bone. People with scoliosis have an abnormal side-to-side curvature of the spine. For some women, these curves produce considerable pain; others feel very little; still others find they have trouble breathing. The most serious type of scoliosis is structural, or true, scoliosis, in which the bones and muscles are abnormally developed. Elise Miller, a yoga teacher specializing in scoliosis therapy, says true scoliosis can develop from birth trauma, a congenital predisposition, or disease. Of course, a large number of scoliosis cases are idiopathic, which simply means no one knows what causes them. Although nothing can truly reverse structural scoliosis, yoga can often decrease the curvature dramatically. Elise's curve went from a surgery-threatening forty-nine degrees to a manageable thirty-two degrees. Elise has idiopathic adolescent scoliosis, which means that it began in her teen years (following a growth spurt) and no one knows why.

Functional scoliosis develops for a variety of reasons. One of your legs could be shorter than the other, causing your pelvis to tilt to one side and—as a counterbalance—your spine to curve in the opposite direction. Again, this leg length discrepancy can be either structural or functional. Functional leg length discrepancies stem from postural problems—one foot is flatter or more turned in than the other, a hip joint rotates in slightly, or one knee is more hyperextended. My daughter Sarah, who has had functional scoliosis since she was six years old, gets intense back spasms on the side of her back that is most contracted. They subside as the muscles calm down.

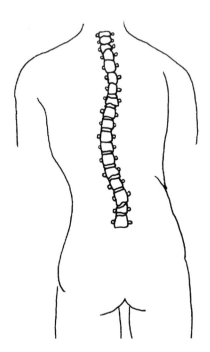

SCOLIOSIS

If you suffer from either structural or functional scoliosis, your back will appear to be lopsided. On one side of a scoliotic spine, the paraspinal muscles are overstretched and weak, forming a convex mound; on the other (concave) side, the muscles are tight and over-worked, creating a sunken hollow area. You can tell whether your scoliosis is structural or functional by bending over. If the lopsided-ness evens out, your curvature is probably functional and caused by misaligned vertebrae, bad postural habits, or muscles pulling on your spine.

According to Elise Miller, there are generally two types of curvature: the S-curve and the C-curve. The S-curve has a major curve to one side (90 percent go to the right), with a compensating, smaller curve to the left. Thoracic scoliosis, for example, has its major curve in the thoracic spine and its smaller curve in the lumbar area. A C-curve begins lower in the thoracic area and continues into the lumbar region. Most scoliotic curves have an element of rotation to them, as well.

Yoga for Scoliosis Yoga poses that lengthen and strengthen the paraspinal muscles work best. The rule of thumb, Elise says, is to lengthen your muscles to decrease the curve, strengthen them to maintain that length, derotate your spine, and realign your posture. Stabilizing and strengthening postures are critical. Yogic breathing also helps by strengthening your lungs—people with scoliosis often have an underdeveloped lung on one side—and by bringing loving attention to your back.

Doing the entire back care sequence at the end of this chapter would be very beneficial, especially the standing poses like Extended Triangle Pose (Utthita Trikonasana) done against a wall. Most women with scoliosis say they benefit from any variation of Downward-Facing Dog Pose (Adho Mukha Svanasana). Elise Miller teaches her students a variation of this pose using a chair. She also teaches a supported Head-on-Knee Pose (Janu Sirsasana), a gentle Simple Seated Twist Pose (Bharadvajasana) on a chair, and supported Shoulderstand (Sarvangasana) on a chair.

As you do these poses, you may experience different sensations from one side of your back to the other, especially if you incorporate twists into your routine. Even if one side is easier to twist than the other, always twist to both sides. Elise Miller explains that twisting to one side derotates your spine; twisting to the other side helps to align it. At the beginning, you'll probably find it's much easier to twist to one side than the other; be patient with yourself and keep working both sides for the best results.

ARTHRITIS

An inflammatory or degenerative condition of the spine, this disease comes in two varieties: rheumatoid arthritis and osteoarthritis. Rheumatoid arthritis is actually an immune system malfunction, which causes your body to turn against itself and destroy the lining of your joints as though that lining were a foreign invader. If that happens in your spine, it's called ankylosing spondylitis. This disease progressively stiffens your spine and causes pain and loss of mobility, first in the core of your body and then throughout your extremities.

According to James Gordon, M.D., director of the Center for Mind-Body Medicine in Washington, D.C., yoga is the hottest new treatment for rheumatoid arthritis. The reason? He believes yoga gives you "all the benefits of range-of-motion exercises. It restores flexibility, improves circulation to your joints, allows more healing nutrition to reach them, forces more oxygen into those joints, and facilitates the release of endorphins, the body's own natural pain-killers." Yoga also brings relief from the tension and stress your body and mind experience. As mentioned before, chronic muscle tension creates more stress, which creates more pain, which causes more muscle tension. Yoga, Dr. Gordon points out, breaks that vicious cycle and brings relaxation and a respite from the pain.

Osteoarthritis is a condition that causes degeneration of the joints. Some doctors believe it is an inevitable side effect of aging; other health experts blame poor posture and bad body alignment; still others believe it can arise from any condition that produces unhealthy demands on the joints—lordosis, kyphosis, or forward head position.

Pam's Story

Pam is literally a walking testimony of what yoga can do. At age twenty-six, she was diagnosed with ankylosing spondylitis, a degenerative form of arthritis. After trying many different drug therapies, she was put on a powerful anti-inflammatory and told that mild exercise would help. Every day was a painful challenge. Her three pregnancies were nightmares. No longer able to walk, she crawled from room to room at home and used two canes in public. For years she went to her local YMCA and swam. At home she clocked thousands of miles on her stationary bike. But she still couldn't touch her toes; her hands only reached her knees. Through exercising she was able to slow the stiffening so that she lost only a few millimeters of movement each year.

At age forty-two, she began massage and Reiki treatments, which gave her lots of pain relief. Then she started yoga—the slow and gentle class—with women in their seventies and eighties who were much more flexible than she was. "Our teacher had us doing forward bends," Pam remembers, "but I couldn't even touch my toes. We did Downward-Facing Dogs, but my back was rounded, my heels miles from the ground." The students were told to bend and to twist, but Pam's arms were too short, her breathing ragged, her ribs aching. As her spine had lost mobility over the years, so had her rib cage, which restricted her breathing. "My teacher told me not to give up," Pam says, "that in ten years I would be more flexible, but I didn't believe her." After only ten weeks, however, Pam did begin to feel more flexible. Although the doctor saw no measurable difference, she was determined to keep going.

Now, after three years, every class is a feast for Pam. She can do forward bends and breathe deeply without pain. Yoga hasn't cured her arthritis, but she's on only a quarter of the medication she was on when she started. Flare-ups happen less often and she actually has days when she's pain-free.

Natural Relief

The following are a few suggestions that may help when you have arthritic flare-ups.

- Anti-inflammatories, such as ginger or curcumin (found in turmeric), can decrease swelling and improve mobility. Cut up a slice of fresh ginger, let it steep in freshly boiled water for five to ten minutes, and drink before bedtime. Use turmeric liberally in cooking or take 400 mg of curcumin (found in tablets at health food stores) to improve mobility and reduce stiffness and swelling. Curcumin, like capsaicin, depletes substance P, a nerve chemical responsible for sending pain signals to your brain, according to James Duke, Ph.D., a well-known herbalist and botanist who was formerly with the U.S. Department of Agriculture.

- Place cold compresses on affected areas to reduce inflammation.

- Take a warm shower first thing in the morning to increase your circulation.

- Increase your daily intake of omega-3 essential fatty acids, either in oil form or by consuming at least one serving of fish a day. The most dramatic improvement, according to C. Leigh Broadhurst, Ph.D., visiting research scientist at the U.S. Department of Agriculture, came for those taking as much as 6g of fish oil a day. Unfortunately, Dr. Broadhurst says you must take fish oil for a few months before you see any results.

- Increase your intake of calcium; selenium; and the antioxidant vitamins C, E, and A. Antioxidants neutralize the systemwide free radicals responsible for making inflammation worse.

- Pay attention to your diet. Some people find their symptoms worsen when they eat tomatoes, potatoes, or eggplant—nightshade vegetables. Others are sensitive to caffeine, white sugar, alcohol, and animal products.

- Do your yoga practice even on days when you have flare-ups. Yoga can keep your joints more mobile and decrease swelling. Most people suffering from rheumatoid arthritis find practicing yoga in the late afternoon or early evening works better than in the morning, when their muscles are stiffer.

Patricia Says

If you have arthritis of any kind, yoga can help. You may feel timid about starting a yoga practice, particularly if you're in pain or very stiff, so it's best to work with a teacher experienced in therapeutic yoga. It's important to increase the space between your joints, provide extension and flexion, and strengthen the surrounding ligaments and tissues. Do poses that encourage movement in your joints. Don't hold a position too long, and keep the joints moving. For example, if you can do Reclining Big Toe Pose I (Supta Padangusthasana I) from the sequence in this chapter, don't hold your leg upright in a fixed position; gently move it back and forth in the socket. Choose poses that take your spine through the full range of motion—very slowly and gently at first—so you can improve blood circulation and gain mobility.

HOW YOGA CAN HELP

A healthy back can exist only when everything works together: when the paraspinals, flexors, extensors, and rotators are balanced; when your spine's natural curvature is maintained; and when your mental and emotional states support a strong, beautiful, and flexible body. Yoga brings both the physiological and the psychological support you need to develop healthy posture, a strong self-image, and a balanced state of mind.

Physical Relief

Although the benefits of yoga extend far beyond prescriptions for pain control, what you want most of all when you're in pain is to feel better, and yoga postures can help you do that. In choosing postures that will help strengthen your back, Elise Miller emphasizes poses that stabilize overly flexible areas and require action from stiff, inflexible ones. Both Patricia and Elise recommend that you do a well-balanced yoga sequence daily to put your back through a complete range of motion.

Don't feel you have to do the complete back care sequence we offer here. Some women find relief by doing standing poses; others notice these poses worsen their pain and they feel better when they lie on their back. Still others need the release they get when they do standing or seated twists. Do whatever makes you feel better and don't worry about following a specific sequence.

Emotional Release

As I mentioned earlier, your posture and your emotions influence one another. As yoga brings balance, flexibility, and alignment to your muscles and bones, it also brings those same qualities to your mind. A more flexible body encourages a more flexible mind and vice versa; a stronger body restores that inner source of strength you thought you had lost.

Mind-Body Awareness

Paying attention to how your body feels as you do your daily sequences will offer you invaluable insight into your physical and emotional needs. Because yoga encompasses so much more than just physical exercises, it engages your mind and spirit in the recovery process. It utilizes your breath to bring an inner awareness to your movements so you can experience not only the source of your pain, but how it connects to your feelings and your expectations. As you increase your body awareness, you'll be able to understand what habits, movements, and attitudes bring about pain and which ones relieve it. This can happen not only on the yoga mat, but out in the everyday world, too. Think of your yoga mat as your practice space, as your laboratory for creating healthy action. As you learn to be present within each pose and move from one to another, you discover what feels good and what doesn't. You can then take this knowledge and apply it to how you sit, stand, and move through your day.

Patricia Says

Western society's emphasis on women being skinny has taken its toll on our backs as well as our psyches. If you feel self-conscious about your breasts, for example, you're more likely to round your shoulders, walk with your head forward, and hunch your upper back. If your abdomen is round and prominent, you may suck it in as you walk, which not only flattens your lower back but impedes circulation to your abdominal and pelvic organs. Yoga not only addresses the physical problems you have created—kyphosis and forward head position—but help you feel better about who you are.

1. Simple Seated Twist Pose
   (Bharadvajasana)
2. Standing Spinal Twist Pose
   (Utthita Marichyasana)
3. Standing Big Toe Pose I
   (Utthita Hasta Padangusthasana I)
4. Standing Big Toe Pose II
   (Utthita Hasta Padangusthasana II)
5. Extended Triangle Pose
   (Utthita Trikonasana)
6. Upward-Facing Dog Pose
   (Urdhva Mukha Svanasana)
7. Reclining Knee-to-Chest Pose
   (Eka Pada Supta Pavanmuktasana)
8. Reclining Big Toe Pose I
   (Supta Padangusthasana I)
9. Upward-Facing Leg Stretch
   (Urdhva Prasarita Padasana)
10. Twisted Stomach Pose
    (Jathara Parivartanasana)
11. Corpse Pose (Savasana)

ADDITIONAL POSES FOR KYPHOSIS

Revolved Triangle Pose
   (Parivrtta Trikonasana)
Hero Pose with Cow-Face Arms
   (Virasana with Gomukhasana Arms)

ADDITIONAL POSES FOR SCOLIOSIS

Downward-Facing Dog Pose
   (Adho Mukha Svanasana)
Head-on-Knee Pose (Janu Sirasana)
Shoulderstand (Sarvangasana)

A SEQUENCE FOR GENERAL BACK PAIN

Remember, do only those postures that make you feel better, and stay away from those that make you feel worse. Your particular type of pain may respond better to standing poses, while other women need the relief of supine postures. Working with a yoga teacher specializing in back care or therapeutic yoga is especially important if you suffer from sacroiliac pain, sciatica, or rheumatoid or osteoarthritis.

1. SIMPLE SEATED TWIST POSE† (**Bharadvajasana**) Sit sideways (to the right) on a chair with your feet on the floor, hip-width apart. Stretch your torso up through the crown of your head. Take one or two breaths in this position. Take another breath and, as you exhale, rotate your torso to the right (toward the back of the chair), initiating the movement from deep in your belly and not from your head or shoulders. Place both hands on the chair back, and turn to look over your right shoulder. Hold this pose for 20 to 30 seconds. Change sides so the chair back is on your left and repeat for your left side.

EFFECTS This pose helps release tension and pain in your lower back, neck, and shoulders.

†CAUTION If you suffer from sacroiliac pain, release your pelvis whenever you twist. Do not practice twists if you have diarrhea.

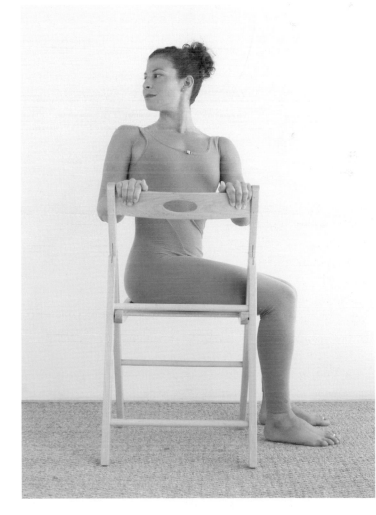

2. STANDING SPINAL TWIST POSE (Utthita Marichyasana) Place a chair with its back legs against the wall. Put a block on the chair at the edge of the seat closest to the wall. (If the chair is slippery, use a sticky mat under the block.) Stand facing the chair with the right side of your body next to the wall. Keeping your left leg firm, put your right foot up on the block and your left hand on your right knee. Putting a block under your left heel increases the rotation of your pelvis. Inhale and stretch up, exhale and turn your whole torso (spine and pelvis together) toward the wall and place your hands on the wall. Continue to breathe in this position for 30 to 60 seconds, stretching up on a deep inhalation and turning your torso a little more on each complete exhalation. (If you are suffering from an acute backache, it is better to hold this pose for a shorter period and repeat it several times.) Release the pose, stand on the other side of the chair, and repeat on your left side. Repeat this pose twice on each side.

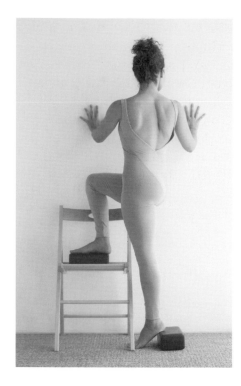

EFFECTS This pose helps release tension and stiffness in your shoulders, neck, and upper back. It also may help alleviate sciatica and pain in your lower back, hips, and sacroiliac joints.

3. STANDING BIG TOE POSE I (Utthita Hasta Padangusthasana I) Place a chair with its back legs against the wall. Stand facing the chair. Bend your right leg; put a strap around the ball of your foot; and, holding the strap with both hands, place your right foot against the wall with your lower leg on the chair back. (If you experience any discomfort in your back, place your foot on a bolster on the chair seat instead.) Straighten both legs and stretch up through your torso. The knee and big toe of your right leg should face the ceiling; push the heel into the wall. Hold this pose for 30 to 60 seconds. Bend your leg to release the strap and stand with your feet together. Repeat the pose with your other leg.

EFFECTS This pose helps alleviate stiffness in your hips and release tension in the backs of your legs.

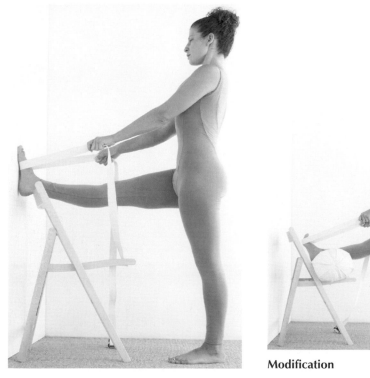

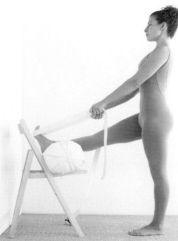

Modification

4. STANDING BIG TOE POSE II (Utthita Hasta Padangusthasana II) Place a chair with its back legs against the wall. Stand with the chair at your right side. Bend your right leg, and put a strap around the ball of your foot. On an exhalation, put your right foot on the wall with your lower leg on the chair back, holding on to the strap with your right hand. (If you experience any discomfort in your back or hamstrings, place your foot on a bolster on the chair seat instead.) Straighten both legs and stretch up through your torso. The knee and big toe of your right leg should face the ceiling; push the heel into the wall. Hold this pose for 30 to 60 seconds. Bend your leg to release the strap and stand with your feet together. Repeat the pose with your other leg.

EFFECTS This pose is good when you need to alleviate stiffness in your hips and release tension in the backs of your legs.

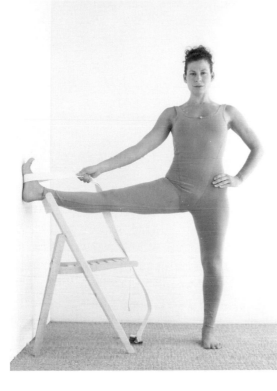

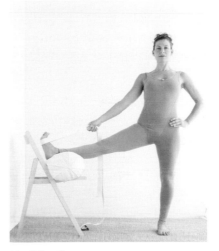

Modification

5. EXTENDED TRIANGLE POSE (Utthita Trikonasana) Stand about 3 inches away from the wall with your feet 3 to 3½ feet apart. Place a block vertically against the wall behind your left foot. Turn your left foot out 90 degrees and your right foot slightly inward; for extra stability brace your right foot against another wall. Raise your arms out to your sides in line with your shoulders. Keep your legs firm. Inhale, stretch up through your torso, and as you exhale bend your trunk to the left, bringing your left palm down to the block. Stretch your right arm over your head and lean your buttocks and torso against the wall. Gently turn your head to look up at your right hand or straight ahead. Continue in this pose for 30 to 60 seconds. To come out of the pose, bend both knees and press against the wall as you come up. Repeat the pose on your right side.

If this pose is too difficult, try the modified version described in chapter 14 (page 335).

EFFECTS This pose helps alleviate stiffness in your neck, shoulders, and knees. It is also excellent for improving your posture.

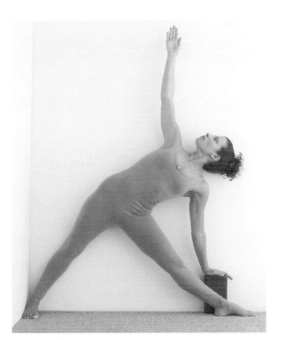

6. UPWARD-FACING DOG POSE (Urdhva Mukha Svanasana) Place a chair with the front edge of its seat against the wall. Stand about a foot away from the chair (depending on your flexibility). Holding the top of the chair and keeping your legs firm, arch up and forward until the tops of your thighs touch the top of the chair back and you are standing on tiptoe. Press down on the top of the chair; arch and lift your sternum (breastbone) and collarbone. Hold this pose for 30 to 60 seconds while breathing evenly. Return to a regular standing position. Repeat this pose two or three times.

NOTE It is important to realize that you're trying to arch your spine while keeping the two ends moving away from each other. Therefore, be sure to keep your legs and tailbone firm while you stretch up with your chest.

EFFECTS This pose helps relieve stiffness and pain in your shoulders, upper back, and neck.

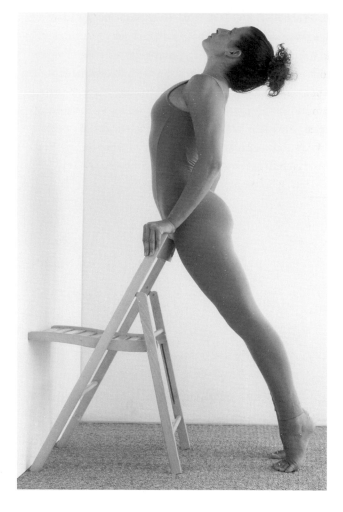

7. RECLINING KNEE-TO-CHEST POSE (Eka Pada Supta Pavanmuktasana) Lie on your back and press your feet into the wall, keeping your heels and big toes together. Press your thighs down toward the floor. Keeping your right leg straight, bend your left leg and use your arms to pull your left knee as close to your chest as possible without disturbing your other leg. Hold this position for 30 to 60 seconds. Release your left leg and return to your starting position, again pressing your feet into the wall; change legs. Repeat two to three times on each side.

EFFECTS This pose is good when you need to relieve pain and release tension in your lower back.

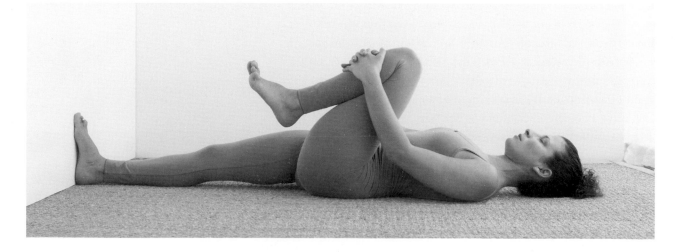

8. RECLINING BIG TOE POSE I (Supta Padangusthasana I)
Lie on your back and press your feet into the wall, keeping your heels and big toes together. Place a looped long strap around your left upper thigh. Bend your right knee slightly and place the other end of the looped strap around your right foot. Raise your left leg, bend your knee, and place a second, shorter, strap around your left foot. Tighten the long strap so that when you straighten your right leg it will create traction in your left leg and hip. Straighten both legs simultaneously. Press into both straps and flex your left foot so you feel a good stretch throughout the back of your leg. Hold this pose for 1 to 2 minutes. Bend both legs to release the straps, then straighten them out in front of you. Lie still, breathing evenly for several breaths. Repeat twice on each side.

EFFECTS This pose helps ease stiffness in your lower back and realign your pelvic area. It also stretches the backs of your legs, your hips, and your calves. It may be beneficial if you suffer from sciatica.

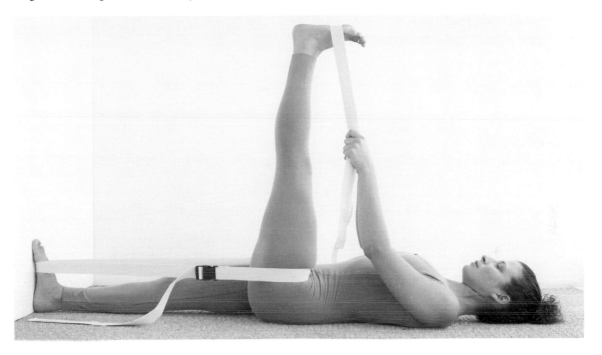

9. UPWARD-FACING LEG STRETCH (Urdhva Prasarita Padasana) Lie on your back and stretch your legs up the wall. Bring your buttocks as close to the wall as possible. Keep your sacrum on the floor and your legs straight. Stretch the bones in your buttocks toward the wall and press your thighs into the wall as you stretch your arms over head. After stretching for about 30 to 60 seconds, relax your arms into any comfortable position, close your eyes, and rest while breathing normally. Stay in this pose for 5 minutes, releasing your lower back into the floor.

EFFECTS This pose relieves stiffness in your lower back and hamstrings.

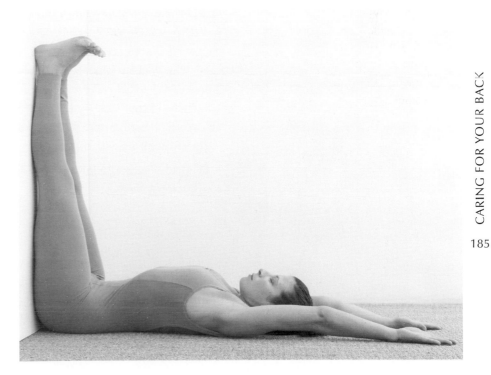

10. TWISTED STOMACH POSE† **(Jathara Parivartanasana)** Lie on your back and bend your knees so your feet are flat on the floor. (If you experience any strain or compression in your neck, place a blanket or rolled-up towel under your neck.) Keeping your knees together, reach your arms straight out to the sides with your palms up. Engage your abdominal muscles, pressing your navel back toward your spine. As you exhale, rock your knees to the left as far as possible, keeping your right shoulder blade on the floor. Pause, then as you inhale, lift them up to center; then smoothly exhale and lower them to the right, keeping your left shoulder blade on the floor. It's critical that you use your abdominal muscles in this pose and not rely on your lower back, especially if you suffer from sacroiliac pain. (It sometimes helps to place your hands underneath your sacrum for more support.) Repeat this several times to relieve tension in your spinal muscles.

EFFECTS This pose helps tone your abdominal muscles and strengthen your lower back muscles.

†CAUTION If you feel any pain while doing this pose, skip it entirely.

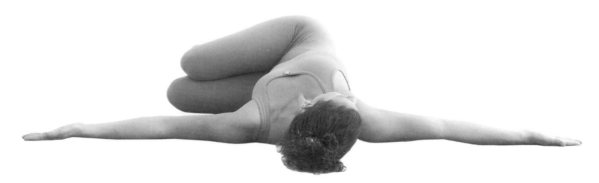

11. CORPSE POSE (Savasana) Place a chair in front of you with its seat facing you and padded with a folded blanket. Lie on a folded blanket or two on your back with your calves on the chair and the rest of you on the blanket. Relax your arms out to the sides with your palms up. Close your eyes, breathe normally, and relax completely. Stay in this position for at least 10 minutes and allow your back to relax into the blankets. If you feel any tension, exhale more deeply to help release it. To come out of the pose, open your eyes slowly, bend your knees into your chest, and roll to the side. Rest on your side for several breaths before coming to a seated position, using your arms to help you come up without strain.

EFFECTS This pose allows you to relax completely by taking pressure off your lower back.

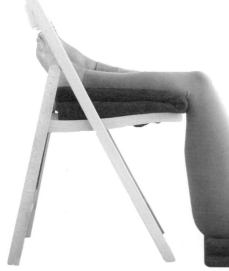

ADDITIONAL POSES FOR KYPHOSIS

Revolved Triangle Pose
    (Parivrtta Trikonasana)
Hero Pose with Cow-Face Arms
    (Virasana with Gomukhasana Arms)

Practice the sequence for general back pain, but add the following two poses after Extended Triangle Pose (Utthita Trikonasana).

REVOLVED TRIANGLE POSE (Parivrtta Trikonasana) Stand facing a wall, with a chair on your right. Step your feet about 3 feet apart; turn your right foot out 90 degrees (so the inner edge is parallel to the wall and your foot slides under the front of the chair) and your left foot in 60 degrees. Keeping your legs firm, stretch up through your torso. On an exhalation, turn your torso toward the chair and place your left hand on the seat and your right hand on your lower back. Relax your shoulders, neck, and facial muscles, and breathe normally for 30 to 60 seconds. (If this is too difficult, come in and out of the pose several times.) Release the pose and move the chair to the other side so your left foot is turned out 90 degrees and your right is in 60 degrees. Do this pose twice on each side.

If you are comfortable doing this pose without using a chair, refer to the instructions in the Woman's Essential Sequence (page 9).

EFFECTS This pose opens your chest and helps strengthen your upper back. It also helps correct the effects of forward head position, as well as those of kyphosis.

HERO POSE† WITH COW-FACE ARMS (Virasana with Gomukhasana Arms) Kneel on the floor with your knees together, your feet pointing straight back, and your calves slightly wider than hip-width apart. Sit between your feet on the floor (or on a block or bolster if you feel any pressure on your knees). Put your left arm behind you and stretch the forearm up your back as far as you can, with the back of your hand against your back. Reach your right arm over your head, bend it at the elbow, and reach down your back toward your left hand. Grasp the fingers of both hands together (or lower a strap in your right hand if your hands won't meet). Keep your right elbow pointing toward the ceiling and your head up. Roll your shoulders back and open your chest. Breathe normally and hold this pose for 30 seconds to 1 minute. Repeat on the other side.

EFFECTS This pose opens your chest, broadens your upper back, and releases tension in your shoulders. It is especially good for arthritic shoulders.

†CAUTION If you feel any strain in your knees, separate them slightly and sit on a bolster or block. If you are a beginner, don't stay in this pose longer than 1 minute.

ADDITIONAL POSES FOR SCOLIOSIS

Downward-Facing Dog Pose
(Adho Mukha Svanasana)
Head-on-Knee Pose (Janu Sirasana)
Shoulderstand (Sarvangasana)

Practice the sequence for general back pain, but add the following three poses after Extended Triangle Pose (Utthita Trikonasana).

DOWNWARD-FACING DOG POSE (Adho Mukha Svanasana) Place a chair with its back against the wall, and stand about 3 feet in front of it. As you inhale, extend up through the crown of your head; as you exhale, bend forward at your hip joints, resting your hands on the chair seat. Walk your feet back, placing them hip-width apart, until they are in line with your hips. Exhale while you press your heels into the floor and your hands into the chair. Raise your buttocks slightly by straightening your knees and pulling your thighs back, but do not arch your lower back. Extend your chest back toward your thighs and lengthen the back of your neck.

Keep your elbows and knees straight; keep pressing back through your heels into the floor. Keep your buttocks extending upward. Stay in this pose for 1 to 2 minutes, breathing deeply. If you cannot hold it that long, come out of it and repeat once.

If you are flexible enough, practice Downward-Facing Dog as described in the Woman's Essential Sequence (page 15) instead.

EFFECTS This pose lengthens and strengthens your paraspinal muscles.

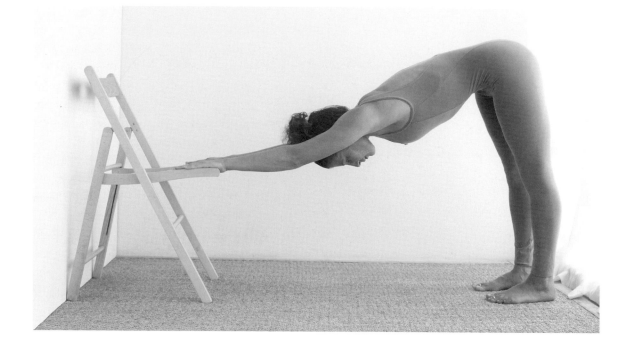

HEAD-ON-KNEE POSE (Janu Sirsasana) Sit with your legs stretched out in front of you. Bend your right knee to the side so your right heel is near your perineum and your right knee is at a 45-degree angle to your left leg. Turn your torso and chest to the left so your sternum is in line with the center of your left leg. Loop a strap around the ball of your foot and straighten your leg. On an exhalation, bend forward from your hips while pulling gently on the strap. Inhale and lift your trunk up from the base of your pelvis. Look forward over your outstretched leg and keep your back slightly concave. Hold for 10 seconds, breathing normally, then release and switch legs.

EFFECTS This pose helps to lengthen and derotate your spine.

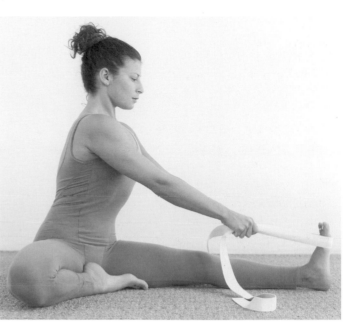

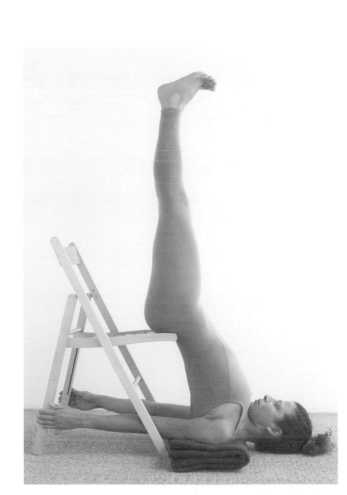

SHOULDERSTAND† (Sarvangasana) (Before beginning, see page 50.) Place a chair about 8 to 10 inches away from the wall and pad the seat with a folded blanket to protect your sacrum (not shown). Put two folded blankets in front of the chair. Sit backward on the chair with your legs bent over the back; move your buttocks into the center of the chair seat.

Holding the sides and then the front legs of the chair, slowly lower your torso so your shoulders are on the blankets and your head is on the floor. You must extend your spine and open your chest while doing this to get the proper position. Move your hands, one at a time, to hold the back legs of the chair; your arms should be between the front legs. Stretch your legs straight up, keeping your sacrum on the chair seat. Rotate your thighs in and extend from your groin to your heels. Close your eyes, bring your chest to your chin, and breathe normally for 3 to 5 minutes, or as long as you're comfortable.

To release from the pose, bend your knees, place your feet on the chair back, release your hands, and slide down until your sacrum rests on the blankets and your calves are on the chair seat. Rest here a moment, then roll to your side and sit up slowly.

EFFECTS This pose lengthens and strengthens your spine, improving flexibility in your back.

†CAUTION Do not do this pose if you have neck or shoulder problems, if you have high blood pressure, if you are menstruating, or if you have a headache.

Chapter 9 *Relieving Headaches*

HAS ANYONE EVER SAID TO YOU, "GEE, I'D LOVE TO, BUT I HAVE A headache"? Did you believe her, or did you wonder whether she was just making up some lame excuse? After all, haven't you, at one time or another, played hooky from work or school and cited this well-worn malady as your alibi? Unfortunately, for the more than 40 million Americans who suffer from them, headaches are more than a feeble excuse to get out of social or professional responsibilities. They are painful, debilitating, and unrelenting. According to the National Headache Foundation's Web site, sick leave and medical expenses for headaches account for $50 billion in lost revenues to American corporations every year; 157 million sick days; and over $4 billion worth of over-the-counter (OTC) pain relievers—the majority of which don't work. For many women, yoga has presented blessed relief—not just from tension headaches, but from migraines and other vascular headaches as well.

Why do we get headaches anyway? And why do women get more than their fair share (70 percent of all migraine sufferers are women)? And how can yoga help?

CATEGORIZING THE PAIN

Almost as many theories exist to explain headaches as there are different types of pain. In fact, researchers can't even agree on how to categorize them. The National Headache Foundation describes headaches in three ways: tension type (with head, neck, and shoulder tightness), vascular (which includes migraines), and organic (evidence of brain tumors or infection). Robert Milne, M.D., offers 11 subcategories to choose from in his *Definitive Guide to Headaches*, including sinus, food sensitivity, eyestrain, trauma, cluster, and exertion headaches. Other physicians dismiss labels altogether, saying that all headaches are basically vascular—that is, they involve changes in the size of the arteries around your head. Still others say poor posture is the culprit for most headaches, even migraines. Most sufferers don't care what category their headache falls into, they just want to know what causes the pain and how to get rid of it.

In order to determine the cause and appropriate action, however, it's important to understand what's going on in your body. It appears that most of Robert Milne's subcategories can be classified as either tension (muscle contraction) headaches or vascular ones, both of which we'll talk about here. Organic headaches, the rarest and most serious type, are beyond the scope of this book. The good news about organic headaches is that they encompass only about 1 to 2 percent of all head pain. The bad news, of course, is that they can be deadly if not treated right away. Brain tumors, hemorrhages, brain infections like encephalitis and meningitis, and concussions are examples of organic headache causes. If your headache begins suddenly; doesn't go away after a few days; awakens you at night; gets worse when you exert yourself; or is accompanied by bleeding from your eyes, nose, or ears, you should seek medical advice immediately.

Tension Headaches

Everyone gets tension headaches from time to time; in fact, roughly 90 percent of all headaches can be classified this way. Tension headache pain can feel oppressive, as though a heavy weight were bearing down on you. Your head feels squeezed, your neck muscles clenched, and your temples sore. The pain is usually constant, not throbbing, and affects your forehead, temples, and the back of your head and neck. These headaches can last from a couple of hours to a few days. Most people get them occasionally and can often pinpoint the stressor that caused them; others suffer from chronic headaches that never truly go away.

If you get a headache no more than once or twice a week, you have episodic tension headaches; if they plague you more than fifteen times per month, you're a chronic sufferer. Also called muscular contraction headaches, this type of headache generally responds well to yoga, chiropractic or osteopathic manipulations, relaxation techniques, and even ultrasound therapy. If you are a chronic sufferer, seek out alternatives to over-the-counter remedies, which you should take only on occasion. An overdependency on analgesics, such as ibuprofen or acetaminophen, or any other pain relievers can result in rebound headaches (explained later in this chapter).

What causes tension headaches? Anything that puts stress on your body and makes it difficult for it to function optimally. The stress can come from emotional challenges such as repressed anger, resentment, fear, and sadness, as well as physical ones—including food allergies, insomnia, chemical sensitivities, poor posture, misalignment of your jaw or teeth, muscle tension or strain, constipation and other digestive disorders, or eyestrain.

H. R. Nagendra, M.D., the director of the Vivekananda Yoga Therapy and Research Foundation and coauthor of *Yoga for Common Ailments*, believes tension headaches are caused by constant overcontraction of the neck and head muscles. In a 1999 article by Ellen Serber published

Food Culprits

Food can be one of the most common triggers of headache pain. Although not all migraine sufferers react to the same food triggers, the following are some well-known culprits.

• Preservatives like MSG (found in lots of prepared foods, salad dressings, Chinese food, and lunch meats) and nitrates and nitrites (found in bacon, hot dogs, and other cured meats)

• Caffeine in coffee, soda, chocolate, and tea

• Aspartame, the artificial sweetener found in diet drinks and sugar-free foods

• Alcohol, including wine, beer, and hard liquor

• The amino acid tyramine (found in aged cheese, pickled herring, figs, dates, raisins, baked goods made with yeast, lima beans, lentils, peanuts, sunflower seeds, sesame seeds, and red wine

• Other amines such as histamines (in fish, cheese, and beer), phenylethylamine (in chocolate and cheese), and octopamine (in citrus fruits)

in *Yoga Journal*, Tomas Brofeldt, M.D., agrees. He says the vast majority of headaches comes from muscle fatigue, especially in the semispinalis capitis and temporalis (which he calls the headache muscles), found in the back of the neck. If you habitually walk or sit with your head forward, these muscles must work extra hard to hold you up. This extra work throws them into overdrive, exhausting them and making them spasm. The resultant pain may show up in the back of your neck or gravitate behind your eyes or across your forehead. You may also feel generally exhausted, spacey, and nauseated.

For most women, the first warning signs of a tension headache show up across the back of the neck or the tops of the shoulders. I hardly ever got headaches until I started spending most of my workday in front of a computer. Now I've discovered that as soon as the upper part of my neck starts to stiffen, I have to take a break and do some yoga. If I don't, my neck goes into spasms and I have a full-blown headache within the hour.

Tomas Brofeldt says that when you keep your muscles in a constant state of contraction, you reduce blood flow to your head. Your sympathetic nervous system senses a problem and rushes blood to the muscles. To help out, the blood vessels in the neighboring tissues constrict, using less blood. If the contracted muscles still don't respond, your body releases certain chemicals that forcibly dilate the blood vessels, allowing blood to flow to the area. This sudden dilation and blood flow bring with them sharp, piercing pain. At that point, your tension headache has become a migraine.

The Migraine Monster

Throbbing, blinding, unrelenting pain, usually along one side of your face, often coupled with nausea, vomiting, and sensitivity to light and sound, characterizes the common migraine. According to Robert Milne's research, this vascular headache affects nearly 18 percent of all women (and 6 percent of all men) in America. Classic migraines—or migraines with aura—bring on similar symptoms, but include warning signs about ten minutes to an hour before the headache strikes. Heather, a musician in her mid-twenties, knows a migraine is coming when her left eye begins to water and she starts feeling light-headed. Kathryn, a twenty-eight-year-old graphic artist, isn't lucky enough to get consistent warning signs, but knows that if she's under a lot of emotional stress and is bombarded with a lot of external noise—like the demolition work going on outside her office—a migraine is sure to surface.

According to information from the National Headache Foundation, before a migraine begins, the blood vessels in and around your skull begin to constrict. The pain comes when these same blood vessels suddenly dilate, pushing blood rapidly through the area and becoming swollen and inflamed. The throbbing you feel is caused by both the inflammation and the pressure on the walls of the vessels themselves.

Anything can trigger a migraine, depending on your sensitivities. For some it can be food, including chocolate; aged cheese; red meat; alcohol, particularly red wine and beer; or any processed foods containing monosodium glutamate (MSG), nitrites, or nitrates. Oral contraceptives bring on migraines for many women, as do fluctuations in estrogen. Other women get them during their period instead of cramps, while still others blame ovulation. If you let your blood sugar dip too low, you could wind up with a migraine. Environmental toxins, bright or flashing lights, loud noises, lack of sleep, and digestive disturbances can all contribute to the problem.

Dr. Karandikar, an Indian physician and yoga practitioner from Pune, India, took part in a symposium on headaches and yoga, which was translated by B. K. S. Iyengar in *Seventy Glorious Years of Yogacharya*. Karandikar believes that vascular headaches have a direct psychological connection. He argues that dilation and contraction of blood vessels depend on the weather outside and the emotions inside. He explains that your body's autonomic nervous system regulates the contraction and dilation of blood vessels, based on a fixed diameter for each vessel, without your knowledge or help. When it's hot outside, the blood vessels dilate to allow you to sweat and cool down. If you walk into an air-conditioned room, the blood vessels will contract. If your emotions interfere with this process, you risk overburdening your blood vessels and interfering with their natural size and shape (anger dilates them; tension constricts them).

There's some evidence to indicate that migraine sufferers inherit at least the tendency to get these headaches. Doctors say if both of your parents get migraines, there's a 75 percent chance you'll suffer, too. It's not unusual for women with migraines to suffer from anxiety and depression, both symptoms of an overwrought nervous system, according to a study from Yale University.

Anyone can get a migraine, although there appears to be such a thing as a migraine personality, according to literature from the National Headache Foundation. The typical migraine sufferer is a woman in her mid-twenties to mid-thirties, a high-strung, compulsive worker who is hypersensitive to the stimuli around her. She is extraordinarily organized, a perfectionist who values order and can be very self-critical. Highly emotional, she reacts quickly to stress and has a tendency to get angry easily, either blowing up at the slightest provocation or holding her emotions inside for fear of exploding. One theory suggests that her throbbing headaches come as she begins to relax the muscles in her head, neck, and shoulders. These muscles, as Robert Milne explains in his book, have been squeezing the arteries and restricting the blood flow. As they relax, blood circulation

Dietary Supplements

Dietary supplements and herbal medicines provide help for some sufferers. Here are a few remedies to try.

• Increase your daily intake of magnesium and calcium to keep serotonin levels normal.

• Increase your dosage of vitamin B$_2$ (riboflavin) to about 400 mg/day to decrease migraine pain.

• Use feverfew, willow bark, or valerian root, which are all good Western herbs to relieve tension headaches. For vascular headaches, try vervain, black cohosh, cayenne, elder flower, feverfew, garlic, ginkgo, rosemary, or lavender.

• Try ginger, cayenne, garlic, or fennel ayurvedic remedies for tension headaches associated with your menstrual cycle, insomnia, anxiety, or constipation. Headaches that come on because of anger, stress, or overwork and that produce stabbing pain (like migraines) may benefit from a liver cleanse using gotu kola and passion flower. David Frawley, an ayurvedic expert, recommends that you put sandalwood oil on your head; take slow, cooling walks in the moonlight; and inhale fragrances of rose and lotus.

increases suddenly and dramatically, putting intense pressure on the blood vessels and causing excruciating pain.

So, why do women get more migraines then men? Most experts believe our hormones play a role. Although fluctuations in serotonin, the neurotransmitter that regulates the size of the blood vessels, may be responsible for migraines in both men and women, it's quite possible that serotonin interacts in a unique way with estrogen to make women more susceptible to vascular pain. Nearly 70 percent of women who get migraines have them during or around their periods. But the mere presence of estrogen doesn't seem to cause migraines, because migraine sufferers generally have few if any attacks when they're pregnant (when their hormones are at an all-time high). As in the onset of puberty and during perimenopause, what causes symptoms appears to be the fluctuation of hormones, not the fact that you have them. Migraines during PMS may be more difficult to diagnose, because they are often associated with other symptoms such as bloating, fatigue, acne, joint pain, and emotional upheavals.

Some women find that menopause lessens the severity of their migraines; the end of menstruation can even mean the end of their head pain. Alas, other women get migraines for the first time in their lives after their menses stops. Most sufferers find hormone replacement therapy makes their headaches worse, but a small percentage actually find relief.

Other Types of Headaches

Cluster headaches are vascular, like migraines, but even more painful. Luckily, they don't last as long. Groups of them occur in close proximity over the course of a few days or weeks and are characterized by intense pain over one eye. For some reason, more men than women suffer from this type of pain.

Rebound headaches come on between migraines or chronic tension headaches. They're generally caused by taking too many over-the-counter pain relievers or drinking too much caffeine. Withdrawal headaches are similar—if you're a coffee drinker, you will recognize this as the pain you experience when you stop drinking coffee for a day or two.

Some chronic headache sufferers have discovered that one type of headache can trigger another. Muscle contractions in the neck and head, if chronic and severe enough, can bring on a migraine; and the anxiety migraine sufferers feel can precipitate a tension headache.

KEEPING TRACK OF YOUR HEADACHES

Because so many things can cause headaches to flare up, discovering what triggers yours could take some detective work. But make the effort, because it's pretty difficult to rid yourself of the pain if you don't know what provokes it in the first place. Start by keeping a headache diary. Write down what you eat, even on pain-free days.

Greta, a thirty-five-year-old yoga student, was surprised to discover that her symptoms don't always follow the trigger immediately. By keeping a daily food log, she was able to see that eating chocolate on Monday would invariably produce a migraine by Wednesday.

Lifestyle Changes That Can Make a Difference

You'll also probably need to address your personal and work lives to find emotional stressors. This list gives some general ideas of ways to counteract the most common of these stressors.

• Reduce your stress level. That may mean working fewer hours, taking time for yourself when you're not working, writing in a journal, exercising more, practicing deep breathing, or seeing a therapist.

• Engage the energy of the migraine itself. Graphic designer Kathryn says she goes inside herself and explores the pain. She lets go, cries, even holds her own hand. Her tears bring the pain, toxins, and everything that's stuck inside up and out, and she feels clear again.

• Stay in touch with your emotions. Christiane Northrup, M.D., says migraines could well be the end result of emotions that have been repressed for years. They are your body's way of getting your attention.

Note your daily activities and your emotions in your diary, too. Did you have an argument with someone? Did anything out of the ordinary happen at or going to and from work? Were you particularly worried, stressed out, angry, or sad? Did you have an allergic reaction to pollen, environmental pollution, or other toxins? Kathryn, the graphic designer, notices that her migraines come on when she feels bombarded by both external and internal stress. She can cope pretty well when she's feeling highly emotional; but if she must also contend with loud noises, an angry boss, or a lot of confusion, her body rebels and she gets a screaming headache. Kathryn, like Greta, also reacts to caffeine, but only just before her period or if she's been under a lot of stress at work.

HOW YOGA CAN HELP

Practicing yoga regularly can help relieve tension headaches and lessen the severity and frequency of migraines. Obviously, since so many headaches appear to be caused by stress, a daily yoga session provides the perfect prescription for releasing pent-up tension and preventing or relieving pain. But it goes deeper than that.

Yogis believe that asanas and pranayama (the physical poses and breathing exercises) balance your endocrine and nervous systems, two interrelated systems that take an active role in producing headache pain. B. K. S. Iyengar, one of the fathers of American yoga, says yoga "drains the brain system and gives rest for the pineal and pituitary glands." Since these glands—and the adrenal glands—play a significant role in how you deal with pain, temperature fluctuations, low blood pressure, stress, and danger, they must stay healthy and calm. Patricia says yoga poses like Bridge Pose (Setu Bandha Sarvangasana) give your pituitary gland and pineal body time to rest and rejuvenate, while supporting and strengthening your adrenals.

Yoga, particularly inversions, helps regulate the blood flow in and around your head. If you practice inversions before you get a headache, they may help stabilize the flow of blood to your head and relax your nervous system, preventing constriction and dilation of the blood vessels.

Through proper deep breathing exercises and restorative poses, yoga offers your body the state of complete rest it craves and needs to restore balance and stop your headache muscles from firing. The poses also help release tension in your shoulders, calm your stomach, and ease estrogen and serotonin fluctuations. Always end your practice with Corpse Pose (Savasana), which Patricia says is a form of conscious sleep that can help your body and mind achieve profound rest.

Standing poses focus on postural alignment, which is critical for relieving headaches. Forward extensions are also important to lengthen and release your neck muscles. According to most chiropractors, poor posture—particularly the forward head position and rounded shoulders so common among computer users—contributes to a large percentage of headache pain. Even wearing the wrong size shoe can cause misalignments in your spine, which in turn can pinch the nerves in your neck.

Patricia Says

Do not try Headstand (Sirsasana) or any other unsupported inversion when you have a headache. Doing them improperly could make your headache worse.

Geeta Iyengar says forward bends in particular can calm the chronic dilation of blood vessels and prevent blood from rushing toward your head too rapidly. Depending on your flexibility, you may benefit from Head-on-Knee Pose (Janu Sirsasana), Seated Forward Bend (Paschimottanasana), or even Easy Seated Forward Bend (Adho Mukha Sukhasana) with your head resting on a bolster or a padded chair. Patricia says these poses should completely relax you, and you should feel no strain anywhere. Remember, now is not the time to try to improve the technical aspects of your practice. It's the time to use yoga to improve your headache situation.

Following forward bends, Geeta advises lying in Half-Plough Pose (Ardha Halasana) with your upper thighs resting completely on a chair or low table. This relieves any tension in the front part of your head, but also controls the blood flow to your brain through the chin lock. If you include supported inversions in your headache practice (and this is especially true for migraine sufferers), Patricia says to begin with forward bends and end with forward bends so you don't increase blood flow too rapidly. Otherwise you may find your practice makes your headaches worse! The combination of forward bends and Half-Plough Pose regulates the hormonal release from your pituitary and adrenals.

Dr. Karandikar says that headaches can result from an outburst of stored-up energy in your body that upsets the balance of contraction and dilation in the blood vessels. Patricia suggests Bridge Pose (Setu Bandha Sarvangasana) and Shoulderstand (Sarvangasana) to distribute the stored, blocked energy evenly. Bridge Pose also helps open your chest and shoulders, which in turn releases those muscles and provides more oxygen and fresh blood to the area. These poses are excellent additions to a preventive practice.

Using an eyebag during restorative poses further relaxes your senses. If you can allow your eyes to sink back into their sockets, you can stop the chatter in your mind and quell the activity in your nervous system. Two of the best restorative poses for headaches are Legs-Up-the-Wall Pose (Viparita Karani) and Corpse Pose (Savasana). Practice these poses with an eyebag over your eyes and a ten-pound weight on your forehead to release your neck. Legs-Up-the-Wall Pose is especially helpful in relieving hypertensive headaches and those caused by intense emotions.

If your headache is in full swing, try the poses we've provided here, but play with the order in which you do them. According to Patricia, most people benefit from beginning with the forward bends, moving to Half-Plough Pose (Ardha Halasana), and ending with Legs-Up-the-Wall Pose (Viparita Karani) and Corpse Pose (Savasana). Others, like yoga teacher Elise Miller, find Half-Plough Pose the only thing that saves them from torture. Still others stay in Legs-Up-the-Wall Pose for half an hour before moving into Half-Plough Pose, then to a supported forward bend, and finishing in Corpse Pose. You may find you want to do only one or two of these poses when you have a headache. Do only those postures that help relieve your pain; avoid those that put any strain on your muscles.

Patricia Says

Gentle breathing brings deep relaxation. Do not practice pranayama—especially pranayama with breath retention such as Interval Breathing (Viloma) —when you have a headache. In fact, taking deep, powerful inhalations or holding your breath can make you feel even worse. But calming, rhythmic breathing that emphasizes the exhalation signals your body that it should relax and helps restore equilibrium to your mind.

A SEQUENCE FOR TENSION HEADACHES

1. Child's Pose (Adho Mukha Virasana)
2. Head-on-Knee Pose (Janu Sirsasana)
3. Seated Forward Bend
   (Paschimottanasana)
4. Standing Forward Bend (Uttanasana)
5. Half-Plough Pose (Ardha Halasana)
6. Reclining Bound Angle Pose
   (Supta Baddha Konasana)
7. Bridge Pose (Setu Bandha Sarvangasana)
8. Legs-Up-the-Wall Pose (Viparita Karani)
9. Corpse Pose (Savasana)

1. CHILD'S POSE (Adho Mukha Virasana) Kneel on the floor with a horizontal bolster in front of you. Spread your knees wide, bringing your toes together. Bend forward and stretch your arms and trunk so you can rest your forehead on the bolster. Fold your arms over your head and relax completely. Release your neck, jaw, and shoulders. Allow your eyes to close and breathe evenly. Stay in this pose for several minutes. To come out, sit up slowly, allowing your head to come up last.

EFFECTS This pose helps relieve headache pain, as well as tension in your neck and upper back. It also stretches and tones your spine and back.

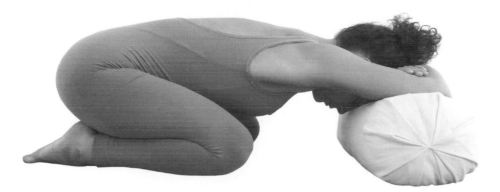

2. HEAD-ON-KNEE POSE (Janu Sirsasana) Sit on the floor with your legs stretched out in front of you, your feet between the front legs of a chair with a folded blanket on the seat. Bend your right knee to the side so it is at a 45-degree angle to your left leg and your right heel is near the right side of your groin. Push your right knee as far back as you comfortably can; keep your left leg straight.

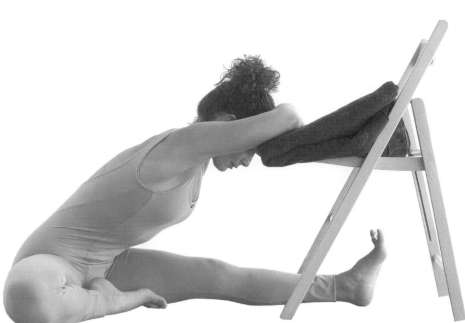

Turn your abdomen and chest so your sternum (breastbone) is in line with the center of your left leg. As you inhale, lift your trunk up from the base of your pelvis; as you exhale, bend forward to rest your head on the chair. (If you feel any strain in your neck, shoulders, or hamstrings, add more blankets to the chair seat. If your hips, back, or legs hurt, simply cross your legs in front of you and lean forward on your support.) Stay in this pose for at least 3 minutes, resting your head, the base of your skull, your eyes, and your brain. Inhale while coming up, straighten your right leg, and reverse sides by bending your left knee. Repeat pose twice on each side.

EFFECTS This pose helps relieve chronic tension headaches and migraines.

3. SEATED FORWARD BEND (Paschimottanasana) Sit on your mat (or on one or two folded blankets) with your legs stretched out in front of you. Place a bolster or folded blanket across your lower legs to support your head. Take a full, deep breath in, stretching up through your spine and lifting your sternum and head. As you exhale, bend forward and rest your forehead on your support. Clasp your hands around the balls of your feet, or cradle your head in your arms. (If you feel strain in your back or legs, add more height to your support or rest your head on a padded chair seat.) Do not allow your buttocks to lift off the floor (or blankets). Breathe softly, releasing any tension with a little-longer-than-normal exhalation. Stay in this pose for 2 to 5 minutes, using your breath to help you release forward without straining. Keep your abdomen soft and relaxed. Rise up slowly on an inhalation.

EFFECTS Try this pose to quiet your sympathetic nervous system and relieve headaches, eye strain, and tension in your throat.

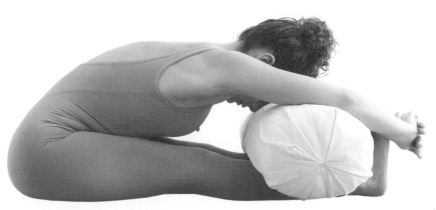

4. STANDING FORWARD BEND

(**Uttanasana**) Place a padded chair about 2 feet in front of you to support your head. Stand facing the chair with your feet together; distribute your weight evenly between the front of your feet and your heels. Tighten your knees by pulling up with your quadriceps (front thigh muscles). Raise your sternum and broaden your chest by rolling your shoulders back and drawing your shoulder blades in. Lift your abdomen and pull your tailbone in without pushing your thighs forward. Put your hands on your hips, and as you exhale extend your spine and bend forward from your hips. Rest your forehead on the chair seat and close your eyes. Fold your arms over your head or let them dangle by your sides. Relax the base of your skull, your neck, your shoulders, and your abdomen. Relax in this position for 1 to 2 minutes, or as long as you like. Release your arms and slowly stand up. Your head should come up last.

EFFECTS You can use this pose to help soothe your mind and quiet the fight-or-flight response.

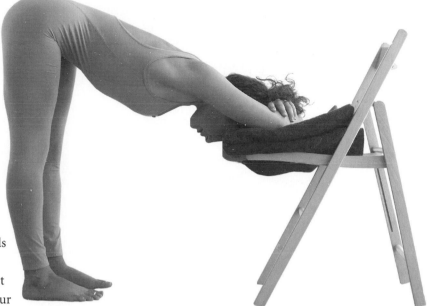

5. HALF-PLOUGH POSE† (**Ardha Halasana**) Place two folded blankets on the floor with the rounded edges near the legs of a chair. Lie on your back, legs outstretched, with your neck and shoulders on the blankets and your head beneath the chair seat. As you exhale, bend your knees and lift your buttocks and legs, so your thighs rest completely on the chair seat. (Pad the seat with blankets if you need more height for your legs to be parallel to the floor.) Move your chest in toward your chin. Bend your elbows at right angles to your body and relax with your palms up and your eyes closed. Rest here for as long as you like breathing deeply to relax and quiet your mind. To come out, place your hands on your back and slowly roll down, one vertebra at a time. Roll to one side and sit up.

EFFECTS This pose may help relieve tension-related or migraine headaches.

†CAUTION Do not do this pose if you suffer from neck or shoulder problems, or if you have your period.

6. RECLINING BOUND ANGLE POSE (Supta Baddha Konasana) Place a bolster vertically behind you and sit just in front of it with your knees bent and your sacrum touching the bolster's edge. Place a strap behind your back, at your sacrum; draw it forward over your hips, across your shins, and under your feet (see page xv). Put the soles of your feet together and let your knees and thighs fall to the sides. Cinch the strap securely under your feet. Lie back so your head and torso rest comfortably on the bolster and your buttocks and legs are on the floor. (If you feel any discomfort in your lower back, add some height to your support with a folded blanket or two. If you feel any strain in your neck, place a folded blanket under your head and neck. If you feel any muscle tension in your legs, roll two blankets vertically and place one under the top of each thigh.) Rest in this pose for as long as you like, breathing deeply.

To come out, draw your knees together, slip the strap off, and slowly roll to one side. Use your hands to push yourself up to a seated position.

EFFECTS This is an extremely relaxing pose that helps quiet your sympathetic nervous system, ease tension, and regulate your blood pressure.

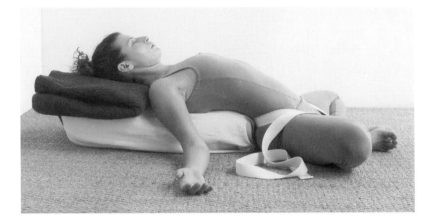

7. BRIDGE POSE (Setu Bandha Sarvangasana) Place one bolster horizontally against the wall and the other vertically, forming a T shape. Sit on the end of the vertical bolster that is closest to the wall. Keeping your knees bent, lie back over the bolster. Slide down until the end of the bolster is in the middle of your back and your shoulders just reach the floor. Rest your shoulders and head on the floor. Keeping your feet and heels together, stretch your legs toward the wall and put your heels on the horizontal bolster so your feet touch the wall. Your legs should be straight out in front of you. Rest your arms in any comfortable position. Close your eyes and relax completely, softening your abdomen and breathing deeply. Stay in this position for 5 to 10 minutes, or as long as you like.

To come out, bend your knees and slowly roll to one side. Using your hands, push yourself up to a seated position.

EFFECTS Try this pose to help relieve eyestrain, tension or migraine headaches, neck strain, and backaches.

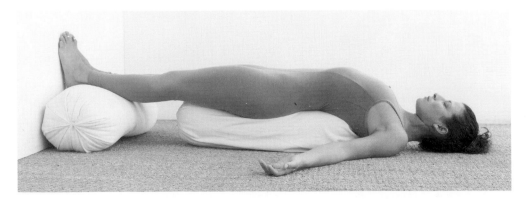

8. LEGS-UP-THE-WALL POSE†

(Viparita Karani) Place a bolster about 3 inches from the wall. Have a bolster draped with a 10-pound soft weight behind you. Sit on the bolster so your right hip and side are touching the wall. Using your hands to support you, lean back and swivel your body around, taking your right leg and then your left leg up the wall. Keep your buttocks against the wall or move them slightly away from the wall if you feel discomfort in your legs or back. Lie down so your lower back and ribs are supported by the bolster and your shoulders and head are on the floor. (If your neck is uncomfortable, put a folded towel or blanket under it.) Pull the second bolster close to you so it is just above your head; move just enough of the weight forward so it rests on your forehead (not on your eyes) and applies steady pressure. Extend through your legs and place your arms out at your sides, elbows bent and palms up. Rest in this position, eyes closed, for at least 5 minutes.

EFFECTS This pose helps alleviate nervous exhaustion, tension related headaches, and migraines.

†CAUTION Do not do this pose when you are menstruating.

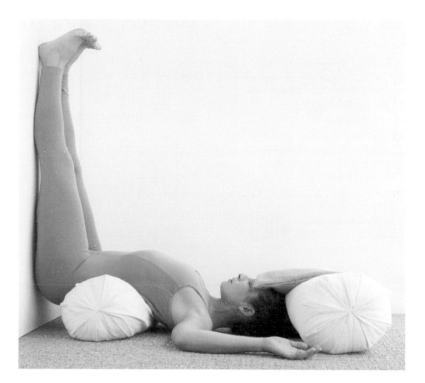

9. CORPSE POSE (Savasana) Position a padded chair at one end of two folded blankets (or a sticky mat, if you prefer) with the chair seat closest to you. Have a bolster and a 10-pound soft weight stacked at the other end. Lie on your back on the blankets and rest your calves on the chair. If your neck is uncomfortable, place a folded towel or blanket under it. Move the weight forward on the bolster just enough so it rests on your forehead (not on your eyes) and applies steady pressure. Place your arms at your sides, elbows relaxed, palms up. Breathe normally, with a slight emphasis on your exhalations. Let go of all tension and relax completely. Rest in this position, eyes closed, for at least 5 minutes.

EFFECTS This deeply relaxing pose helps alleviate nervous tension and balances your sympathetic nervous system.

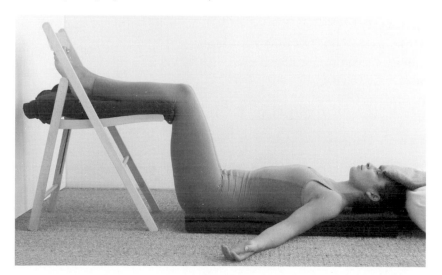

A SEQUENCE FOR MIGRAINE HEADACHES

1. Child's Pose (Adho Mukha Virasana)
2. Bridge Pose (Setu Bandha Sarvangasana)
3. Head-on-Knee Pose (Janu Sirsasana)
4. Seated Forward Bend
   (Paschimottanasana)
5. Standing Forward Bend (Uttanasana)
6. Half-Plough Pose (Ardha Halasana)
7. Head-on-Knee Pose (Janu Sirsasana)
8. Seated Forward Bend
   (Paschimottanasana)
9. Reclining Bound Angle Pose
   (Supta Baddha Konasana)
10. Legs-Up-the-Wall Pose (Viparita Karani)
11. Corpse Pose (Savasana)

1. CHILD'S POSE (Adho Mukha Virasana) Do Child's Pose as described on page 197. Remain in the pose for several minutes, as long as you are comfortable.

EFFECTS This restful pose helps soothe your nerves and calm your mind.

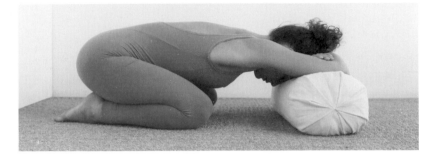

2. BRIDGE POSE (Setu Bandha Sarvangasana) Do Bridge Pose as described on page 200. Use an eyebag or eyewrap to cover your eyes and help keep out any external distractions.

EFFECTS Try this pose to help relieve eyestrain, tension or migraine headaches, neck strain, and backaches.

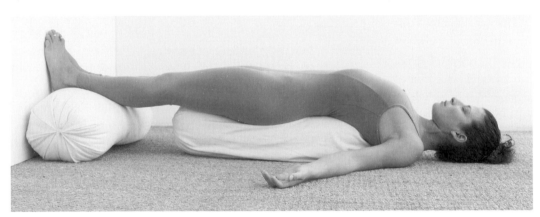

3. HEAD-ON-KNEE POSE† (Janu Sirsasana) Do Head-on-Knee Pose as described on page 198, using a padded chair for support. Stay in this pose for 30 seconds to 2 minutes.

EFFECTS This pose helps relieve chronic tension headaches and migraines.

†CAUTION Do not do this pose if you have diarrhea or feel nauseous.

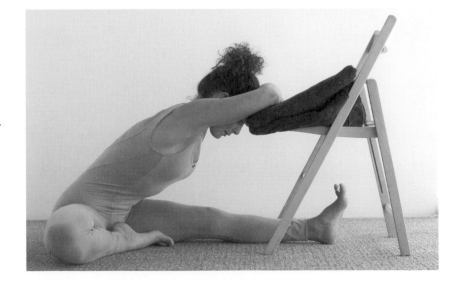

4. SEATED FORWARD BEND†

(Paschimottanasana) Do Seated Forward Bend as described on page 198, placing a bolster across your shins to support your head. (If you feel strain in your back or hamstrings, add more height to your support or rest your head on a padded chair seat as in Head-on-Knee Pose on page 198). Stay in this pose for 2 to 5 minutes. Your body should feel completely relaxed.

EFFECTS This pose can be beneficial for quieting your sympathetic nervous system and relieving headaches, eyestrain, and tension in your throat. It promotes a sense of safety and peace.

†CAUTION Do not do this pose if you have diarrhea.

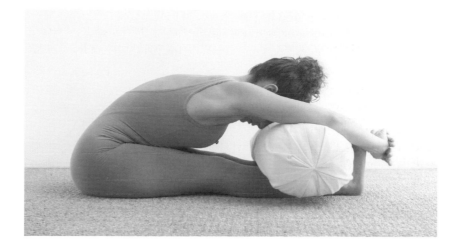

5. STANDING FORWARD BEND

(Uttanasana) Do Standing Forward Bend as described on page 199. If you feel tension anywhere—especially in the backs of your legs, your lower back, or your shoulders—add more support on the chair. Stay in the pose for about 1 minute, or as long as you're comfortable. To come out of the pose, use your hands to push yourself up from the chair and slowly stand up. Your head should come up last.

EFFECTS This pose helps soothes your mind and sympathetic nervous system, quieting the fight-or-flight response and easing feelings of stress. It's beneficial for relieving tension or migraine headaches.

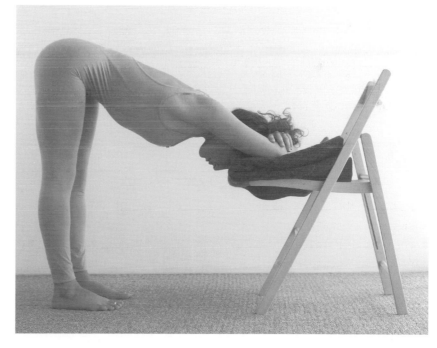

6. HALF-PLOUGH POSE† **(Ardha Halasana)** Do Half-Plough Pose as described on page 199. Stay in the posture for 2 to 3 minutes, breathing normally, with a slight emphasis on the exhalation.

EFFECTS This pose helps reduce anxiety and irritability.

†CAUTION Do not do this pose if you suffer from neck or shoulder problems, or if you have your period.

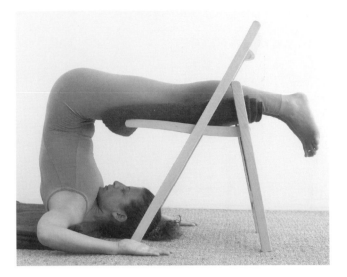

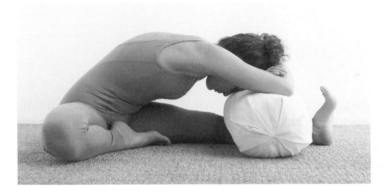

7. HEAD-ON-KNEE POSE† **(Janu Sirsasana)** Repeat Head-on-Knee Pose (see page 198) with your head completely relaxed on either a bolster (or two) or a chair, depending on your flexibility. Stay in the pose for about 1 minute, breathing normally.

†CAUTION Do not do this pose if you have diarrhea.

8. SEATED FORWARD BEND† **(Paschimottanasana)** Repeat Seated Forward Bend (see page 198). Remain in the pose for about a minute or two, breathing normally.

†CAUTION Do not do this pose if you have diarrhea.

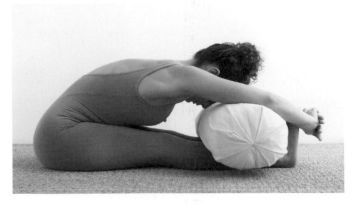

9. RECLINING BOUND ANGLE POSE (Supta Baddha Konasana) Do Reclining Bound Angle Pose as described on page 200. Rest in the pose for as long as you like and breathe normally, gently emphasizing your exhalations.

EFFECTS This extremely relaxing pose helps quiet your sympathetic nervous system and regulate your blood pressure.

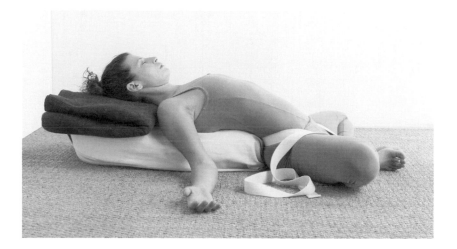

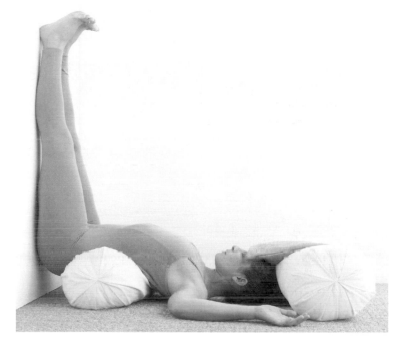

10. LEGS-UP-THE-WALL POSE† (Viparita Karani) Do Legs-Up-the-Wall Pose as described on page 201. Rest in the pose, eyes closed, for at least 5 minutes.

EFFECTS Try this pose to ease nervous exhaustion and all types of headaches.

†CAUTION Do not do this pose when you are menstruating.

11. CORPSE POSE (Savasana) Do Corpse Pose as described on page 201. Rest in this position, eyes closed, for at least 5 minutes.

EFFECTS This form of Corpse Pose blocks out all distractions and allows you to relax deeply. It is beneficial for all types of headache pain.

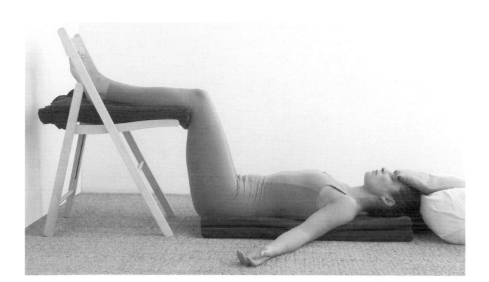

PART FOUR

Speaking the Truth

Introduction

For many women, the time from their late forties to their late fifties is not unlike going through puberty all over again. It is a time of great fluctuation, heralding the death of what is comfortable and the birth of uncertainty (just like when you were thirteen years old), followed by a resurgence of creativity and comfort. In fact, there are really two or three times in a woman's life when she feels her whole world is being turned upside down and presented anew: puberty, pregnancy, and menopause. All this fluctuation reminds me of what I learned in a seventh-grade science project, that nothing changes without a catalyst. In fact, most people will agree that what got them to change their behavior, their jobs, or their relationships was dissatisfaction, anxiety, anger, or frustration, in other words, some form of emotional heat that pushed them to make decisions.

And so it seems for the body. In order to effect a change (chemical, emotional, spiritual), a woman's hormones must heat up, causing great agitation and discomfort. All of a sudden her normal routine doesn't work anymore. She can't sleep the way she used to; she gets angry at things she once tolerated; her body shape is changing and she hates it; she craves the attention of her peers, her husband, her lover, and yet she wants to be left alone. When everything calms down, the body gives birth to something new and stronger—a young woman capable of creating life (postpuberty), a mother capable of nurturing life (postpartum), or a wise woman capable of guiding life all around her (postmenopause). If women honor themselves during these times and take care of one another, then each metamorphosis gives rise to a new, more powerful voice.

Besides typical perimenopausal complaints like hot flashes, fatigue, insomnia, irritability, and vaginal dryness, the most common disorders women shared with us were depression, anxiety, and digestive complaints. It's not surprising, given society's obsession with young, thin, beautiful women who are smart (but not too vocal), agreeable, sexy, and loving, that women whose bodies are softening and widening, who can no longer bear children, and who increasingly feel less agreeable and more critical, would succumb to depression. Furthermore, mourning the end of an era is a natural stepping-stone toward the next. Women at this age bid a tearful farewell to their ability to bear children but look toward nurturing in a much larger context.

A woman's yoga practice during this time has much to offer. Physiologically, yoga can keep your endocrine system in balance (or bring it into balance, if it is stressed). The adrenal glands must now produce the small amount of estrogen the body needs to function properly, but if they are depleted through stress, smoking, poor eating habits, or compromised immunity, they can't do their job. A variety of yoga poses, most specifically forward bends, twists, and backbends, work to pacify and then activate the adrenals. Yoga also helps you overcome the fatigue, insomnia, anxiety, and hot flashes that often characterize perimenopause. Patricia, who teaches regular workshops on menopause and depression, tells her students that through daily practice they can lift their spirits, regain valuable energy, and equally important, get the time they need for contemplation, so they can make thoughtful, careful choices.

Yoga can help a woman get to know her body again and feel comfortable with the way she looks, the way she moves, and how she's feeling. This time of life, just like puberty, challenges a woman to accept her body and its changing shape. She can read all the books and articles she wants, telling her that women naturally gain weight as they get older, reminding her that bigger, softer bellies and breasts are not unusual, in fact they're healthy and beautiful. But if she's heard all her life that thin is desirable, she may have a hard time embracing her new look. Patricia says yoga is extremely beneficial in helping women celebrate their softer, more sensuous appearance.

Patricia stresses again and again the importance of women reaching out to each other, women in community, women practicing yoga. Women need to talk together, share their fears, discomforts, and joys. Women must empower one another, she reminds us all, mentor and support one another with a clarity of intent and a purity of heart. By joining together, women create a collective voice that is more beautiful, more powerful, one that has the ability to change the world. You can fulfill such promise only by starting with yourself. Once you are "self-full, soul-full," as Borysenko says, then you can move toward compassionate action. A commitment to practicing yoga can help you develop the confidence and the passion you need to stand up for what you think is right. Yoga won't get rid of all that hormonal heat, nor do I think it should; but it will help you direct it in a positive, passionate, and effective way.

Chapter 10 Working with Depression

A COUPLE OF YEARS AGO, I WENT TO VISIT MY FRIEND KENDRA, who had just turned forty-three. I happened to be in her neighborhood, hadn't seen her in a long time, and on a whim, thought I would take her out for a cup of tea. When I showed up at her house, I found her sitting on her living room floor sobbing. Her Labrador retriever lay next to her, doing his best to cheer her up. I thought someone had died. "No," she assured me, "everyone is alive. It's just this huge funk I'm in. I can't shake it and I don't know what's causing it." Lots of women get depressed, I thought, but not Kendra. After all, she had remarried about a year before—happily, too. She had what I thought was a thriving business as a freelance seamstress, and her daughter had just gone off to the school of her dreams. What was there to be unhappy about? "You're right," she cried. "I should be happy. So, why aren't I?" She went on to explain that she suddenly felt overwhelmed by so many things she used to take in stride. And she lamented that she was forty-three but still doing the same job she had done since she was twenty-three. What she really wanted to do was write a novel, but she had no energy or confidence to start. What if she were too old to start anything new? On top of it all, her only daughter had left home, her husband worked long hours, and she didn't feel needed. Her low spirits and even lower sense of self-worth had affected her ability to get her work done, and as a result, her workload had diminished.

Kendra struggled with her depression for another year before things got better. During that time her emotional state worsened; she could barely function and admitted she didn't care "two hoots about myself— or anybody else, for that matter." Her doctor prescribed Paxil, an antidepressant. It helped her sleep, but she hated the way it made her feel during the day—sluggish, apathetic, and "puffy." Finally, at the insistence of several friends, Kendra agreed to look into alternative therapies. Luckily, her depression responded well to these noninvasive means. She went to a nutritionist, who helped her adjust her diet and explained that although the cookies, breads, and chocolates Kendra was consuming gave her short-term relief from her depression, they actually exacerbated it in the long run. Kendra also worked with a therapist who not only encouraged her to talk, but also insisted that she get outside, walk her dog, get some exercise. And I took her to her first yoga class. She loved it and started going several times a week. She found her practice profoundly nourishing and relaxing. "As I started to care about myself in a deep and gentle way, my health problems began to disappear, and the fog finally lifted," she confided not long ago.

Kendra's condition is far from unusual. In fact, the U.S. Center for Mental Health Services says that at least 5 percent of American adults suffer from depression every year. Other researchers believe it's more like 20 percent. In *Women's Bodies, Women's Wisdom*, Christiane Northrup, M.D., estimates that at least a quarter of all women in the United States battle serious depression sometime in their lives. How can you tell whether you're one of the 25 percent or just feel blue?

HOW BLUE IS BLUE?

Just because you experience occasional PMS, rage and cry at the end of a long-term relationship, or occasionally feel overwhelmed and paralyzed by the sheer magnitude of your responsibilities, it doesn't mean you're clinically depressed. These small bouts of depression may simply be your body's (and your mind's) way of getting you to pay attention to what's going on and make some changes. Apparently you haven't been listening, and now it's time to turn up the volume.

Some therapists define depression as unexpressed anger or rage turned inward. Others say depression is the result of unhealed feelings buried deep within us, years of broken and bruised emotions that not only damage our psyches but make us sick. Marion Woodman, a Jungian psychotherapist and prolific author, says depression arises when we become disconnected from our dreams and our souls. Joel Robertson, coauthor of *Natural Prozac*, sees depression as "an imbalance in our approach to life, an imbalance that gives rise to chemical changes in the brain and the central nervous system." The National Institute of Mental Health (NIMH) describes clinical depression as a sense of profound hopelessness and helplessness; the feeling that life is horrible and it will never get any better. All experts agree that if you are constantly plagued by thoughts of suicide and have become incapacitated by your depression, you need to seek medical advice as soon as possible.

Most women think of depression as incapacitating: The world presses down on them; there's a weight on their chest; their breathing feels shallow; they've lost the ability or desire to do anything. This is one type of depression (chronic depression); it grips your entire being and leaves you feeling as empty as a deflated balloon. But thousands of women suffer from another, equally insidious type of depression that is masked by high levels of anxiety and is thus called anxiety-driven depression. The high-stress lifestyle these women insist on keeps them from experiencing the feelings beneath their tension and fear; it keeps them from recognizing what's really going on inside. They feel anxious all the time and find themselves easily agitated, quick to anger, and very impatient. Some suffer from menstrual irregularities, digestive disorders, and even chest pains.

MESSENGERS OF GLAD (OR SAD) TIDINGS

The brain and the endocrine, nervous, and immune systems all contribute to emotional well-being. They communicate on a cellular level through a complex system of messengers and receptors. Candace B. Pert, a pioneer in the relatively new field of biophysics called psychoneuro-immunology (PNI) describes this process in her groundbreaking book *Molecules of Emotion: Why You Feel the Way You Feel.* She explains that when you have a thought or emotion, your brain releases neuropeptides, which translate that thought or feeling into a physical state. The neuropeptides circulate throughout your body, looking for cells whose receptors match the messenger (kind of like two pieces of a jigsaw puzzle). When they find a match (for example, in your intestines, hypothalamus, pituitary gland, or heart), the neuropeptides grab on to the receptors and deposit their information. The receptors push that information—the thought or emotion you've just had—farther into the cell, transforming it dramatically. These cellular changes deeply affect your physiology, your behavior, and even your moods.

Pert explains that your brain also has neurotransmitters working for it, shepherding information to and from brain cells. Each neurotransmitter takes information from one neuron (or brain cell), moves it, and binds it to the receptor of another neuron, which, upon receiving the information, makes physiological changes. Researchers believe that this movement from one neuron to another influences emotional as well as physical responses. If a neuron gives off too many neurotransmitters, the other cell uses what it needs and the excess gets reabsorbed by a "reuptake mechanism" in the original neuron. If you have enough neurotransmitters traveling between your cells, you feel healthy, happy, and energized. If you lack the right balance—either too few or too many—you may suffer from depression or anxiety attacks.

The three most important neurotransmitters governing your emotional health are serotonin, dopamine, and its derivative norepinephrine. Sufficient serotonin boosts your sense of well-being, self-esteem, calm, and security. You have no trouble sleeping soundly, concentrating, or digesting your food easily. Norepinephrine and dopamine together give you strength, vitality, and a sense of power. You feel alert, feel in command of any situation, and can work quickly and efficiently. These two neurotransmitters join with adrenaline to produce the fight-or-flight response that helps you through emergency situations.

If your body produces too little serotonin (or it gets reabsorbed too quickly), you feel depressed and insecure and suffer from an overall "What's the use?" attitude. You may lose interest in eating and begin to lose weight or, conversely, eat compulsively and gain too much. Your sexual appetite plummets, and you can't concentrate. You feel confused and basically worthless. (Hardly anyone has serotonin levels that are too high.)

According to Joel Robertson, an imbalance in dopamine/norepinephrine tends to affect the psyche and give rise to either suicidal tendencies or violent behavior. If dopamine and norepinephrine levels soar too high, you have too much nervous energy and may feel overly anxious, fearful, and aggressive. You could have trouble falling and staying asleep, and your sexual appetite increases dramatically. If the levels plummet, you may experience depression ranging from mild to severe.

WHAT ABOUT MEDICATION?

If the pharmaceutical companies had their way, everyone complaining about dark, relentless moods would have a prescription for any of a number of antidepressants available today.

Antidepressants work in a very logical way. If the serotonin that resides in the pathways between brain cells increases your feelings of well-being and self-esteem, then why not find a way to keep more of it there longer so you feel better? Researchers created drugs that could do just that. They called these drugs selective serotonin reuptake inhibitors (SSRIs); we know them by their brand names, such as Prozac, Zoloft, and Paxil. As their generic name implies, they prevent reabsorption of serotonin by the brain cells that produce it.

Another group of antidepressants—the tricyclics (Triavil, Elavil, and Doxepin are some examples)—not only raise your serotonin level, but increase the amount of time dopamine and norepinephrine stay in your system. This theoretically creates feelings of well-being and self-esteem, while increasing energy, a sense of control, and assertiveness. Antipsychotic drugs like Thorazine and Haldol work like SSRIs except that they prevent dopamine and norepinephrine from being reabsorbed too quickly.

It all sounds good on paper, but does it work? According to a meta-analysis (a comprehensive look at various studies and clinical trials) conducted by R. P. Greenberg and published in the *Journal of Nervous and Mental Diseases* (1994), Prozac had only a moderate effect on depression. However, SSRIs, tricyclics, and antipsychotics produce an impressive list of side effects severe enough to spur many women to look for alternatives. These side effects include digestive disorders, insomnia, anxiety, headaches, dry mouth, heart palpitations, an inability to concentrate, fatigue, loss of strength, dizziness, and an inability to achieve orgasm.

SUGGESTIONS TO ALLEVIATE DEPRESSION

Although I'm not suggesting that prescription antidepressants are never an option, it may be wise to think of them as a last resort and focus on gentler alternatives first. Certainly, if you currently take Prozac or another antidepressant, don't stop taking it without consulting your health practitioner. You can, however, employ many of the alternatives described in this section as adjuncts to your medication. After all, although antidepressants may temporarily boost your feel-good neurotransmitters, they never get to the root of the problem; they never fix what made you depressed in the first place. Nor do antidepressants correct what causes too little serotonin—or too much norepinephrine—in the system.

Pay Attention to Your Body

In *Women's Bodies, Women's Wisdom*, Christiane Northrup writes that emotions "help us participate fully in our own lives." Sometimes, if

Patricia Says

Restorative yoga poses offer the best way to be fully present in the moment, to allow your body and your emotions to express themselves. With no place to go, nothing to prove, and nobody to impress, you can completely let go. For those who like to retreat, Child's Pose with a bolster works well. Other women find they feel closed in when they do forward bends and prefer fully supported reclining poses like Reclining Bound Angle Pose (Supta Baddha Konasana) or inversions like Legs-Up-the-Wall Pose (Viparita Karani). If you're particularly anxious, using a yoga audiotape with instructions or playing soft music can help you stay focused. Expanding Life Force Energy Breathing (Ujjayi Pranayama) can help stabilize your energy as you rest in the poses.

Yoga can also show you that what you do with your body has a profound impact on your emotions. Standing tall with dignity, opening and broadening your chest, and walking confidently announce to the world—and, most important to your own mind—that you are grounded, happy, and in tune with your surroundings.

you don't pay attention to your emotions, your body and mind have to shout. Crying jags, crippling fatigue, and panic attacks are all ways your body tells you to take a look at what's really going on. Don't be so quick to repress those feelings or medicate those emotions. Stay with them; hear what they have to say; write them down in your journal. Allow your feelings to come up and out of you.

Northrup believes crying is one of the ways you can rid your body of toxins. She says it helps you "move energy around [your] body and sometimes rechannel it or understand it in a different way." Tears, in this case, are the messengers that carry toxins out of the cells and out of your body. Kathryn, a graphic designer who suffers from acute migraine headaches, says weeping helps her stay present with her feelings; it allows her to participate fully in her own healing process and not ignore feelings or stuff them away where they can do more damage. Jungian analyst Marion Woodman calls tears "the connection to our souls." Give your soul some time each day: meditate, practice yoga, write down your dreams—which Woodman says "are the bridge between your body and your soul."

Feelings of depression could be your body and mind's way of pouting, of telling you they feel left out, sad, and neglected. You've drifted too far from your center, your passions. Treat yourself with loving kindness, the same way you would care for a friend who is suffering. Ask yourself what you need to feel better; be patient and gentle.

Psychoneuroimmunology experts, such as Candace Pert, teach that your body and mind have the tools they need to heal themselves. Antidepressants (pharmaceutical, food-based, or herbal) work because your body manufactures similar chemicals that it needs to stay healthy. These chemicals are created as a physiological response to your thoughts, feelings, behaviors, and actions.

Have Your Thyroid Checked

Hypothyroidism (an underactive thyroid gland) can often mimic depression. Not only does this condition slow down the functioning of your thyroid gland, it causes many other systems in your body to slack off. For example, many hypothyroidic women suffer from constipation, difficult periods, low blood pressure, and fatigue. They tend to "hold on" to their weight, feel spacey, and suffer from low-grade depression. Even postpartum depression could be a sign of a skewed thyroid or parathyroid gland.

One simple way of checking thyroid function is to monitor your basal temperature for three or four days. Place a thermometer under your armpit before you get out of bed in the morning. Keep it there for ten minutes; if your temperature is lower than normal (97.7°F or below), talk to your doctor. Your thyroid might be sluggish.

Yoga practitioners claim that yoga works well to regulate the thyroid gland. The best poses, like Shoulderstand (Sarvangasana) and Plough Pose (Halasana), employ a chin lock that presses your chin down toward your chest. This action compresses and massages the thyroid and parathyroid glands, which first calms and then energizes them. By isolating the glands in this way, the pose squeezes out toxins and stagnant blood; as you release the pose, fresh oxygenated blood can circulate more freely in and around the area, activating the glands. Stay in either pose for eight to ten minutes to get the full effect. Backbend poses also stimulate both glands.

Monitor Your Blood Sugar

Some studies suggest that low blood sugar may contribute to low energy, fatigue, and high levels of anxiety or agitation. One reason is that insulin, which is produced by the pancreas, not only helps your body control glucose or blood sugar but also transports tryptophan to your brain. Tryptophan is an amino acid your brain needs to manufacture serotonin, the neurotransmitter responsible for your feelings of well-being and calm. If your brain doesn't get enough tryptophan, it demands more sugar, which will (at least temporarily) elevate your insulin levels. That, in turn, increases the amount of tryptophan reaching your brain, which then causes your serotonin levels to soar. Generally someone with depression caused by low blood sugar will feel drastic changes in mood—from euphoria to dark anger to overwhelming fatigue.

Yoga works well to help balance pancreatic function. Twisting postures like Spinal Twist Pose (Marichyasana III) and Seated Forward Bend (Paschimottanasana) squeeze and massage the pancreas. Backbends like Bridge Pose (Setu Bandha Sarvangasana) and Inverted Staff Pose (Viparita Dandasana) rinse the pancreas with blood, which may help it function better and prevent atrophy.

Review Your Diet

What you eat—or don't eat—could be affecting your moods. First, rule out any food allergies. Some people find that a sensitivity to wheat, sugar, dairy products, aspartame (sugar substitute), caffeine, or overprocessed or pesticide-laden foods contributes to their depression.

Elson Haas, M.D., director of the Preventive Medical Center in San Rafael, California, recommends a cleansing program of steamed vegetables, oils, and whole grains in his book *A Diet for All Seasons.* Although carbohydrates boost serotonin levels, Haas warns against eating the wrong kind. Whole grains and whole-grain flour products increase serotonin slowly, because they release their sugars gradually into the bloodstream. As a result, they have a longer-lasting effect than simple carbohydrates (such as refined sugar and white flour products).

Protein-rich foods increase levels of dopamine and norepinephrine (arousal chemicals), so go easy on meats if you are prone to anxiety-driven depression. Also, cut back on (or give up) caffeinated beverages, eliminate white sugar and alcohol from your diet, and stop smoking.

Consider Supplements

Increase your intake of essential fatty acids (EFAs) like flaxseed or borage oil. Remember that information is being shared among your body's cells. For that material to flow smoothly from one place to another, your body needs fat to keep things fluid. Vitamins C, B_1, B_6, and B_{12} help convert EFAs into the essential hormones you need to stay healthy. In a seminar she gave at the International Herbalists Symposium in Massachusetts in June 1998, Tierona Low Dog, M.D., a herbalist and medical doctor practicing in New Mexico, suggested taking vitamin B_{12} in nasal drops or in liquid form under the tongue; both methods work better than pills.

Your liver rids your body of excess toxins and hormones that contribute to depression. You can strengthen your liver by taking milk thistle, dandelion root, or turmeric in pill (powdered) form or tincture (liquid).

Try Alternative Antidepressants

St. John's Wort is the alternative drug of choice for women suffering from mild to moderate depression. It acts like an SSRI by preventing the reuptake of serotonin, but it does this much more gently than Prozac or other pharmaceuticals. Check with your holistic health care practitioner to find a dosage that works for you. If you already take a synthetic antidepressant, check with your physician before you try St. John's Wort or any other herbal alternative.

If you suffer from debilitating anxiety, have trouble shutting your mind down at the end of the day, and experience muscle pain and tension, a combination of valerian, black cohosh, and cramp bark can sometimes help. Again, check with your health care practitioner for dosage.

Get the Right Amount of Sleep

It's imperative for women with anxiety-driven depression to get enough sleep. Without adequate rest, Joel Robertson warns, your body has no time to heal itself and your immune system weakens. Marion Woodman says the psyche restores itself through a woman's dreams; if you don't sleep, you get disconnected from your unconscious, your core, which can bring on depression. Restorative yoga poses, meditation, and relaxing aromatherapy baths generally help if you suffer from anxious insomnia, but not before you've treated yourself to something more energizing like vigorous exercise or more strenuous yoga poses to burn off the excess agitation.

Patricia Says

If you suffer from chronic depression, doing yoga with these suggestions in mind may help:

• Keep your eyes open throughout the poses, so you engage your senses and don't drop back into the dark pool of your emotions.

• Concentrate on each inhalation, the bringer of life force, to lift feelings of despondency.

• Be sensitive to mind-body reactions. If you start to feel anxious or experience strain, pause or stop and just relax with focused exhalations to reduce the feeling.

• If you come face-to-face with difficult thoughts or feelings, direct your mind as well as your body to balance negative thoughts with positive ones.

• Remember to take an action, no matter how small; do anything as long as you do something.

• From space comes quiet; within the silence, look to your heart to find peace.

Conversely, sleeping all day because you feel so sad you want to escape from life also poses a health problem. This type of depression is caused by low serotonin and very low dopamine and norepinephrine levels. Although sleep does increase serotonin (but only while you are sleeping), it diminishes the other two neurotransmitters, which are needed for any activity that involves your neuromuscular system. If you want to get out of the doldrums, reduce the number of hours you sleep every day so you gradually increase your dopamine and norepinephrine.

Make Time for Vigorous Exercise

It's hard to stay blue when you're exercising. First of all, physical activity takes your mind off your troubles, and it also changes your brain chemistry fairly rapidly. A rousing game of tennis, a brisk walk, or a moderate jog can raise serotonin levels, increase your body's endorphins (natural pain relievers), and clear out toxins. Because dopamine and norepinephrine respond to changes in respiration, muscle activity, and heart rate, vigorous exercise raises the levels of these neurochemicals dramatically. Once you stop exercising, dopamine and norepinephrine burn off, serotonin levels rise, and you feel relaxed and pleased with yourself. Women suffering from either type of depression benefit from working out.

THE PAIN OF DEPRESSION

You can take all the St. John's Wort (or Prozac) you want, eat better, and increase your intake of vitamins and herbal supplements, but eventually you'll have to confront the underlying pain that created your depression in the first place. In a May 1999 talk at Kripalu Yoga Center, Marion Woodman said that women often get ill when a conflict too unbearable to face remains in the body. She explained that the psyche tries to protect you by burying the pain deep inside; your body then holds on to that pain as long as possible. Finally, it becomes too difficult to bear and you break down. Don't wait until you get to this point to seek help from a qualified therapist or a trusted friend.

HOW YOGA CAN HELP

The gift yoga brings to someone who's depressed is not just physical— yoga soothes the mind and spirit as well. Obviously, it's impossible to separate the physiological benefits from the emotional and spiritual ones. We've already discussed how thoughts affect feelings which, in turn, affect physiology. In yoga, the reverse is also true. For example, Inverted Staff Pose (Viparita Dandasana) is a backbending chest opener. The mere act of lifting your chest can elevate your emotions and lead your mind to a clearer state. It creates space for your breath to move more freely, and freer breath brings lighter feelings. Backbends further release any blockage in and around your heart that could be contributing to your rounded shoulders and sunken chest.

Seated forward bends, on the other hand, can quiet a nervous system that goes into overdrive when you become anxious, fearful, or nervous. Inversions allow oxygenated blood to circulate more freely, which soothes and then energizes the glands in and around your head and throat. Standing poses can also elevate your mood, making you feel stronger and more capable (literally, "standing on your own two feet").

Corpse Pose (Savasana) and other restorative poses provide conscious rest to your sympathetic nervous system—and your whole body—so healing can take place. They take you to a place of repose, to a state of complete relaxation, so your brain can restore and rebalance its neurotransmitters. They also give you an opportunity to look deeper inside and discover where the tensions are or where the pain resides, and they send the gift of breath to help push some of the tension and pain out.

Yoga can teach you to pay attention to what's going on in your body, to feel your emotions, and to let go. If you've ever struggled to master a difficult pose, you know that mastery doesn't come until you stop working so hard. Yoga also reminds you that nothing is permanent, that you are not your feelings. By staying present in a pose, especially one that challenges you at first, you learn that you can be uncomfortable, even unhappy, and still be all right. You come to see that what was impossible last week is doable today.

Working with your breath in the physical poses and during breathing (pranayama) practice can be a wonderful aid. Patricia says that deep, healing inhalations lift your spirits and long, slow exhalations soothe your nerves. Don't be surprised if feelings of sadness, anger, or even fear well up inside you during your practice. Acknowledge them and then let them go. They've been waiting to get out for a long time. A Tibetan friend of mine, composer and didgeridoo player Nawang Khechog, once described the breath as the bridge between the body and the mind, the link that brings the body, mind, and spirit together.

The sequences we've provided here are for two different types of depression: chronic depression and depression coupled with anxiety. You'll notice that the sequence for chronic depression gradually moves from quiet, chest-opening poses to more active, energizing postures. The sequence for anxiety-driven depression reverses the order, starting with more active poses to get rid of excess nervous energy, then moving to restorative poses to calm you.

Regardless of which sequence you choose, don't be afraid to explore all the postures—some may work better than others. If your

Patricia Says

Besides the physiological benefits of a consistent yoga practice, incorporating a full-range of poses can help you emotionally in the following ways:

• Standing poses help ground you, literally and figuratively, connecting you to the Earth through your legs. They are confidence builders, which not only energize you but focus that energy.

• Backbends give you a feeling of hope as they invigorate you and open your chest.

• Inversions help balance your endocrine system and even out your emotions—by turning everything upside down, they help you get "unstuck."

depression brings paralyzing fatigue, the standing poses might prove too taxing; just skip them, or do them with your back against the wall. Some days you may feel like staying in Reclining Bound Angle Pose (Supta Baddha Konasana) for twenty minutes; other days going from Plough Pose (Halasana) to Seated Forward Bend (Paschimottanasana) and back again several times may be the only thing that works.

The PMS sequence in chapter 5 works well for depression resulting from your period or perimenopause. Patricia says forward bends often work better for hormone-based depression than they do for chronic depression. Bending forward when you feel grief or deep despair can heighten the sense of loss and give you the feeling that everything is closing in on you. Instead you need to open your chest, bathe your body in the healing power of deep inhalations, and reenergize yourself.

A SEQUENCE FOR CHRONIC DEPRESSION

1. Cross Bolsters Pose or Reclining Easy Seated Pose (Supta Sukhasana)
2. Downward-Facing Dog Pose (Adho Mukha Svanasana)
3. Headstand (Sirsasana)
4. Inverted Staff Pose (Viparita Dandasana)
5. Upward-Facing Bow Pose (Urdhva Dhanurasana)
6. Simple Seated Twist Pose (Bharadvajasana)
7. Downward-Facing Dog Pose (Adho Mukha Svanasana)
8. Shoulderstand (Sarvangasana)
9. Plough Pose (Halasana)
10. Bridge Pose (Setu Bandha Sarvangasana)
11. Reclining Bound Angle Pose (Supta Baddha Konasana)
12. Corpse Pose (Savasana)

1. CROSS BOLSTERS POSE or RECLINING EASY SEATED POSE (Supta Sukhasana) Place a bolster on your mat and lay another one across the center of the first to form a cross. Sit on the middle of the top bolster and carefully lie back so your spine is supported on the bolster and the back of your head touches the floor. (If that is too much of a stretch or puts strain on your neck, place a folded blanket underneath your head.) Place your arms on either side of your head, palms up, elbows bent, and relax completely. (If you feel any strain in your lower back, raise your feet on a block.) Relax in this pose for several minutes, softening your abdominals and breathing deeply. To come out of the pose, bend your knees and roll to one side. Help yourself up using your hands.

EFFECTS This supported backbend opens your chest, improves respiration and circulation, helps balance adrenal and thyroid function, and helps alleviate depression and fatigue.

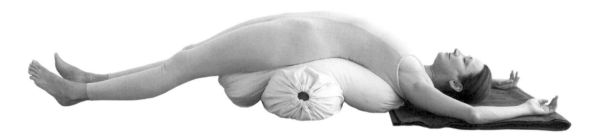

ALTERNATIVE: RECLINING EASY SEATED POSE (Supta Sukhasana) If Cross Bolsters Pose is difficult or uncomfortable, do this one instead. Place a bolster vertically on the floor behind you and sit just in front of it with your knees bent and your sacrum touching the bolster's edge. You may put a folded blanket on the bolster to support your head. Cross your legs comfortably at your shins and extend up through your spine. Using your hands to support you, lie back on the bolster. Rest your arms out to the sides, bring your shoulder blades into your back ribs, and lift your chest. This should be a restful pose and you should feel no discomfort anywhere. (If you feel any strain in your back, add more height to your support.) To come out, uncross your legs, place your feet flat on the floor, and roll slowly to one side. Use your hands to push yourself up to a sitting position.

2. DOWNWARD-FACING DOG POSE (Adho Mukha Svanasana) Lie facedown on your sticky mat. Place your palms on the floor by each side of your chest with your fingers well spread and pointing straight ahead. Come up on your hands and knees. That's your position. Now place a bolster or one or two folded blankets so your support is in line with your sternum. It should be high enough to support your head, but low enough so that you can lengthen your neck. Return to your hands-and-knees position, and turn your toes under.

Exhale, press your hands firmly into the mat and extend up through your inner arms. As you exhale, raise your buttocks high into the air and move your thighs up and back. Keep stretching through your legs and bring your heels toward the floor. Keep your legs firm and your elbows straight as you lift your buttocks upward and release the crown of your head onto your support. The action of the arms and legs serves to elongate your spine and release your head. Hold this pose for 30 seconds to 1 minute, breathing deeply. Let your head rest completely and release the base of your neck. To come out, return to your hands and knees and sit back on your heels.

EFFECTS This is a wonderful pose to combat depression because it helps increase circulation to your chest, improve respiration, and calm your mind.

3. HEADSTAND† **(Sirsasana)** Place a folded blanket against the wall. Kneel in front of it with your feet and knees together. Interlace your fingers firmly, thumbs touching and your hands cupped. Position your hands no more than 3 inches from the wall, your elbows shoulder-width apart. Your wrists, forearms, and elbows form the foundation for this pose.

Lengthen your neck and place the crown of your head on the blanket. The back of your head should be in contact with your hands. Press your forearms into the floor and lift your shoulders away from the floor. Maintain this action throughout the pose. Straighten your legs, raise your hips toward the ceiling, and walk your feet in until your spine is almost perpendicular to the floor. As you exhale, lift one leg at a time, and bring your feet to the wall.

Keep your heels and buttocks against the wall. Roll your thighs in, lift your tailbone, lengthen your legs upward, and keep your feet together. Balance on the crown of your head, press your forearms into the floor, and continue to lift your shoulders away from your ears. Keep your breathing even, your eyes and throat soft, and your abdomen relaxed. With regular practice, you can learn to bring your buttocks and heels away from the wall. Hold the pose as long as you can, up to 5 minutes.

To come out, exhale and bring your legs down to the floor one at a time. Bend your knees, sit back on your heels, and rest for a few breaths before raising your head. .

EFFECTS This is a wonderful pose if you feel agitated, depressed, or spacey. It encourages freshly oxygenated blood to circulate more freely throughout your head and chest, balancing your neuroendocrine system and rejuvenating your entire body.

†CAUTION Do this pose only if it is already part of your yoga practice. Do not do this pose if you have high blood pressure, have your period, or suffer from neck or back problems or migraines.

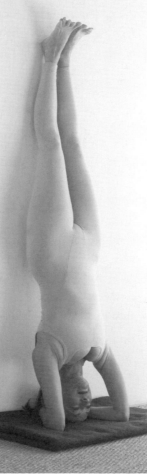

4. INVERTED STAFF POSE† **(Viparita Dandasana)** (Before beginning, see pages 34–35.) Place a folded blanket on a chair that has been placed about 2 feet from the wall—far enough away so your feet can press into the wall when your legs are outstretched. Sit backward on the chair, facing the wall, with your feet through the chair back. Letting your hands slide down the sides of the chair and supporting yourself on your elbows, lean back slowly so your head and neck extend past the front of the chair seat.

Still holding the sides of the chair, arch back so your shoulder blades are at the front edge of the seat. (You may need to scoot your buttocks farther toward the back edge of the seat.) Take your feet to the wall, legs slightly bent, and hold the back legs or sides of the chair. Lengthen your legs, pressing the chair away from the wall, and roll your thighs in toward each other. Keep your hands on the chair sides or legs. (If you have neck problems, rest your head on a bolster. If you feel any pain in your lower back, elevate your feet on a block or bolsters placed against the wall.) Breathe quietly for 1 to 2 minutes. If you can't maintain the pose that long, do it for 30 seconds, sit up, and repeat a couple of times.

To come out, bend your knees and place your feet flat on the floor. Hold on to the sides of the chair back and carefully come up, lifting from your sternum. Lean over the chair back for a few breaths to release your back.

EFFECTS This pose helps your whole body feel invigorated, opens your chest (improving circulation and respiration), and lifts your spirits.

†CAUTION Seek the advice of an experienced teacher if you have neck problems. Do not do this pose if you have a migraine or tension headache or diarrhea.

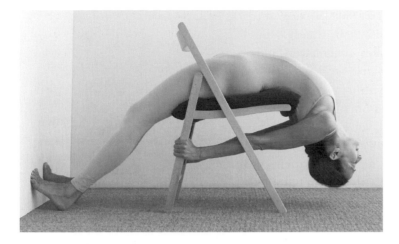

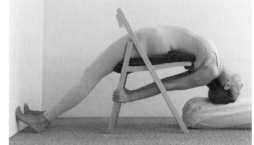

Modification

5. UPWARD-FACING BOW POSE† (Urdhva Dhanurasana) Position two blocks against the wall, shoulder-width apart. Lie on your back with your head between the blocks, your knees bent, your feet hip-width apart, and your heels close to your buttocks. (If you need more support, lie on a bolster.) Bend your elbows and place your hands on the blocks, fingers pointing toward your feet. As you exhale, raise your hips and chest, straighten your arms, and stretch your legs. Lift your tailbone and move the backs of your thighs toward your buttocks. Hold the pose for 5 to 10 seconds, if you can. If not, come in and out of it two or three times. To come out of the pose, bend your knees and elbows, and slowly lower your body to the floor.

EFFECTS This full backbend stimulates your entire body and leaves you with an overall feeling of elation and well-being.

†CAUTION Do the unsupported version of this pose only if it's already part of your yoga practice; if you have trouble pushing up into a backbend, try the modification on page 37 of the Women's Energizing Sequence. Seek the advice of an experienced teacher if you have neck problems. Do not do this pose if you have a migraine or tension headache, suffer from heart trouble or any serious illness, or are pregnant. If it is too difficult, substitute Cross Bolsters Pose (see page 220). Don't be afraid to give it a try, however, even if you can get up only a little bit. It gets easier with practice.

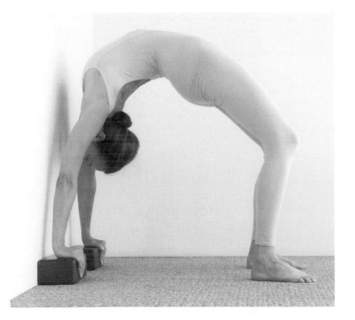

6. SIMPLE SEATED TWIST POSE†
(**Bharadvajasana**) Sit up straight with your legs stretched out in front of you and your left hip elevated on two folded blankets. Bend both legs to the right so your feet are next to your right hip. Keeping your thighs and knees facing forward, make sure your right ankle rests on the arch of your left foot and your buttocks are not on your foot. Draw your shoulder blades into your back, broaden your chest, and extend your spine upward. On an exhalation, turn your abdomen, ribs, chest, and shoulders (in that order) to the left; place your right hand on the outside of your left thigh and your left hand on the blankets behind you. Remain in this pose for 10 to 20 seconds. Come back to the center position, straighten your legs, and change sides.

EFFECTS This gentle twist helps lift your spirits as it opens and broadens your chest, increases circulation and respiration, and releases the muscles in your shoulders and back.

†CAUTION Do not practice twists if you have diarrhea or feel nauseous. Do not do this pose if you have arthritis in your knees. If you suffer from sacroiliac pain, release your pelvis whenever you twist.

7. DOWNWARD-FACING DOG POSE
(**Adho Mukha Svanasana**) Repeat Downward-Facing Dog Pose (see page 221), this time without supporting your head. Remain in the pose for 10 to 20 seconds.

EFFECTS This is a good pose to do after backbends to stretch out your back.

8. SHOULDERSTAND† (**Sarvangasana**) (Before beginning see pages 18–19.) Lie on your back with two folded blankets supporting your shoulders and your arms stretched out beside you. On an exhalation, bend your knees and raise your legs toward your chest. Pressing your hands into the floor, swing your bent legs over your head; support your back with your hands and press your elbows firmly into the blankets. Raise your torso up until it is perpendicular to the floor and your knees are close to your chest. Supporting your back, raise your legs until your thighs are parallel to the floor; raise them some more until your knees point toward the ceiling. Now raise your legs completely and extend up through your heels until your whole body is perpendicular to the floor. Move your tailbone up and in and use your hands to lift your back ribs. Feel that your whole body is long and straight. Move your shoulders away from your ears. Hold this pose as long as you can, at least 2 minutes. To come out, bend your knees. Slowly roll down.

EFFECTS This pose helps calm anxiety and irritability, bringing strength, peace, and a renewed sense of resolve when your spirits are low.

†CAUTION Do not do this pose if you suffer from neck or shoulder problems, if you have high blood pressure, if you are menstruating, or if you have a headache.

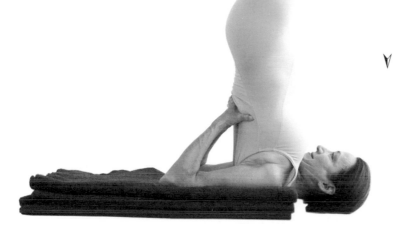

9. PLOUGH POSE† (Halasana) Lie on your back with two folded blankets supporting your neck and shoulders; your head is on the floor and your arms are down by your sides. Your legs should be straight out in front of you, feet together and knees tightened. As you exhale, bend your knees and bring your thighs in to your chest. Roll your shoulders away from your head and expand your chest. On another exhalation, swing or lift your buttocks and legs up, supporting your back with your hands, and extend your legs over your head, placing your toes on the floor behind you. (To keep your elbows in, you can use a strap around both arms, just above your elbows, before you begin.) Keep your thighs active by tightening your knees to create space between your face and your legs. Stay in this pose, breathing deeply and slowly, for several minutes or as long as you're comfortable. To come out, slowly roll down one vertebra at a time. Rest with your back flat on the floor, breathing deeply, for several breaths.

EFFECTS This pose helps balance your endocrine system and quiet your nervous system, bringing your body and mind to a state of complete relaxation. It is ideal for taming irritability and anxiety.

†CAUTION Do not do this pose if you have neck problems or if you are menstruating.

10. BRIDGE POSE (Setu Bandha Sarvangasana) Place one bolster horizontally against the wall and the other vertically, forming a T shape. Spread a folded blanket on the floor at the end of the vertical bolster that is farthest from the wall (for your head). Sit on the end of the vertical bolster that is closest to the wall. Keeping your knees bent, lie back over the bolster. Slide down until the end of the bolster is in the middle of your back and your shoulders just reach the floor. Rest your shoulders and head on the blanket. Keeping your feet and heels together, stretch your legs toward the wall and put your heels on the horizontal bolster so your feet touch the wall. Your legs should be straight out in front of you, hip-width apart. Rest your arms in any comfortable position—over your head or out by your sides. Close your eyes and relax completely, breathing deeply. Stay in this position for at least 1 or 2 minutes, or as long as you like.

To come out, bend your knees and slowly roll to one side. Using your hands, push yourself up to a seated position.

EFFECTS This lovely, relaxing pose is great if you need to quell anxiety, calm your nervous system, and relieve irritability.

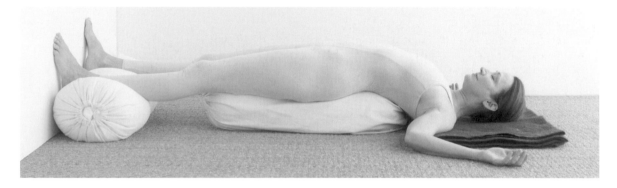

11. RECLINING BOUND ANGLE POSE (Supta Baddha Konasana) Place a bolster vertically behind you and sit just in front of it with your knees bent and your sacrum touching the bolster's edge. Place a strap behind your back, at your sacrum; draw it forward over your hips, across your shins, and under your feet (see page xv). Put the soles of your feet together and let your knees and thighs fall to the sides. Cinch the strap securely under your feet. Lie back so your head and torso rest comfortably on the bolster and your buttocks and legs are on the floor. (If you feel any discomfort in your lower back, add some height to your support with a folded blanket or two. If you feel any strain in your neck, place a folded blanket under your head and neck. If you feel any muscle tension in your legs, roll two blankets vertically and place one under the top of each thigh.) Rest in this pose for as long as you like, breathing deeply.

To come out, draw your knees together, slip the strap off, and slowly roll to one side. Use your hands to push yourself up to a seated position.

EFFECTS This quintessential "because I'm worth it" pose opens your chest, improves respiration and circulation, and helps lift your spirits while completely supporting your body, mind, and spirit.

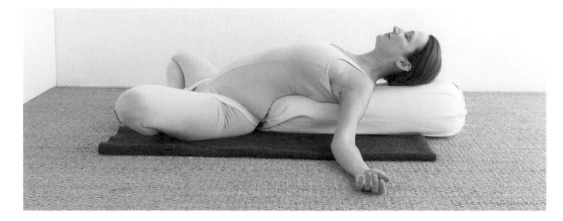

12. CORPSE POSE (Savasana) Lie on your back with your legs stretched out in front of you. Place your arms comfortably at your sides, slightly away from your torso, with your palms facing upward. Actively stretch your arms and legs away from you, then allow them to release completely. Close your eyes and let everything relax. Take a few deep breaths, inhaling into your chest without tensing your throat, neck, or diaphragm. Exhale your body into the floor, releasing your shoulders, neck, and facial muscles. Keep your abdomen soft and relaxed, and release your lower back. Keep your eyes still and your mind quiet, and surrender yourself completely to the pose. Breathe normally for at least 5 to 10 minutes, taking in energy and releasing tension. To come out of the pose, bend your knees, roll slowly to one side, and after a few breaths, gently push yourself to a seated position.

EFFECTS This pose is good when you want to soothe your nerves and calm your mind through total relaxation—and through relaxation comes renewed energy and determination.

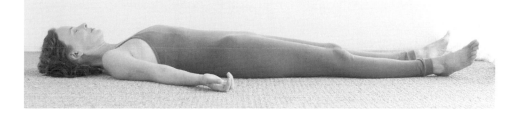

A SEQUENCE FOR ANXIETY-DRIVEN DEPRESSION

1. Downward-Facing Dog Pose (Adho Mukha Svanasana)
2. Standing Forward Bend (Uttanasana)
3. Wide-Angle Standing Forward Bend (Prasarita Padottanasana)
4. Downward-Facing Dog Pose (Adho Mukha Svanasana)
5. Inverted Staff Pose (Viparita Dandasana)
6. Upward-Facing Bow Pose (Urdhva Dhanurasana)
7. Child's Pose (Adho Mukha Virasana)
8. Shoulderstand (Sarvangasana)
9. Plough Pose (Halasana)
10. Seated Forward Bend (Paschimottanasana) to Plough Pose (Halasana)
11. Bridge Pose (Setu Bandha Sarvangasana)
12. Corpse Pose (Savasana)

*NOTE If you feel agitated or anxious this sequence can help ground your energy, taking you out of your head and into your body. You can begin by moving from Mountain Pose (Tadasana) to Standing Forward Bend (Uttanasana) to Downward-Facing Dog (Adho Mukha Svanasana) and back again several times before going on to the backbends. By the time you reach the supported poses, you should feel calmer and ready to receive their healing benefits.

1. DOWNWARD-FACING DOG POSE (Adho Mukha Svanasana)
Do Downward-Facing Dog Pose as described on page 221. Remain in the pose for 1 to 2 minutes.

EFFECTS Resting your head on a support helps calm your mind and relieve anxiety and nervous tension, while increasing circulation to your chest.

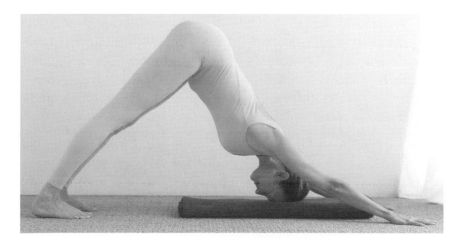

2. STANDING FORWARD BEND (Uttanasana) Stand up straight facing a padded chair placed about 2 feet in front of you; distribute your weight evenly between the front of your feet and your heels. Tighten your knees by pulling up with your quadriceps (front thigh muscles). Raise your sternum and roll your shoulders back, drawing your shoulder blades in. Lift your abdomen and pull your tailbone in without pushing your thighs forward. As you inhale, extend your spine, stretching your whole body. Exhale and bend forward, resting your head on the chair seat. Fold your arms over your head. Breathe normally for 1 minute. Release your arms and slowly stand up. Your head should come up last.

EFFECTS This pose helps calm and rejuvenate your body and mind.

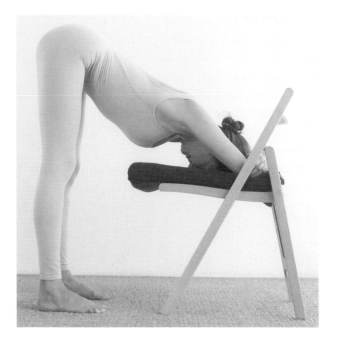

3. WIDE-ANGLE STANDING FORWARD BEND (Prasarita Padottanasana) Place a folded blanket or a bolster vertically in front of you. Step your feet wide apart (about 4 feet or so), keeping the outer edges of your feet parallel. Tighten your quadriceps to draw your kneecaps up and keep your thighs well lifted. On an exhalation, bend forward from your hips, place your hands on the floor between your feet. Lift your hips toward the ceiling, draw your shoulder blades into your back. Look up and extend your trunk forward, arching your back slightly. (See page 11.) Remain this way for 5 to 10 seconds.

Keeping your trunk extended, exhale, bend your elbows, and release the crown of your head onto your support. Keep your legs firm, but relax your shoulders and neck. Breathe deeply and let your trunk release downward. Stay in this pose for 1 minute. To come out, return to the concave back position, bring your hands to your hips, and raise your trunk. Step your feet together.

EFFECTS This pose is excellent for calming anxiety, jittery nerves, and mental or physical tension, as well as for combatting fatigue.

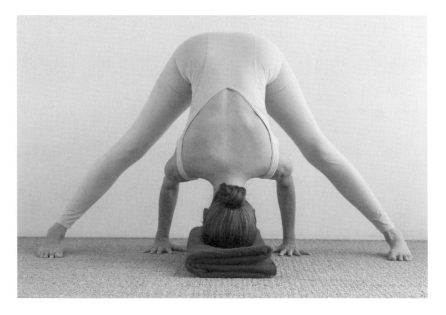

4. DOWNWARD-FACING DOG POSE (Adho Mukha Svanasana) Repeat Downward-Facing Dog Pose (see page 221), this time without supporting your head. Stay in the pose for 15 to 20 seconds.

EFFECTS This active variation of the pose helps increase circulation to your head and chest.

5. INVERTED STAFF POSE† (**Viparita** ➤
Dandasana) (Before beginning, see
pages 34–35.) Place a folded blanket
on a chair that has been placed
about 2 feet from the wall—far
enough away so your feet can press
into the wall when your legs are
outstretched. Place a bolster (or two,
depending on your flexibility) in
front of the chair to support your
head. Sit backward on the chair,
facing the wall, with your feet
through the chair back. Letting your
hands slide down the sides of the
chair and supporting yourself on
your elbows, lean back slowly so
your head and neck extend past the
front of the chair seat.

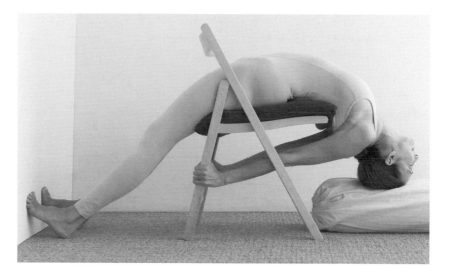

Still holding the sides of the chair, arch
back so your shoulder blades are at the front
edge of the seat. (You may need to scoot
your buttocks farther toward the back of the
seat.) Take your feet to the wall, legs slightly
bent, and move your hands to the back legs
of the chair (your arms should be between
the front legs). Lengthen your legs, pressing
the chair away from the wall, and roll your
thighs in toward each other. (If you feel
strain in your lower back, rest your feet on
bolsters or a low stool.) Rest your head on
your support and breathe quietly for 1 to 2
minutes. If you can't maintain the pose that
long, do it a couple of times for 30 seconds.

To come out, bend your knees and place
your feet flat on the floor. Hold on to the
sides of the chair back and carefully come
up, lifting from your sternum. Lean over the
chair back for a few breaths to release your
back.

EFFECTS Placing your head on a bolster
creates a cooling, calming effect for your
mind, which helps restore your equilibrium
and calm agitation.

†CAUTION Seek the advice of an experienced
teacher if you have neck problems. Do not do
this pose if you have a migraine or tension
headache or diarrhea.

6. UPWARD-FACING BOW POSE† (**Urdhva Dhanurasana**)
Do Upward-Facing Bow Pose as described on page 223. Try
to stay in the pose for 5 to 10 seconds; if this isn't possible,
come in and out of the pose two or three times.

EFFECTS This full backbend stimulates your entire body and
leaves you with an overall feeling of elation and well-being.

†CAUTION Do the unsupported version of this pose only if it is
already part of your yoga practice; if you have trouble pushing
up into a backbend, try the modification on page 37 of the
Woman's Energizing Sequence. Seek the advice of an experienced teacher if you have neck problems. Do not do this pose if
you have a migraine or tension headache, suffer from heart
trouble or any serious illness, or are pregnant.

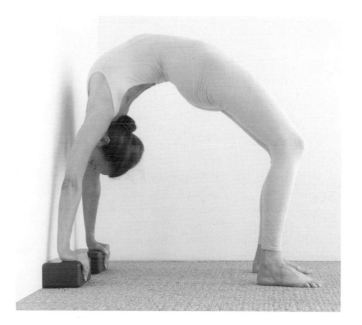

7. CHILD'S POSE (Adho Mukha Virasana) Kneel on the floor with your knees slightly wider than your hips and bring your big toes together. Bend forward and stretch your arms and trunk forward. Rest your head on the floor or a blanket.

EFFECTS This pose stretches your back after backbends and helps calm your nerves.

8. SHOULDERSTAND† (Sarvangasana) Do Shoulderstand as described on page 224. Remain in the pose for several minutes, if you can.

EFFECTS This pose helps calm anxiety and irritability, bringing you a feeling of strength and peace and a renewed sense of resolve when your spirits are low.

†CAUTION Do not do this pose if you suffer from neck or shoulder problems, if you have high blood pressure, if you are menstruating, or if you have a headache.

230

9. PLOUGH POSE† (Halasana) Do Plough Pose as described on page 225. Remain in the pose for as long as you're comfortable.

EFFECTS This pose can lift your spirits and help calm agitation by quieting your sympathetic nervous system.

†CAUTION Do not do this pose if you have neck problems or if you are menstruating.

10. SEATED FORWARD BEND (Paschimottanasana) to PLOUGH POSE† (Halasana) Sit on your mat or on one or two folded blankets with your legs stretched out in front of you. Take a full, deep breath; as you exhale, bend forward and extend your arms beyond your feet, placing your hands on the floor. On an inhalation, stretch up through your spine and lift your sternum and head, keeping your back slightly concave. Exhale and extend your torso over your legs; rest your head just beyond your knees, if you can (A). Do not allow your buttocks to come off the floor (or blankets).

Come out of the forward bend, curling your back and pulling your knees up to roll backward into Plough Pose (Halasana). Raise your hands overhead to meet your feet (B). (If you feel strain in your neck, support your back with your hands. Release your hands to the floor as you roll down.) Go back and forth between the two poses 15 to 20 times.

NOTE In order to practice this sequence effectively, you must be able to do both poses without the use of chairs or bolsters.

EFFECTS This sequence brings relief from despondency or anxiety, energizes your whole body, and makes you feel more alive.

†CAUTION Do not do this sequence if you have back or neck problems, high blood pressure, or heart problems; if you are menstruating or pregnant; or if you have diarrhea or feel nauseous.

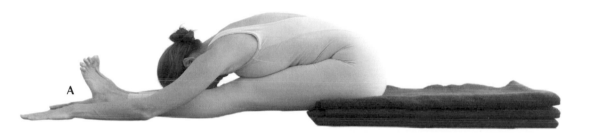

A

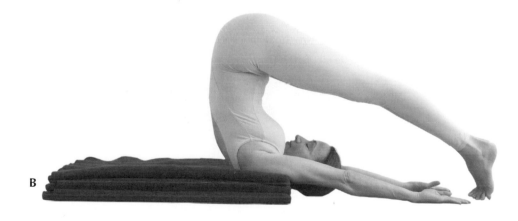

B

11. BRIDGE POSE (Setu Bandha Sarvangasana) Do Bridge Pose as described on page 226. Remain in the pose for at least 1 to 2 minutes.

EFFECTS This lovely, relaxing pose quells anxiety, calms your nervous system, and relieves irritability.

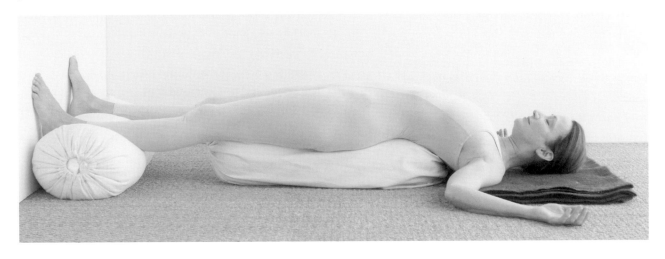

12. CORPSE POSE (Savasana) Do Corpse Pose as described on page 227. Remain in the pose for at least 5 to 10 minutes, taking in energy and releasing tension. If you have trouble lying still with your eyes closed, skip this pose and end your practice with Bridge Pose (Setu Bandha Sarvangasana).

EFFECTS This pose is good when you want to soothe your nerves and calm your mind through total relaxation.

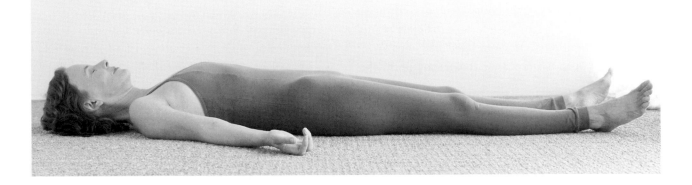

Chapter 11 *Easing into Menopause*

JUST WHEN YOU'RE FEELING PRETTY GOOD ABOUT YOUR BODY, IN control of your emotions, and in tune with your spiritual side, something happens to set your head spinning. Out of the blue, you experience waves of anxiety, bouts of paranoia, and a week of insomnia. You can't concentrate; at times, you can't even string two sentences together. And to top it all off, just yesterday as you sat in a meeting, you suddenly felt a wave of heat surge through your body that left you sweaty, clammy, and mildly disoriented. That's menopause for you: a roller-coaster ride of unpredictable speed and duration filled with highs and lows, bumps and bruises along the way. But, if you hang on, menopause will leave you wiser and more complete when it finally sets you down.

WHAT IS MENOPAUSE, AND HOW CAN I TELL WHETHER I'M IN IT?

Menopause literally means the cessation of menses. It's as natural a fact of life for women as puberty or pregnancy. You stop ovulating, and you stop bleeding. Estrogen and androgen production shifts to the adrenals, body fat, and muscles. Progesterone production, on the other hand, stops completely once you stop ovulating.

Menopause generally happens when you're in your late forties to early fifties, although it can happen earlier or later. Most women start around the same age their mothers and grandmothers did. If menopause happens before you turn forty, it's called premature menopause, which often has more severe symptoms.

Although menopause itself means that moment in which menstruation stops, the transition can take several years. During these years, called perimenopause, your ovaries and pituitary gland perform a little dance, which can alternately seem sweet and lyrical or frenetic and out of control. Tired of producing eggs, your ovaries want to retire and turn hormone manufacturing over to your adrenal glands and other organs. So they prefer the waltz—unhurried and gentle, until the music slows to a sleepy rhythm. Your pituitary gland, on the other hand, wants to keep going. It prefers the fox trot, and to get things moving, it sends down even more follicle-stimulating hormone (FSH) and luteinizing hormone (LH) to shake the ovaries out of their doldrums and encourage them to make more estrogen and progesterone.

This rather schizophrenic pas de deux can bring on symptoms that are annoying at best and debilitating at worst. These symptoms are

233

not generally caused by the decline in hormonal production per se, but by the unpredictable hormonal fluctuations created by the argument taking place between your ovaries and pituitary. A surge of estrogen can cause fibroid tumors and sore breasts; a decline in estrogen and a spike in progesterone, on the other hand, bring bouts of depression and profound lethargy. But, as you may remember from puberty, once the hormone producers figure out what they're supposed to do, your body usually finds a balance point and many of your complaints disappear. Once your ovaries win the fight and level off their production of estrogen and androgen, your pituitary gland also allows other organs to step in and take over. Your adrenal glands, skin, muscle, brain, pineal body, hair follicles, and body fat all manufacture the androgenic hormones your body needs to function effectively.

The key here is that your body eventually adjusts to these changes in hormone levels and regains its balance. As Nancy Lonsdorf, coauthor of *A Woman's Best Medicine: Health, Happiness, and Long Life through Ayurveda*, writes, "The issue for each of us is whether the adjustment comes easily or with difficulty." When your reproductive years wind down, your body no longer needs the same amount of estrogen and progesterone it once did. It can survive, even thrive, on much less. But if your body has grown used to a certain hormone level, Lonsdorf explains, it will go through a period of withdrawal and imbalance before it achieves equilibrium. When girls go through puberty, no one suggests preventing it; no one labels the inevitable mood fluctuations and, for some, temporary craziness that ensues as symptoms of a disease needing therapy. Parents simply roll their eyes, grit their teeth, and wait out the storm; most teenagers do the same.

Society has been slow to show the menopausal woman the same patience. On the contrary, instead of celebrating a woman's "coming of age," our culture bombards her—and the fifty million other women who will enter menopause within the next fifteen years or so—with images of barrenness, of stooped women who are brittle of bone but could come alive and be young again with the help of pharmaceuticals and elective surgery. Luckily, women who refuse to accept this prognosis can weather the menopausal storm with simple lifestyle and dietary changes—and, of course, yoga.

Going into your menopausal years with a healthy attitude about who you are makes a huge difference. Experts in complementary medicine who specialize in women's health point out that Western women struggle much more than their counterparts in cultures where the wisdom and beauty of older women are celebrated. The Japanese, for example, don't even have a translation for hot flashes, the symptom Western women complain about most. Is that because Western women are the only ones who get intense heat surging through their bodies? Maybe. Clearly Japanese women, who eat more soy and less meat, suffer less than most American women. But our society's attitude toward menopausal symptoms—that they signal the loss of youth, beauty, and a woman's usefulness in society—could also contribute to the pain and shame many women feel about menopause.

If Western culture supported women as they made the transition from childbearing to wisdom years, you might welcome your rising temperature as a power surge and take comfort in your graying hair and thickened waistline. You might learn to focus your anger constructively to enact changes in your community and the environment. And imagine: Your family would sustain you—with love and good humor—when you felt fatigued or fuzzy, and you would embrace the extra rest time you deserve for reflection and renewal. But as long as youth represents opportunity, hope, and health in our society, those attitudes, coupled with the stressful lifestyles most women maintain, will continue to fuel the discomfort women feel about their bodies as they approach their mid-forties and fifties.

So, is there anything you can do about all this? Do you suffer silently, figuring the incapacitating hot flashes, the terrible anxieties and self-doubt, and the sleepless nights are bound to go away eventually? Or is there something you can do to improve your quality of life now so you can reach your wisdom years with your sanity intact?

The most important thing you can do for yourself is to head into your menopausal years as healthy as possible—in body, mind, and spirit. If your diet has included nutrient-deficient fast foods, white sugar, and lots of animal proteins laced with hormones and antibiotics; if you've exercised sporadically or not at all; if you work at a high-stress job; and if you laugh very little, chances are you will enter the transition years with seriously depleted adrenals, an overloaded sympathetic nervous system, and an imbalanced endocrine system. Not a good way to deal with the hormonal fluctuations and emotional roller coasters that await you.

Yoga can help you pay attention to what your body and its changes have to tell you. It can realign your focus inward and teach you to love yourself and the process you're going through as it all unfolds. Modifying your diet, exercise routine, and lifestyle will also help your body adjust to the changes it's going through. In this chapter, you'll find many suggestions, organized by specific symptom, that can help you prepare for your menopausal journey even before it begins.

HOT FLASHES

No one knows for sure what causes the unpredictable power surges that visit perimenopausal—and even some postmenopausal—women when they least expect it. Conventional wisdom suggests that they stem from a malfunction or imbalance in the body's temperature control center, located in the hypothalamus, as a woman's hormones fluctuate. Another theory states that the fluctuation in hormones irritates the blood vessels and nerve endings, causing the vessels to dilate too much, and producing a hot, flushed feeling.

The American medical establishment believes hot flashes are the result of estrogen deprivation. Although that observation is scientifically accurate, I much prefer herbalist and author Susun Weed's explanation. In her book *Menopausal Years: The Wise Woman Way*, she describes a hot flash as "a release of kundalini electricity, which rewires the nervous system, making it capable of transferring and moving powerful healing energies for the entire community." It is prana, chi, your life force rushing through you, "flashing, flushing, pulsating." Joan Borysenko, in *A Woman's Book of Life: The Biology, Psychology, and Spirituality of the Feminine Life Cycle*, likens hot flashes to a woman's inner sacrificial fires, in which she burns her offerings of troubles, worries, stress, and destructive attachments.

Hot flashes are a fact of menopausal life. Most experts agree that nearly 80 percent of all women have them sometime during their perimenopausal years, and a small percentage continue to get them for several years after menopause. Fewer than 20 percent of women find hot flashes debilitating, and not all women experience them the same way. Some flash at regular intervals—every hour or so, some only at night or only during the early morning. For others, it's more erratic. They may get flashes every day for three weeks and then nothing at all for a time, only to have them come back unexpectedly a month or two later.

Just in case you're wondering if you've experienced your first one, a hot flash is a sudden, intense feeling of heat in your body. Most women feel a rapid blushing that begins in the chest and spreads quickly up their neck and face, and even down their arms. Their body temperature rises, their pulse speeds up, and they break out in a visible sweat. To cap it off, many women, who have just taken off layers of clothing to cool down, suddenly experience a brief but intense chill as their body struggles to correct the temperature fluctuations.

Patricia has two types of hot flashes—the first is like the conventional type we just discussed; the second actually begins at the back of her knees and creeps up her body and spine and into her face. The few flashes I've experienced have been coupled with intense anxiety, heart palpitations, and an almost hypoglycemic sensation of hunger—when I suddenly feel so hungry I get shaky.

Night sweats are hot flashes that wake you up, so it's easy to see why they bring on fatigue and make you feel edgier and more out of control. Women experience night sweats differently as well. Some say they sweat so profusely they not only throw off everything they're wearing but must then get up (sometimes two or three times a night) to change the soaking sheets. A lot of women keep a towel by the bedside to wipe themselves off before trying to go back to sleep.

Hot flashes and night sweats generally stop once hormone fluctuations calm down and your body adjusts to lower estrogen levels. But not always. Patricia still has them regularly even though she stopped menstruating four years ago, and Susan, a well-known yoga teacher in Colorado, figures her hot flashes should have stopped at least five years ago when her menses did.

What Makes Them Worse

Just about the time women begin experiencing hot flashes, they inexplicably find themselves with what some refer to as "middle-age spread."

Although it can feel like adding insult to injury, the added weight actually helps regulate hot flashes. Thinner women, according to Susun Weed, experience more rapid changes in their estrogen and FSH/LH levels than women with more fat in their bodies. These rapid changes can increase the frequency and severity of hot flashes. Fat cells contain estrogen and, as a result, help slow down the production of FSH/LH in the pituitary gland and calm hot flashes. However, Dr. Susan Love, author of *Dr. Susan Love's Hormone Book: Making Informed Choices About Menopause*, says if you're naturally thin and physically fit, you shouldn't have any more trouble than someone more substantial. Generally it's women who have a history of strict dieting to keep their weight unnaturally low who have more hot flashes.

Many experts believe stress plays a big part in bringing on hot flashes. In fact, most women I talked to felt that not being able to handle the stress in their lives contributed greatly to hot flashes and other menopausal symptoms.

Anything that affects your central nervous system has the potential to increase the frequency and intensity of hot flashes. Smoking not only stimulates the sympathetic nervous system, it also appears to effect hormonal output in the ovaries. Caffeine, alcohol, over-the-counter decongestants, and diet pills all have the added disadvantage of interrupting your sleep. And as perimenopausal women everywhere can attest, lack of sleep exacerbates many of the symptoms they face, including hot flashes. Some women react to anything that will increase heat in their bodies, including spicy foods, hot baths (especially before bedtime), and unrelenting stress.

How to Stop Flashing

Most women report that once they've experienced their first hot flash, nothing except time works to completely get rid of them. But there are several steps you can take to minimize their frequency and severity.

1. *Awareness.* Before you attempt to alter your diet and your lifestyle drastically, try to pinpoint your hot flash agitators. Does drinking coffee, eating chocolate, or having a steak bring on a flash? Do you feel hot, constricted, and claustrophobic when you wear clothing that fits snugly around your abdomen or chest? Did your last flash coincide with a heated argument with your boss or daughter?

2. *Attitude.* How do you feel about having hot flashes, especially in public? Try allowing the heat to flow up and out of you instead of fighting it or panicking. If you view flashes as power surges or heightened prana or chi energy, instead of a horrific reminder that you've lost your youth, you may be able to endure them with more patience and some gentle humor.

3. *Diet.* If you discover that caffeine, alcohol, red meat, and white sugar aggravate your symptoms, remove them from your diet. Add plenty of soy to the menu—especially soy nuts, tempeh, or

sea vegetables. Women who eat animal products often get relief from salmon, which is high in omega-3 essential fatty acids.

4. *Destressing.* For the majority of women, stress is the number-one cause of recurring hot flashes. Now, more than ever, take time to establish priorities and make conscious, careful choices. It's ironic that as women grow older, they have more freedom, but may lack the energy to act on it. During this perimenopausal transition, take on less and spend more time in reflection.

5. *Complementary therapies.* Many women swear by weekly acupuncture treatments and herbal supplements such as black cohosh, motherwort, dong quai, chaste tree (*Vitex agnus castus*), damiana, fennel, anise, and wild yam root. (Don't use dong quai if you also suffer from heavy bleeding.) Naturopathic doctors often include additional vitamin E (800 mg/day), bioflavonoids (250 mg, five to six times/day), and essential fatty acids. Herbal supplements that tone your liver (like dandelion root and milk thistle) and support and pacify your adrenals (like nettles, Siberian ginseng, and oatstraw) can soothe your neuroendocrine system and possibly lessen the severity of your hot flashes.

6. *Hormone replacement therapy (HRT).* Even though most health care practitioners agree that this shouldn't be your first choice of treatment, many women who suffer from debilitating hot flashes find short-term HRT the only thing that works. Susan Love recommends increasing your soy intake and exercising more (more yoga) if you take estrogen supplements. There doesn't seem to be much evidence to suggest that short-term use of estrogen (one to four years) causes problems, unless you have breast cancer or are at risk of developing it. If that's the case, progestin supplements may work well in the short term. Don't quit taking any hormones abruptly, however. Dr. Love advises tapering off gradually with the help of herbs such as black cohosh. If you stop HRT gradually, you stand a better chance of not getting any more hot flashes. If you quit cold turkey, your hot flashes may come back with a vengeance.

Patricia Says

Here are some tips I've found helpful in dealing with hot flashes or other symptoms.

• Wear loose, comfortable clothing. I can't stand having clothes on that bind me around my abdomen or breasts when I'm having flashes.

• Stress and fatigue make my hot flashes worse. Because of my busy schedule, I am conscious of establishing priorities and boundaries.

• As women, we should support each other, share our experiences—the joys as well as the pain and frustration we go through during this time of our lives. Sharing with other women navigating the same rite of passage helps us put our experiences into perspective.

• Don't allow your commitments to family, career, and friends cause you to lose connection with yourself. To lose that connection is to feel out of control, out of sync. For many women, that feeling causes their symptoms (hot flashes, anxiety, depression) to worsen. Honor yourself each step of the way.

How Yoga Can Help

Yoga, particularly inversions (upside-down poses), has a powerful effect on your neuroendocrine system, especially the pineal body, pituitary gland, hypothalamus, and thyroid and adrenal glands. Patricia says that inversions can either jump-start a sluggish system or calm an overly excited one by allowing fresh, oxygenated blood to flow into your head and neck.

In her book *Relax and Renew: Restful Yoga for Stressful Times*, yoga teacher Judith Hanson Lasater explains that during hot flashes, prana (life force) moves from the center of your body outward, heating your skin. Inversions, she says, draw the prana inward toward your organs and away from the skin surface, cooling everything down.

You don't have to have an advanced practice that includes unsupported inversions like Headstand (Sirsasana) or Shoulderstand (Sarvangasana) to reap the benefits of turning upside down. Putting your legs up against the wall with your pelvis higher than your chest or doing Shoulderstand using a chair and bolsters will give you many of the same benefits without challenging or straining your body. Patricia says doing unsupported Headstand generates too much heat if she's already having hot flashes, but some women swear by it. Geeta Iyengar encourages women in the latter category to do the pose with the soles of their feet together or with their legs spread apart (see page 249). Try supported Shoulderstand, Bridge Pose (Setu Bandha Sarvangasana), or even Downward-Facing Dog (Adho Mukha Svanasana) if Headstand is not part of your usual practice or if it produces too much heat.

Forward bends also work well for Patricia. Because they put little or no strain on her lower back, she often prefers to do them unsupported. But if you feel strain in your lower back or hamstrings when you bend forward, use a prop to take the strain away. These poses should be cooling and restful, not challenging. Supporting your head on a bolster or chair helps cool your brain and calm your nerves. If you like Seated Forward Bend (Paschimottanasana) to cool you off but have a hard time reaching your toes with your hands, use a strap. If even supported forward bends don't feel restful, Child's Pose (Adho Mukha Virasana) or Easy Seated Forward Bend (Adho Mukha Sukhasana) can give you the same cooling benefits.

Since a variety of things can bring on a hot flash—stress, hot weather, spicy foods, fatigue, anger, or agitation—you may have to try a variety of poses to dampen your menopausal fires. Sometimes forward bends prove effective by allowing you to surrender to the sensation; other times, inversions are the ticket. Or you may feel better creating space within yourself, and supine poses are the only postures that cool you off. Don't be afraid to experiment. Remember, relaxation is the most important element; Patricia says any gripping in your body reduces the benefit of the pose.

Patricia found that doing an energizing yoga practice can occasionally cause a flashing flare-up. "There were times during this period when I would start doing a vigorous backbend practice and my nerves would feel very, very shaky," she remembers. "I would have to stop in the middle and do something else." That something else would often be supported backbends (over bolsters or chairs) and forward bends. These cooling poses helped pacify her nervous system, restoring a sense of calm and groundedness, and generating a more balanced sense of energy. Then she could return to her usual routine. Don't be afraid to change your sequence midstream and move into something more calming. Yoga should support, not agitate you. As Patricia discovered, going through perimenopause doesn't mean you have to give up doing a rigorous practice; it only means you have to be more aware of what you need. "What I did when I had symptoms was to internalize my practice more," she explains. "I practiced from the inside out, focusing on breath, concentrating much more on the internal sensations than on the muscles and bones." On days she had no symptoms at all, she would resume her normal practice. But even now, when she does an active sequence, she often begins with cooling poses like Reclining Bound Angle Pose (Supta Baddha Konasana) or Reclining Big Toe Pose (Supta Padangusthasana) to open up her hips, shoulders, and chest, and to get her joints and muscles feeling "juicy" again before moving into the more active, challenging poses.

The postures we show here can also help with other heat-related conditions, such as night sweats and hypersensitive nerve endings in your skin. Sometimes these symptoms—as well as hot flashes—can be preceded by inexplicable anxiety. Yoga poses that pacify your adrenals and tone your liver work well to mitigate these conditions. Again, choose only the poses that work for you on any given day, and don't do the poses that don't feel good when you have symptoms.

HEAVY OR IRREGULAR PERIODS

As many women learned when entering puberty, heavy or erratic bleeding comes with the territory. Most of the time this symptom merely indicates hormonal fluctuation and is benign. Some women find they skip a period one month, have a heavier-than-normal flow the next, and then skip two more cycles. Others find their periods come much closer together than they used to, and they bleed much more than they did in their twenties and thirties. Holly, now in her fifties, began skipping periods—and then bleeding profusely—in her mid-forties. Acupuncture treatments relieved the overflow she experienced and put her periods back on track for a couple more years. Generally speaking, doctors say if you are regular in your irregularity, you probably have nothing to worry about. Nonetheless, if you bleed much more than normal and your periods continue that way for more than a couple of months, see your health care practitioner.

Susan Lark, author of *The Lark Letter* (a newsletter on women's health), says heavy or irregular bleeding can be exacerbated by stress, smoking, alcohol consumption, and poor diet. She recommends that you monitor your intake of vitamin C, iron, and bioflavonoids, because heavy bleeding can deplete these vital nutrients.

How Yoga Can Help

Yoga can have a pronounced effect on regulating erratic bleeding and combatting the fatigue and depression that result from profuse blood loss. If you experience a lot of fatigue with your heavy periods, don't do standing poses—except possibly Half-Moon Pose (Ardha Chandrasana) from the Woman's Essential Sequence—because they may be too taxing.

ERRATIC MOOD SWINGS

Suzanne, a fifty-year-old yoga teacher, found herself in the midst of perimenopause when she was only forty-three. As she told me, "I am pretty even-tempered, but I suddenly found myself enraged at the slightest provocation. I would say and do outrageous and inappropriate things, while I schizophrenically watched myself, unable to stop." She says the pinnacle of craziness happened, of all places, in the frozen food section of her local supermarket. "I threw a tantrum," she remembers. "I felt like my entire world had been turned upside down." Those words triggered something, and she immediately went home and stood on her head. It was her last experience with mood swings. For about a year, she says, "whenever I felt I was losing control, I would stand on my head. My students who don't do Headstand report that Shoulderstand works just as well."

Lots of women see a marked change in their moods during perimenopause. Some, like Suzanne, experience irritability and inexplicable anger; others sink into depression at the slightest provocation; still others have bouts of free-floating anxiety. It appears that fluctuations in progesterone and estrogen contribute to this menopausal mood syndrome (just like during puberty). Too much estrogen produces anxiety, nervousness, and flightiness; too much progesterone brings on depression. Susan Love writes that the hormonal changes by themselves probably don't cause mood swings, but they "change the body's equilibrium, so that a situation that would normally upset you a little upsets you a lot." That could be what's happening to you now.

Relieving the Symptoms

As mentioned earlier, how you feel about entering menopause in general, and getting older in particular, can have an impact on your moods, and for certain women will trigger bouts of depression, anxiety, and anger. In her book *Women's Bodies, Women's Wisdom,* Christiane Northrup reminds women they are preparing to enter a new phase—the wisdom years—and may still have some unfinished business from the first half of their lives that they need to mourn, rebel against, or simply reexamine. If a woman is willing to do this kind of reflection, Northrup says, she will probably have fewer or more manageable symptoms, and she'll at least come to see those symptoms as "messages from her inner guidance system" telling her that "parts of her life need attention."

Just about as many remedies exist to relieve erratic mood swings as there are symptoms. Some women, like Suzanne, couldn't make it through menopause without yoga inversions; other women find support by taking herbal treatments, receiving acupuncture, or even getting weekly massages. Still others know they feel better if they cut out meats and sugar from their diet. The majority of the women I spoke to found the most relief by combining a consistent yoga practice with other lifestyle changes, such as diet, supplements, meditation, and support from other women.

EASING INTO MENOPAUSE

How Yoga Can Help

Yoga is particularly beneficial for balancing unpredictable emotions during menopause. Both standing and seated forward bends soothe and calm your mind and nervous system, pacify your adrenal glands, elongate your spine, and encourage you to surrender completely. As you will see in the sequences at the end of this chapter, you can rest your head completely while applying gentle, squeezing pressure on your abdomen by placing a pillow or bolster on your lap during seated forward bends.

Twists can help invigorate and tone your adrenals as well as calm your sympathetic nervous system, which may go into overdrive due to stress. Twists will also help improve the functioning of your liver and kidneys. Unless you feel fatigue, standing poses can ground erratic moods. (Take a look at the sequences for depression in chapter 10 for more ideas about chest openers and breathing exercises.) Remember, no data exist to suggest that menopause itself causes depression; in fact, most studies indicate that perimenopausal women are no more depressed, on average, than anyone else. If you learn to deal with stress through a daily yoga and meditation practice, this will help enormously should you find yourself depressed or inexplicably moody.

As Suzanne found after that unfortunate incident in the supermarket, inversions can be a woman's best friend. They can help balance your endocrine system and improve circulation to your pituitary, thyroid, parathyroid, and hypothalamus glands and your brain.

Patricia agrees that inversions can help balance mood swings and every woman's practice should include some. Supported inversions and backbends (using a chair or bolster) help to pacify your nerves and cool your brain, but also generate a more balanced energy. Since she began having perimenopausal symptoms several years ago, Patricia begins her daily practice with Bound Angle Pose (Baddha Konasana) and Wide-Angle Seated Pose I (Upavistha Konasana I) and includes the "suptas"—reclining poses like Reclining Bound Angle Pose (Supta Baddha Konasana) and Reclining Hero Pose (Supta Virasana)—and supported Bridge Pose (Setu Bandha Sarvangasana).

If Sirsasana (Headstand) is not part of your practice or makes you feel agitated, Patricia recommends Downward-Facing Dog Pose (Adho Mukha Svanasana) and Wide-Angle Standing Forward Bend (Prasarita Padottanasana) instead. Shoulderstand (Sarvangasana) or a modified version of it, Half-Plough Pose (Ardha Halasana) or full Plough Pose (Halasana), and Legs-Up-the-Wall Pose (Viparita Karani) work well, too. (In addition to the sequences in this chapter, refer to the sequence for PMS in chapter 5.)

Patricia says forward bends can also help alleviate moodiness brought on by perimenopause. However, if you suffer from long-standing depression or deep despair, forward bends may make symptoms worse, giving you the feeling that the world is closing in on you. (For that type of depression, please refer to chapter 10).

INSOMNIA

Not being able to get a good night's sleep can seriously aggravate perimenopausal symptoms. Women generally say they could deal with mood swings a lot easier if they could only sleep through the night. (If night sweats keep you from sleeping, refer to the suggestions for hot flashes on pages 237–238.)

Herbal teas with valerian, hops, and chamomile soothe your mind and promote sleep. If you feel nervous or jittery, a tincture of mother-wort should take the edge off. Balancing your adrenals and calming your sympathetic nervous system also can't hurt. Rosemary Gladstar suggests herbs such as dong quai, St. John's Wort, Siberian ginseng, black cohosh, and sarsaparilla. Check with your herbalist or health care practitioner for doses that work for you.

Of course, nothing will make your insomnia go away unless you change your lifestyle and decrease your stress level. Ayurvedic physicians remind us that we can make a few very simple changes to lessen our stress and promote a good night's sleep:

- Go to bed at the same time each night (preferably by 10:00 PM) and get up early (by 6:00 AM, if possible).
- Eat your main meal at midday and a light dinner by 6:00 PM. Avoid stimulants, such as caffeine and alcohol, after dinner.
- Avoid stimulating activities just before bed.
- Unless it triggers night sweats, take a warm bath scented with sleep-inducing aromatherapy—try lavender essential oil—to promote sleep.
- Exercise early in the day—aerobic activity like walking or jogging, energizing yoga sequences, and pranayama practice.
- Set aside some "worry time" so you can clear your mind before bedtime.
- Drink warm milk/soy milk seasoned with honey and cardamom to calm and relax your nerves.

How Yoga Can Help

A daily yoga practice that combines active standing poses and back-bends with more restorative poses first tires you out and then calms your nerves, quiets your mind, and relaxes your body.

FUZZY THINKING

Short-term memory loss is a common symptom of perimenopause, but you'll be happy to know that, like most of the other symptoms, it is only temporary and does not indicate premature senility. In fact, it appears to be associated with the hormonal fluctuations your body is experiencing. This type of fuzzy thinking is no different from what many women encounter when they go through puberty, pregnancy, or even the postpartum months. Again, it's not the drop in estrogen that befuddles your brain, but the wild hormonal highs and lows that leave you wondering whether you've lost your mind. Take heart. Once the fluctuations subside, your ability to think clearly and rationally should return.

How Yoga Can Help

Not surprisingly, yoga helps you clear your mind and, although it can't promise you'll always remember where you put your keys, it can quiet the chatter and remove the cobwebby feeling that plagues many women during this time. Turning upside down helps increase circulation to your brain and balances your glandular system (which calms fluctuating hormones). Corpse Pose (Savasana) is everyone's favorite resting pose and helps soothe your nerves, calm your mind, and put your body into a complete state of repose. It's particularly beneficial when fuzzy thinking is exacerbated by a lack of sleep or increased agitation.

Incorporating yoga postures into your daily routine may clear the cobwebs, but don't expect it to solve your fuzzy thinking if you don't make other changes to your daily routine. The following sections provide some other suggestions to try.

Diet

Eat a healthy, balanced diet. Avoid alcohol (which can make fuzzy thinking even fuzzier), white sugar, and caffeine. Eat plenty of organic fresh fruits and vegetables, and drink lots of water. Keep your blood sugar under control by eating several small meals throughout the day, rather than three large ones. Anyone who's ever suffered from hypoglycemia (low blood sugar) will acknowledge how it can bring on foggy thinking.

Complementary Medicine

Many studies in Germany and the United States have shown that ginkgo helps increase circulation to your brain and improves oxygen delivery (much like yoga inversions). Herbalist Susun Weed swears by sage, which she says will help bring you not only clarity, but a sense of calm and well-being, too. Rosemary Gladstar recommends American ginseng to slowly replenish the life force (chi or prana) in your body. She says it brings grounded energy, which can help you think more clearly. Be sure to confer with an experienced herbalist who can help you select high-quality ginseng.

Attitude

Above all, remember that your fuzzy thinking is temporary. Think of menopause as the journey into your wisdom years. As a result of that journey, your thought processes may shift to accommodate a more intuitive, heart-based self. That doesn't mean you can no longer think logically and clearly. It only means that you're honing your ability to take in the big picture, to understand the world as a whole. Don't be surprised if your linear, rational thinking takes a backseat for a time while you explore this new side of yourself. Now may be the time for you to think with your heart as well as your head.

FATIGUE

Of all the symptoms women complain about in perimenopause, fatigue is second only to hot flashes. Even women who think of themselves as asymptomatic admit to inexplicable weariness. Although fatigue can result from lack of sleep, hot flashes, and heavier/longer periods, many women can find no real reason for feeling zapped of their usual get-up-and-go. Krishna Raman, in *A Matter of Health*, blames depleted adrenals for the lack of energy. He says women need a daily yoga practice that massages and stimulates their adrenal glands in order to replenish their energy levels.

Patricia warns that you can't tone and invigorate your adrenals without first pacifying them and quieting your sympathetic nervous system. You can use forward bends to do that. Then standing poses like Extended Triangle Pose (Utthita Trikonasana) and Half-Moon Pose (Ardha Chandrasana) performed against a wall will invigorate your glands; backbends will squeeze them and rid them of stale blood; and twists will rinse them with fresh, oxygenated blood. In other words, a well-rounded daily yoga practice is what works.

OTHER SYMPTOMS

Headaches

Some women who experience premenstrual headaches find that they worsen during perimenopause. Menstrual migraine sufferers may not get a break in perimenopause either, especially those whose headaches are sensitive to hormonal fluctuations. Refer to chapter 9 for specific yoga poses to help tension headaches and migraines.

Watch your diet as well. Many women react badly to alcohol, estrogenic foods like meat, and vegetables from the nightshade family such as tomatoes, eggplant, and potatoes. Ayurvedic physicians blame irregular sleep and eating patterns for migraines, and caution that emotional stress doesn't help matters.

Urinary Incontinence

Although some perimenopausal women have trouble with weak bladders or pelvic floor muscles, this symptom is more common among older women who have stopped bleeding. See chapter 13 for a discussion of incontinence and what to do about it.

Heart Palpitations

Many women experience rapid, irregular heartbeats at times and admit they can be scary. Usually associated with hot flashes, palpitations don't mean you're having a heart attack or that you've suddenly developed coronary heart disease. If you have grown up with a mitral valve prolapse or a slight heart murmur—two fairly common conditions for women—you may experience palpitations more frequently during perimenopause. Thinner women complain about these fibrillations more often than their heavier friends. Hot flashes, free-floating anxiety, and agitation can all bring on bouts of erratic heart rhythm. Follow the suggestions for diet, yoga, herb therapy, and stress relief that we described earlier for hot flashes and mood swings. Hypoglycemia and insomnia-induced fatigue can make palpitations worse, so get plenty of rest, eat regular meals, and stay away from caffeine and sugar.

Free-Floating Anxiety

Nervousness or anxiety with no apparent cause, another common complaint among perimenopausal women, generally indicates fluctuating hormones. Many women I spoke to complained that since they've entered perimenopause they worry about things that never would have concerned them before. My own experience bears that out. Too often I have felt like a bundle of nerves just waiting for something to make me anxious.

Do the yoga sequence in this chapter for erratic mood swings or simply choose a few of the poses there. As Patricia says, you'll need to experiment, because some of the poses might be too energizing if you suffer from fatigue as well as anxiety. Restorative poses help mitigate the weariness, but Patricia cautions that sometimes what you need when you feel really tired is the jump-start that standing poses and inversions can provide. Find what works best for you; if Headstand (Sirsasana) makes you feel more agitated or brings on hot flashes, don't do it! The same goes for the standing or seated forward bends—if they generate too much heat or put too much strain on the backs of your legs, support your head with bolsters, as described in the modifications, or omit these poses from your sequence.

A SEQUENCE FOR HOT FLASHES

1. Bound Angle Pose (Baddha Konasana)
2. Wide-Angle Seated Pose I (Upavistha Konasana I)
3. Head-on-Knee Pose (Janu Sirsasana)
4. Wide-Angle Standing Forward Bend (Prasarita Padottanasana)
5. Downward-Facing Dog Pose (Adho Mukha Svanasana)
6. Headstand (Sirsasana)
7. Shoulderstand (Sarvangasana)
8. Half-Plough Pose (Ardha Halasana)
9. Bridge Pose (Setu Bandha Sarvangasana)
10. Reclining Bound Angle Pose (Supta Baddha Konasana)
11. Legs-Up-the-Wall Pose (Viparita Karani)
12. Corpse Pose (Savasana)

1. BOUND ANGLE POSE (Baddha Konasana) Sit against the wall on a block or folded blanket (about 4 inches thick) with your back straight and your abdomen lifted. Bending your legs, open your knees out and bring the soles of your feet together. Hold the tops of your feet and draw your heels in toward your perineum or pubic bone. The outer edges of your feet should remain on the floor. Lengthen your spine upward, leading with the crown of your head. Stretching your inner thighs from the groin to the knee, gently lower your knees as far as possible. Place your hands behind you to sit up straighter, and lift your abdomen. Stay in this position for 1 minute or more, breathing normally. To come out, relax your arms by your sides and bring your knees up one at a time. Stretch your legs out in front of you.

EFFECTS This pose increases circulation to your abdomen and pelvis, toning and improving function in your reproductive organs.

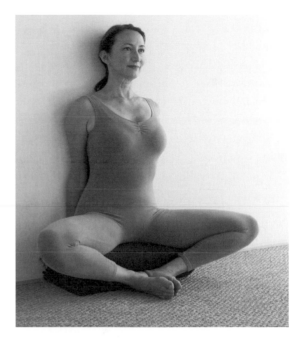

2. WIDE-ANGLE SEATED POSE I (Upavistha Konasana I) Sit against the wall on a block or a folded blanket (about 4 inches thick). Spread your legs wide apart and flex your feet. Adjust the flesh of your buttocks by drawing it behind you and out to the sides. Place your hands on the floor behind you, draw your abdomen and floating ribs up toward your chest, and pull your shoulder blades into your back. Sit up tall, stretching through your legs and keeping the knees straight. Stay in this pose for at least 1 minute. To come out, relax your arms and release your legs.

EFFECTS This pose helps increase circulation to your pelvis, stimulate and improve circulation to your ovaries, and lift and tone your uterus.

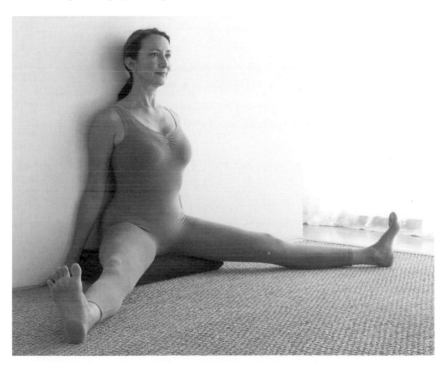

3. HEAD-ON-KNEE POSE (Janu Sirsasana) Sit on the floor in front of a padded chair with your legs stretched out in front of you. Bend your right knee to the side so it is at a 45-degree angle to your left leg and your right heel is near the right side of your groin. Push your right knee as far back as you comfortably can; keep your left leg straight.

Turn your abdomen and chest so your sternum (breastbone) is in line with the center of your left leg. As you inhale, lift your trunk up from the base of your pelvis; as you exhale, lean your trunk forward to rest your head on the chair. Fold your arms to cradle your head. Your head should rest without straining your neck.

Stay in this pose for 1 to 2 minutes, or as long as you're comfortable. Inhale while coming up, straighten your right leg, and reverse sides.

EFFECTS This pose helps revitalize your adrenal glands, which can help mitigate hot flashes.

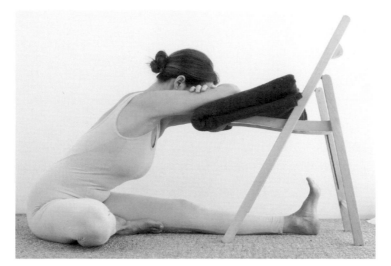

4. WIDE-ANGLE STANDING FORWARD BEND (Prasarita Padottanasana)
Place a folded blanket or a bolster vertically in front of you. Step your feet apart about 4 feet or so, keeping the outer edges of your feet parallel. Tighten your quadriceps (front thigh muscles) to draw your kneecaps up and keep your thighs well lifted. On an exhalation, bend forward from your hips, place your hands on the floor between your feet. Lift your hips toward the ceiling, draw your shoulders blades into your back, and bend your elbows, releasing the crown of your head onto your support. Keep your legs firm, but relax your shoulders and neck. Breathe deeply and let your trunk release downward. Stay in this pose for 1 minute. To come out, bring your hands to your hips, and raise your trunk. Step your feet together.

EFFECTS This pose helps calm your mind and relieve the stress that can cause hot flashes.

5. DOWNWARD-FACING DOG POSE (Adho Mukha Svanasana) Place a bolster or one or two folded blankets vertically so your support is in line with your sternum, and come to your hands and knees, turning your toes under.

Exhale, press your hands firmly into the mat and extend up through your inner arms. Exhale again as you raise your buttocks high in the air and move your thighs up and back. Keep stretching through your legs and bring your heels toward the floor. Keep the legs firm and the elbows straight as you lift your buttocks upward. The action of the arms and legs serves to elongate your spine and release your head. Hold this pose for 30 seconds to

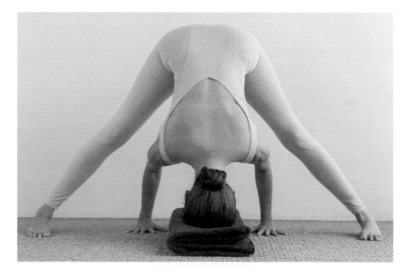

1 minute, breathing deeply. Let your head rest completely and release the base of your neck. To come out, return to your hands and knees. Bring your feet together, keep your knees slightly spread, and sit back on your heels.

EFFECTS Try this pose to relieve anxiety, tone and relax your nervous system, and relieve hot flashes.

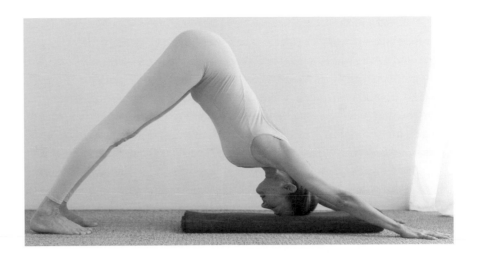

6. HEADSTAND† **(Sirsasana)** (Before beginning, see pages 16–17.) Place a folded blanket against the wall. Kneel in front of it with your feet and knees together. Interlace your fingers firmly, thumbs touching and your hands cupped. Position your hands no more than 3 inches from the wall with your elbows shoulder-width apart and wrists perpendicular to the floor. Your wrists, forearms, and elbows form the foundation for this pose.

Lengthen your neck and place the crown of your head on the blanket. The back of your head should be in contact with your hands. Press your forearms into the floor and lift your shoulders away from the floor. Straighten your legs, raise your hips, and walk your feet in until your spine is almost perpendicular to the floor. Exhale, bend your legs, and bring your feet to the wall.

Straighten your legs and keep your heels and buttocks against the wall. Roll your thighs in, lift your tailbone, lengthen your legs upward, and keep your feet together. Keep your breathing even, your eyes and throat soft, and your abdomen relaxed.

LEG VARIATIONS FOR ADVANCED PRACTITIONERS Spread your legs wide, stretching from your groin to your heels (see page 115). Keeping your legs straight, stretch up through your spine and broaden your chest. Remain this way for 10 to 15 seconds.

Next, bend your legs, spread your knees outward, and press the soles of your feet firmly together. Remain in this position for another 15 to 20 seconds, keeping your knees wide apart, and breathe normally. Straighten your legs and return to the wide-leg position, then to your original Headstand position, before coming down.

To come out, exhale, bend your knees, and bring your feet to the floor. Finish by resting in Child's Pose (Adho Mukha Virasana) (see page 230).

EFFECTS This pose helps stimulate blood flow to your brain. Many women find standing on their heads helps relieve hot flashes.

†CAUTION Do this pose only if it is already part of your yoga practice. Do not do this pose if you have high blood pressure, are menstruating, or suffer from neck or back problems or migraines.

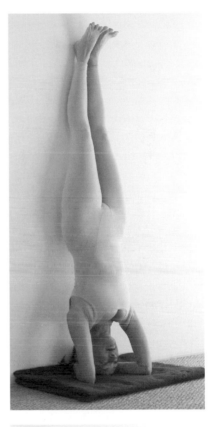

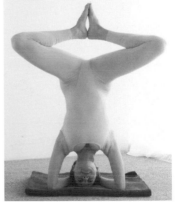

Variation

7. SHOULDERSTAND† **(Sarvangasana)** (Before beginning, see page 50.) Place a chair with its back about 8 to 10 inches away from the wall. Put a folded blanket on the chair seat, and two or three folded blankets in front of the chair. Sit backward on the chair with your legs bent over the top of the back; move your buttocks into the center of the chair seat.

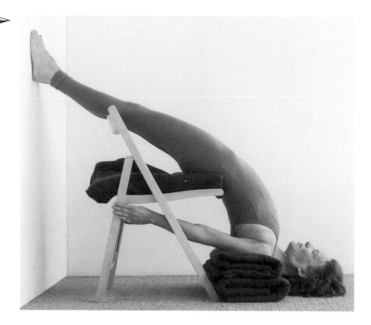

Holding the sides and then the front legs of the chair, slowly lower your torso so your shoulders are on the blankets and your head is on the floor. You must extend your spine and open your chest while doing this to get the proper position. Move your hands, one at a time, to hold the back legs of the chair; your arms should be between the front legs. Stretch your legs, extend from your groin to your heels. Rotate your thighs in, and rest your heels against the wall or lift your legs straight up. Close your eyes, breathe normally, and bring your chest toward your chin. Hold this pose for 3 to 5 minutes, or as long as you're comfortable.

To release from the pose, bend your knees, place your feet on the chair back, and slide down until your sacrum rests on the bolster and your calves are on the chair seat. Roll to your side and sit up slowly.

EFFECTS This pose is calming and soothing for your nervous system and excellent for relieving hot flashes.

†CAUTION Do not do this pose if you suffer from neck or shoulder problems, if you have high blood pressure, if you are menstruating, or if you have a migraine or tension headache.

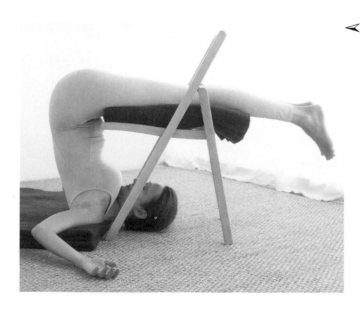

8. HALF-PLOUGH POSE† **(Ardha Halasana)** Place a folded blanket on top of your sticky mat with the rounded edge near the legs of a chair. Lie on your back with your legs outstretched, your shoulders on the blanket, and your head beneath the chair seat. As you exhale, bend your knees and swing or lift your buttocks and legs, so your thighs rest completely on the chair seat. (Pad the seat with blankets if you need more height for your legs to be parallel to the floor.) Move your chest in toward your chin (not your chin toward your chest). Rest here, with your palms up and your eyes closed, for as long as you like—at least 3 to 5 minutes—breathing deeply. To come out, place your hands on your back and slowly roll down, one vertebra at a time. Roll to one side and sit up.

EFFECTS This pose helps calm anxiety and nervousness and relieve hot flashes.

†CAUTION Do not do this pose if you suffer from neck or shoulder problems, or if you have your period.

9. BRIDGE POSE (Setu Bandha Sarvangasana) Place a bolster horizontally against the wall and another vertically, forming a T shape. Spread a folded blanket on the floor at the end of the vertical bolster that is farthest from the wall (for your head). Sit on the end of the vertical bolster that is closest to the wall. Keeping your knees bent, lie back over the bolster. Slide down until the end of the bolster is in the middle of your back and your shoulders just reach the floor. Rest your shoulders and head on the blanket. Stretch your legs toward the wall and put your heels on the horizontal bolster so your feet touch the wall. Your legs should be straight out in front of you, hip-width apart. Rest your

arms in any comfortable position—over your head or out by your sides. Close your eyes and relax completely, breathing deeply. Stay in this position for 5 to 10 minutes, or as long as you like.

To come out, bend your knees and slowly roll to one side. Using your hands, push yourself up to a seated position.

EFFECTS This pose is great if you're trying to cool down your hot flashes and rebalance your thyroid and parathyroid glands.

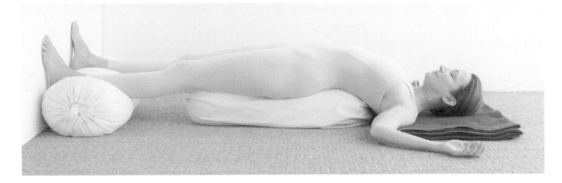

10. RECLINING BOUND ANGLE POSE (Supta Baddha Konasana) Place a bolster vertically behind you and sit just in front of it with your knees bent and your sacrum touching the bolster's edge. Place a strap behind your back, at your sacrum; draw it forward over your hips, across your shins, and under your feet (see page xv). Put the soles of your feet together and let your knees and thighs fall to the sides. Cinch the strap securely under your feet. Lie back so your head and torso rest comfortably on the bolster and your buttocks and legs are on the floor. (If you feel any discomfort in your lower back, add

some height to your support with a folded blanket or two. If you feel any strain in your neck, place a folded blanket under your head and neck. Rest in this pose for as long as you like, breathing deeply.

To come out, draw your knees together, slip the strap off, and slowly roll to one side. Use your hands to push yourself up to a seated position.

EFFECTS This pose is comforting, cooling, and supportive when you have hot flashes.

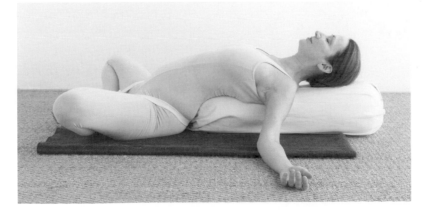

11. LEGS-UP-THE-WALL POSE† (Viparita Karani) Place a bolster about 3 inches from the wall. (If you are tall, you may need a higher support, such as a folded blanket on top of the bolster.) Sit on the bolster so your right hip and side are touching the wall. Using your hands to support you, lean back and swivel your body around, taking your right leg and then your left leg up the wall. Keep your buttocks close to or against the wall. (If you feel stiffness or discomfort in your legs, push your buttocks slightly away from the wall.) Lie down so your lower back and ribs are supported by the bolster and your shoulders and head are on the floor. (If your neck is uncomfortable, put a folded towel or blanket under it.) Extend through your legs and place your arms out at your sides, elbows bent and palms up. Without moving your torso, allow your legs to open out to the sides. Remain in this position, breathing normally, for 3 to 5 minutes. (If you wish, you can drape an eyebag over your eyes to help remove all distractions.)

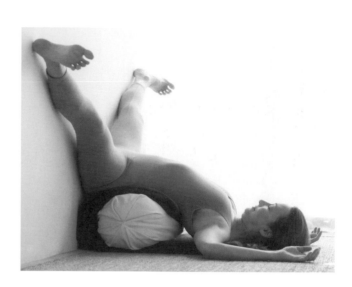

To come out, place your feet on the wall and gently push yourself off the bolster. Slowly roll to one side and push up to a seated position.

EFFECTS If you experience a jittery feeling with your hot flashes, this pose may be all you need to feel more balanced and in control.

†CAUTION This pose may be done during menstruation if you don't use a bolster; your pelvis should not be higher than your chest when you are menstruating.

12. CORPSE POSE (Savasana) Lie on your back with your legs stretched out in front of you. Place a folded blanket under your neck and head, if you wish. Alternatively, if you want to practice Interval Breathing (see sidebar), lie back on a vertical bolster with a folded blanket at one end for your head. Place your arms comfortably at your sides, slightly away from your torso, with your palms facing upward. Actively stretch your arms and legs away from you, then allow them to release completely. Close your eyes and let everything relax. Visualize heat rising up and out of you with every breath you take. An eyebag draped over your eyes will help quiet external distractions. Remain in this pose, breathing normally, for at least 10 minutes.

EFFECTS This pose helps relieve anxiety, nervous tension, and hot flashes. It may also calm your nervous system and relax your mind.

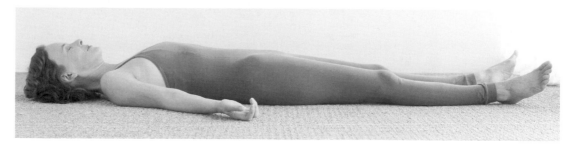

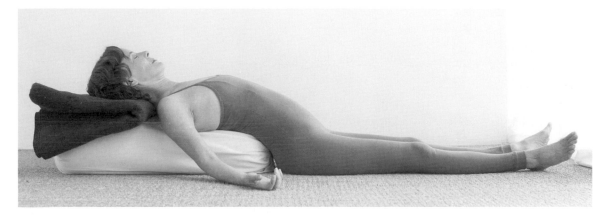

Interval Breathing (Viloma) ʌ

Interval breathing is a wonderful way to bring a sense of lightness to your body and mind. It can also help calm your nervous system and relieve the jittery nerves that sometimes accompany hot flashes.

While you are lying in Corpse Pose (Savasana), with your sternum lifted by a bolster and blanket, begin by inhaling normally, and then exhaling slowly and deeply without force. Your exhalation should last for 2 to 3 seconds. At the end of the exhalation, pause for 2 seconds before beginning inhaling again. This is one complete cycle of Interval Breathing (Viloma).

Repeat this cycle several times, until your breath fades effortlessly at the end of the exhalation and begins easily after the pause. Your exhalations should continue to be longer than your inhalations. Do 15 to 20 cycles over the course of 10 minutes, focusing on the sense of peace and calm that comes in the silence of the pause. Return to your normal breathing and rest in Corpse Pose (Savasana) for several more minutes.

A SEQUENCE FOR HEAVY OR IRREGULAR PERIODS

1. Bound Angle Pose (Baddha Konasana)
2. Wide-Angle Seated Pose I (Upavistha Konasana I)
3. Reclining Bound Angle Pose (Supta Baddha Konasana)
4. Wide-Angle Standing Forward Bend (Prasarita Padottanasana)
5. Bridge Pose (Setu Bandha Sarvangasana)
6. Corpse Pose (Savasana)

1. BOUND ANGLE POSE (Baddha Konasana) Do Bound Angle Pose as described on page 247. Remain in the pose for 30 seconds or more, breathing normally.

EFFECTS This pose helps strengthen your uterus, kidneys, and bladder.

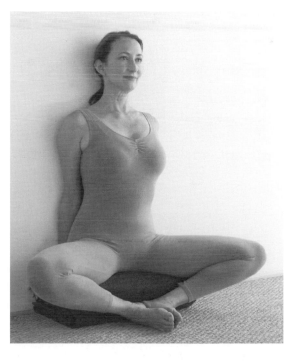

**2. WIDE-ANGLE SEATED POSE I
(Upavistha Konasana I)** Do Wide-Angle
Seated Pose I as described on page 247.
Remain in the pose for at least 30
seconds or more, breathing normally.

EFFECTS Try this pose to help improve
circulation to your reproductive organs
and regulate your menstrual flow.

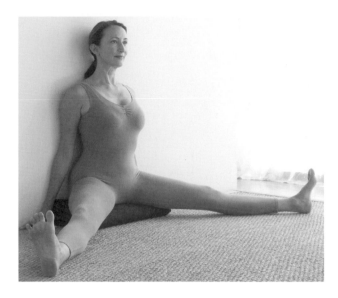

**3. RECLINING BOUND ANGLE POSE (Supta
Baddha Konasana)** Sit in the middle of a vertical
bolster with a folded blanket at the end for your
head. Place a strap behind your back, at your
sacrum; draw it forward over your hips, across
your shins, and under your feet (see page xv). Put
the soles of your feet together and let your knees
and thighs fall to the sides. Cinch the strap
securely under your feet. Lie back so your head
and shoulders are off the bolster. Breathe normally, softening your belly and releasing your
pelvic floor. Remain in this pose at least 5 to 10
minutes. To come out, draw your knees together,
slip the strap off, roll to one side, and sit up.

EFFECTS This pose helps relieve cramping and
spasms associated with heavy bleeding.

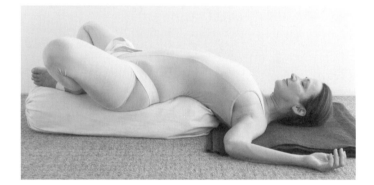

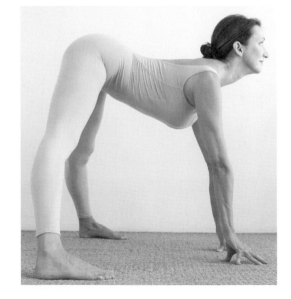

**4. WIDE-ANGLE STANDING FORWARD BEND (Prasarita Padot-
tanasana)** Step your feet about 4 feet apart, keeping the outer
edges of your feet parallel. Tighten your quadriceps to draw your
kneecaps up and keep your thighs well lifted. On an exhalation,
bend forward from your hips and place your hands on the floor
between your feet. (If you feel strain in your lower back, place
your hands on blocks.) Lift your hips toward the ceiling, draw
your shoulder blades into your back, and look up as you extend
your chest forward, keeping your entire spine concave. Remain
this way for 10 to 15 seconds. To come up, bring your hands to
your hips and raise your trunk.

EFFECTS This pose helps lift and strengthen your uterus and may
lessen heavy bleeding. Also relieves fatigue.

5. BRIDGE POSE (Setu Bandha Sarvangasana) Do Bridge Pose as described on page 251. Remain in the pose for as long as you like, but at least 5 to 10 minutes.

EFFECTS Try this pose to help tone and rejuvenate your reproductive organs and relieve fatigue.

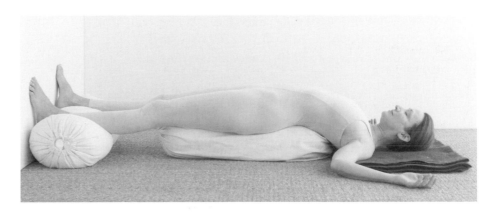

6. CORPSE POSE (Savasana) Do Corpse Pose as described on page 252, taking care to completely relax your belly and pelvic floor. Remain in this pose for at least 5 to 10 minutes, breathing normally.

EFFECTS This is a calming, relaxing pose for your entire body.

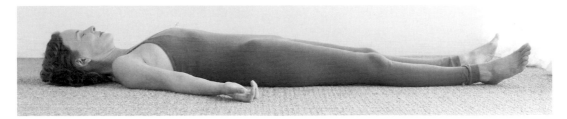

A SEQUENCE FOR ERRATIC MOOD SWINGS

1. Downward-Facing Dog Pose (Adho Mukha Svanasana)
2. Standing Forward Bend (Uttanasana)
3. Wide-Angle Standing Forward Bend (Prasarita Padottanasana)
4. Headstand (Sirsasana)
5. Inverted Staff Pose (Viparita Dandasana)
6. Shoulderstand (Sarvangasana)
7. Half-Plough Pose (Ardha Halasana)
8. Bridge Pose (Setu Bandha Sarvangasana)
9. Legs-Up-the-Wall Pose (Viparita Karani) and Cycle
10. Corpse Pose (Savasana)

1. DOWNWARD-FACING DOG POSE (Adho Mukha Svanasana)
Do Downward-Facing Dog Pose as described on page 248. You can rest your head on folded blankets or a bolster or two, depending on your flexibility. Remain in this position for 1 to 2 minutes, or as long as you are comfortable.

EFFECTS This pose helps calm jittery nerves, relax your mind, and bring a sense of release and relief.

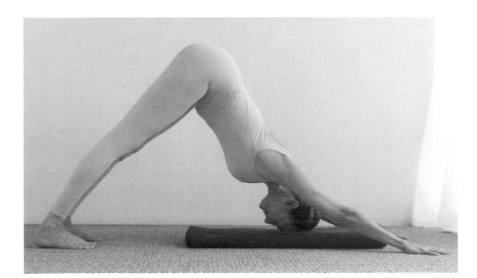

2. STANDING FORWARD BEND (Uttanasana) Stand up straight facing a padded chair; distribute your weight evenly between the front of your feet and your heels. Tighten your knees by pulling your quadriceps up. Raise your sternum and broaden your chest by rolling your shoulders back and drawing your shoulder blades in. Lift your abdomen and pull your tailbone in without pushing your thighs forward. Put your hands on your hips and as you exhale, extend your spine and bend forward from your hips. Rest your forehead on the chair seat and close your eyes. Fold your arms over your head or let them dangle by your sides. Relax the base of your skull, your neck, your shoulders, and your abdomen. Relax in this position for 1 to 2 minutes, or as long as you like. Release your arms and slowly stand up. Your head should come up last.

EFFECTS This calming, stabilizing pose is good for your nervous system, may increase circulation to your brain, and helps relieve agitation.

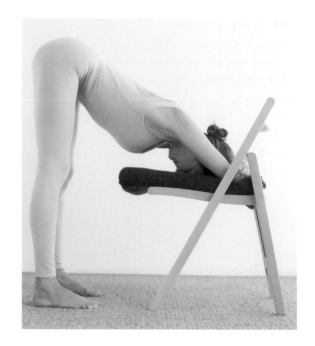

3. WIDE-ANGLE STANDING FORWARD BEND (Prasarita Padottanasana) Do this pose as described on page 248, remaining at least 1 to 2 minutes.

EFFECTS This pose offers many of the same benefits as Headstand (Sirsasana), if the latter is not part of your practice.

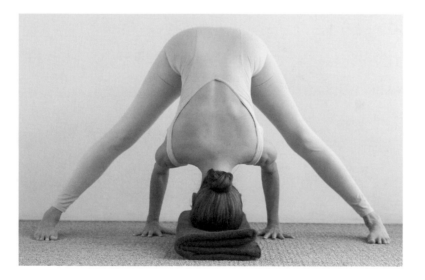

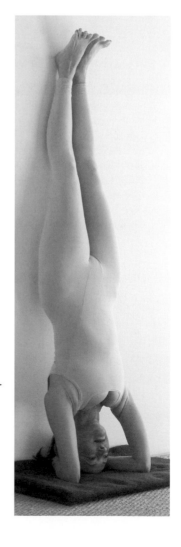

4. HEADSTAND† (Sirsasana) Do Headstand as described on page 249.

EFFECTS You may use this pose to help clear your mind, increase blood flow to your brain, and revitalize your whole body so you can think and act more clearly.

†CAUTION Do this pose only if it is already part of your yoga practice. Do not do this pose if you have high blood pressure, have your period, or suffer from neck or back problems or migraines.

5. INVERTED STAFF POSE† (Viparita Dandasana) (Before beginning, see pages 34–35.) Place a folded blanket on a chair that has been placed about 2 feet from the wall— far enough away so your feet can press into the wall when your legs are outstretched. Place a bolster (or two, depending on your flexibility) in front of the chair to support your head. Sit backward on the chair, facing the wall, with your feet through the chair back. Letting your hands slide down the sides of the chair, lean back slowly until your head and neck extend past the front of the chair seat.

Still holding the sides of the chair, arch back so your shoulder blades are at the front edge of the seat. (You may need to scoot your buttocks farther toward the back of the seat.) Take your feet to the wall, legs slightly bent, and move your hands to the back legs of the chair (your arms should be between the front legs). Rest your head on your support. Lengthen your legs, pressing the chair away from the wall, and roll your thighs in toward each other. (If you feel strain in your lower back, rest your feet on bolsters or a low stool.) Breathe quietly for 1 to 2 minutes. If you can't maintain the pose that long, do it for 30 seconds, sit up, and repeat a couple of times.

To come out, bend your knees and place your feet flat on the floor. Hold on to the sides of the chair back and carefully come up, lifting from your sternum. Lean over the chair back for a few breaths to release your back.

EFFECTS Placing your head on a bolster creates a more cooling, calming effect for your mind, which helps restore equilibrium when you suffer from erratic mood swings.

†CAUTION Do not do this pose if you have neck problems, a migraine or tension headache, or diarrhea. If this pose is too difficult, substitute Cross Bolsters Pose (see page 220).

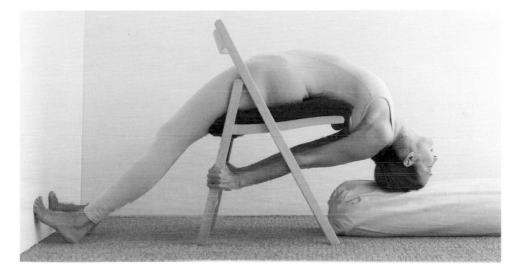

6. SHOULDERSTAND† (Sarvangasana)
Do Shoulderstand as described on page 50. Remain in the pose, breathing normally, for several minutes.

EFFECTS This pose helps soothe your nerves and restore balance to your mind. Some women find it helps cultivate patience and emotional stability.

†CAUTION Do not do this pose if you suffer from neck or shoulder problems, if you have high blood pressure, if you are menstruating, or if you have a migraine or tension headache.

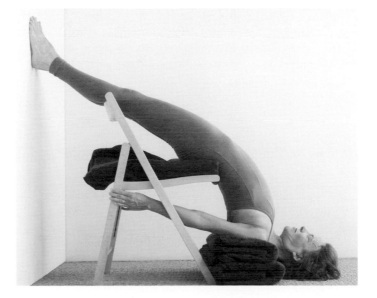

7. HALF-PLOUGH POSE† **(Ardha Halasana)** Do Half-Plough Pose as described on page 250. Stay in the pose for 3 to 5 minutes, breathing calming, nurturing energy into your whole body.

EFFECTS This pose helps to calm anxiety and jittery nerves and to relieve tension headaches, while bringing clarity and peace to erratic emotions.

†CAUTION Do not do this pose if you suffer from neck or shoulder problems, or if you have your period.

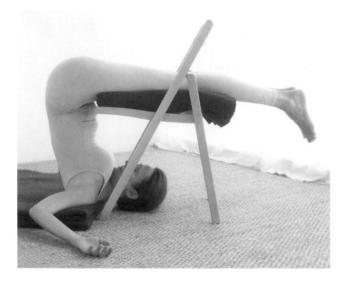

8. BRIDGE POSE (Setu Bandha Sarvangasana) Do Bridge Pose as described on page 251. Breathe normally, with a slight emphasis on the exhalation for a calming effect. Remain in this pose as long as you like, at least 3 to 5 minutes.

9. LEGS-UP-THE-WALL POSE† **(Viparita Karani) AND CYCLE** Place a bolster about 3 inches from the wall. (If you are tall, you may need a higher support, such as a folded blanket on top of the bolster.) Sit on the bolster so your right hip and side are touching the wall. Using your hands to support you, lean back and swivel your body around, taking your right leg and then your left leg up the wall. Keep your buttocks close to or against the wall. (If you feel stiffness or discomfort in your legs, push your buttocks slightly away from the wall.) Lie down so your lower back and ribs are supported by the bolster, and your shoulders and head are on the floor (A). (If your neck is uncomfortable, put a folded towel or blanket under it.) Extend through your legs and place your arms out at your sides, elbows bent and palms up. Rest in this position, eyes closed, for 5 minutes.

CYCLE Without moving your torso, open your legs out to the sides (B). Remain in this position, breathing normally, for 3 to 5 minutes.

Bend your knees, cross your legs at the ankles, and continue for another 3 to 5 minutes (C).

Push away from the wall until your buttocks are just off the bolster and resting on the floor; the backs of your thighs rest on the bolster (D). Remain in this position for 5 minutes, or as long as you like.

To come out of the pose, uncross your legs, push gently away from the bolster, and roll to one side. Then use your arms to help you to a seated position.

EFFECTS This calming cycle helps restore your body, mind, and spirit, leaving you feeling refreshed.

†CAUTION This pose may be done during menstruation if you don't use a bolster; your pelvis should not be higher than your chest when you are menstruating.

EFFECTS Supporting your body with bolsters and your head and neck with a blanket allows you to relax completely into the pose. Creating space in your abdomen and chest helps when you feel irritable.

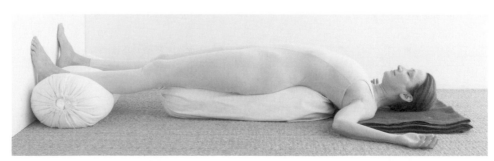

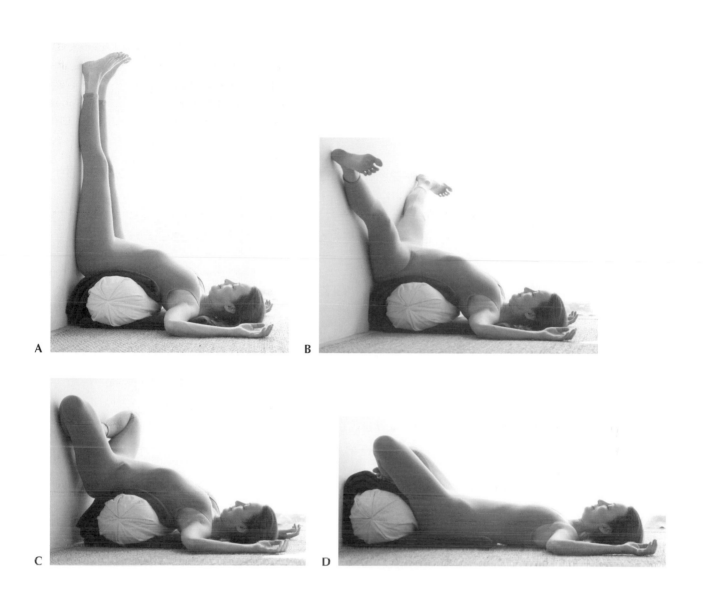

A

B

C

D

10. CORPSE POSE (Savasana) Do Corpse Pose as described on page 252. Remain in this pose for at least 5 to 10 minutes, breathing normally.

EFFECTS This wonderfully rejuvenating pose helps calm and restore your mind and body, bringing balance to your sympathetic nervous system.

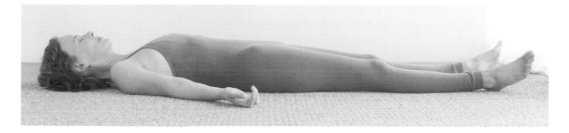

A SEQUENCE FOR INSOMNIA

1. Reclining Bound Angle Pose (Supta Baddha Konasana)
2. Downward-Facing Dog Pose (Adho Mukha Svanasana)
3. Standing Forward Bend (Uttanasana)
4. Headstand (Sirsasana)
5. Shoulderstand (Sarvangasana)
6. Half-Plough Pose (Ardha Halasana)
7. Bridge Pose (Setu Bandha Sarvangasana)
8. Easy Seated Forward Bend (Adho Mukha Sukhasana)
9. Corpse Pose (Savasana)

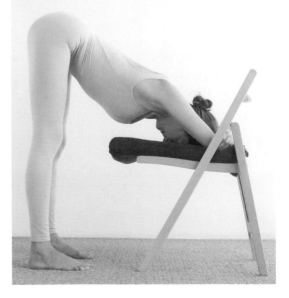

1. RECLINING BOUND ANGLE POSE (Supta Baddha Konasana) Do this pose as described on page 251. Rest quietly and breathe with emphasis on your exhalations for at least 5 minutes.

EFFECTS This pose improves circulation in your abdomen, helping to calm your nerves.

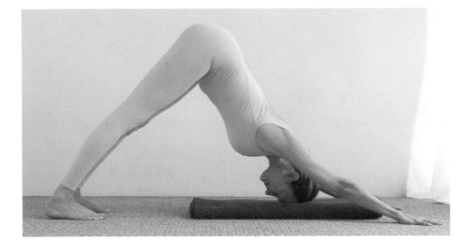

2. DOWNWARD-FACING DOG POSE (Adho Mukha Svanasana) Do Downward-Facing Dog Pose as described on page 248. Stay in the pose for as long as you like.

EFFECTS This pose relaxes your nervous system, relieving anxiety and tension.

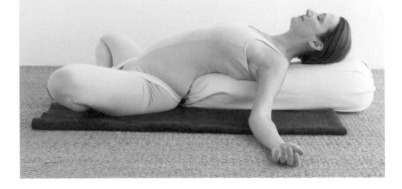

3. STANDING FORWARD BEND (Uttanasana) Do Standing Forward Bend as described on page 256. Remain in the pose for 1 to 2 minutes, if possible.

EFFECTS By soothing your sympathetic nervous system and easing tension, this pose can help combat insomnia.

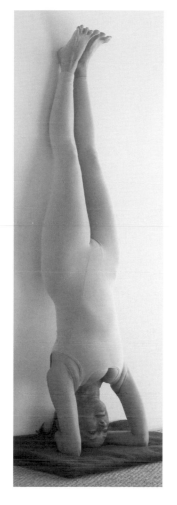

4. HEADSTAND† (Sirsasana) Do Headstand as described on page 249.

EFFECTS You can use this pose to help balance your endocrine system and relieve insomnia and nervous energy.

†CAUTION Do this pose only if it is already part of your yoga practice. Do not do this pose if you have high blood pressure, have your period, or suffer from neck or back problems or migraines.

5. SHOULDERSTAND† (Sarvangasana) Do Shoulderstand as described on page 250. Remain in this position for 5 to 10 minutes, keeping your breath calm and steady.

EFFECTS This pose helps soothe your nervous system and is especially useful in fighting insomnia, emotional distress, and irritability.

†CAUTION Do not do this pose if you suffer from neck or shoulder problems, if you have high blood pressure, if you are menstruating, or if you have a migraine or tension headache.

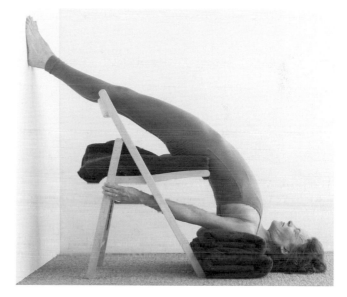

6. HALF-PLOUGH POSE† (Ardha Halasana) Do Half-Plough Pose as described on page 250. This modification allows you to maintain an internal focus and use your breath as a way of winding down.

EFFECTS Try this pose to help bring a sense of calm and clarity to your mind and body, balance your energy, and relieve anxiety.

†CAUTION Do not do this pose if you suffer from neck or shoulder problems, or if you have your period.

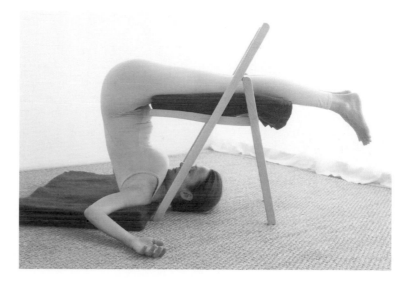

7. BRIDGE POSE (Setu Bandha Sarvangasana) Do Bridge Pose as described on page 251. Remain in the pose for 5 to 10 minutes, or as long as you like.

EFFECTS This pose can help calm nervousness and relieve anxiety to help you sleep.

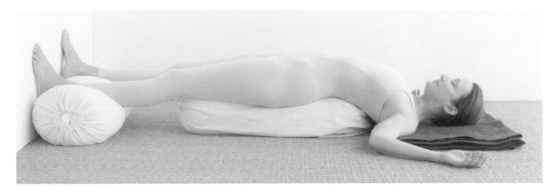

8. EASY SEATED FORWARD BEND (Adho Mukha Sukhasana) Sit in front of a vertical bolster or two (or a padded chair, depending on your flexibility) and cross your legs in front of you. On an inhalation, lift up from the base of your pelvis. As you exhale, bend your elbows and lean forward onto your support. Fold your arms above your head, turn your head to one side, and relax completely. Remain in the pose, breathing normally, up to 5 minutes.

EFFECTS This restful pose helps calm your nerves and prepare your body and mind for sleep.

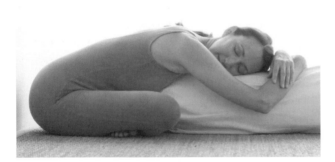

9. CORPSE POSE (Savasana) Do Corpse Pose as described on page 252. Remain in this pose for at least 5 to 10 minutes, focusing on your exhalations.

EFFECTS Relaxing, nourishing, and calming, this pose helps prepare your mind and body for a restful sleep.

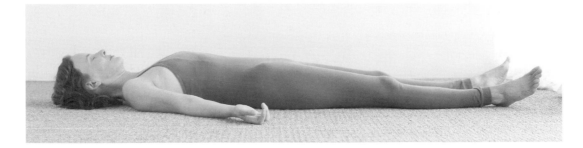

A SEQUENCE FOR FUZZY THINKING

1. Downward-Facing Dog Pose (Adho Mukha Svanasana)
2. Standing Forward Bend (Uttanasana)
3. Headstand (Sirsasana)
4. Shoulderstand (Sarvangasana)
5. Plough Pose (Halasana)
6. Bridge Pose (Setu Bandha Sarvangasana)
7. Legs-Up-the-Wall Pose (Viparita Karani)
8. Corpse Pose (Savasana)

Patricia Says

If you can, do these poses the way we present them here. You'll find they will engage your energy and keep you grounded in your body and in the moment, which may help get the cobwebs out. Of course, if any of the poses feel too challenging, either omit them or use the modifications appearing in the Woman's Restorative Sequence (see page 43).

1. DOWNWARD-FACING DOG POSE (Adho Mukha Svanasana) Lie face-down on your sticky mat. Place your palms on the floor by each side of your chest with your fingers well spread and pointing straight ahead. Come up on your hands and knees, and turn your toes under.

Exhale, press your hands firmly into the mat and extend up through your inner arms. Exhale again as you raise your buttocks high in the air and move your thighs up and back. Keep stretching through your legs and bring your heels toward the floor. Keep the legs firm and the elbows straight as you lift your buttocks upward. The action of the arms and legs serves to elongate your spine and release your head. Hold this pose for 30 seconds to 1 minute, breathing deeply. Let your head rest completely and release the base of your neck. To come out, either return to your hands and knees and sit back on your heels or step the feet forward into Standing Forward Bend (Uttanasana) and slowly stand up.

EFFECTS Doing this pose unsupported brings a sense of accomplishment and helps to ground you in the moment, calming and soothing your mind, relieving anxiety, and balancing your nervous system.

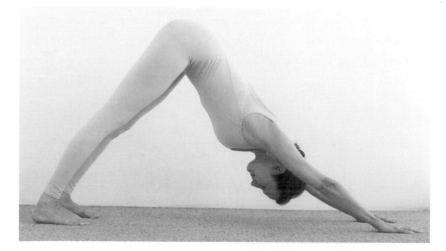

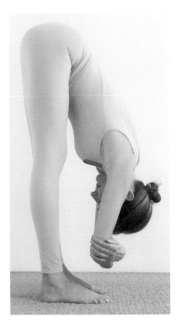

2. STANDING FORWARD BEND

(Uttanasana) Stand in Mountain Pose (Tadasana). Balance the weight evenly between your feet, lengthen up through your inner thighs, and roll your thighs in. Keep your legs firm as you lift your arms overhead, stretching up through your waist and ribs. Fold your arms and cup your elbows with your hands. As you exhale, bend forward from your hips with straight legs, and release your side body down. Continue to hold your elbows and release your spine. Breathe normally for 30 to 60 seconds. To come out, release your arms, and keeping your legs active, lift up slowly.

EFFECTS This pose can help increase blood flow to your brain and soothe your sympathetic nervous system, relieving anxiety and clearing foggy thoughts.

4. SHOULDERSTAND† (Sarvangasana) ➤

(Before beginning see pages 18–19.) Lie on your back with two folded blankets supporting your shoulders and your arms stretched out beside you. On an exhalation, bend your knees and raise your legs toward your chest. Pressing your hands into the floor, swing your bent legs over your head; support your back with your hands and press your elbows firmly into the blankets. Raise your torso up until it is perpendicular to the floor and your knees are close to your chest. Supporting your back, raise your legs until your thighs are parallel to the floor; raise them some more until your knees point toward the ceiling. Now raise your legs completely and extend up through your heels until your whole body is perpendicular to the floor. Move your tailbone up and in and use your hands to lift your back ribs. Feel that your whole body is long and straight. Move your shoulders away from your ears. Hold this pose as long as you can, at least 2 minutes. To come out, bend your knees and slowly roll down.

EFFECTS Like all inversions, this pose brings fresh blood to your endocrine glands and brain, helping to clear your thinking and reenergize you.

†CAUTION Do not do this pose if you suffer from neck or shoulder problems, if you have high blood pressure, or if you are menstruating.

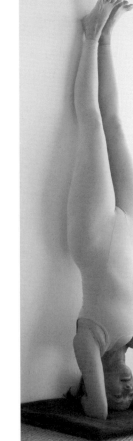

3. HEADSTAND† **(Sirsasana)** Do Headstand as described on page 249.

EFFECTS This balancing, energizing pose helps bring freshly oxygenated blood to your head and focus to your mind.

†CAUTION Do this pose only if it is already part of your yoga practice. Do not do this pose if you have high blood pressure, have your period, or suffer from neck or back problems or migraines.

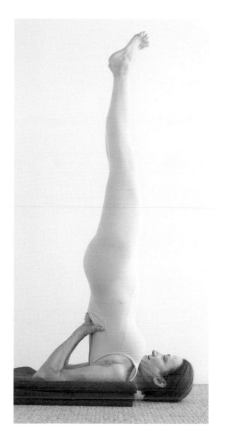

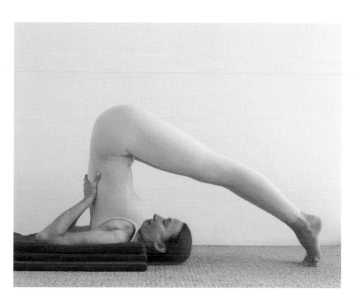

Λ **5. PLOUGH POSE**† **(Halasana)** From Shoulderstand (Sarvangasana), still supporting your back with your hands, extend your legs down over your head, placing your toes on the floor behind you. Keep your thighs active by tightening your knees to create space between your face and your legs. Remain in the pose for 1 to 2 minutes, breathing normally. To come out, slowly roll down one vertebra at a time.

EFFECTS This pose helps calm anxiety and nervousness and helps you think more clearly by bringing freshly oxygenated blood to your head.

†CAUTION Do not do this pose if you have neck problems or if you are menstruating.

6. BRIDGE POSE (Setu Bandha Sarvangasana)
Do Bridge Pose as described on page 251.

EFFECTS Supporting your body with bolsters and using a blanket for your head and neck allows you to relax completely into the pose. Your steady, comforting breath will help calm you if you feel anxious.

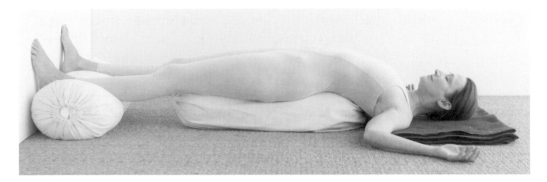

7. LEGS-UP-THE-WALL POSE† **(Viparita Karani)** Do Legs-Up-the-Wall Pose as described on page 258. Remain in this pose, with your eyes closed, for at least 5 to 10 minutes. Draping an eyebag over your eyes helps reduce outside distractions, bringing you a deeper feeling of calm and relaxation.

EFFECTS This restorative pose helps relieve agitation and anxiety, helping you to focus and think more clearly.

†CAUTION This pose may be done during menstruation if you don't use a bolster; your pelvis should not be higher than your chest when you are menstruating.

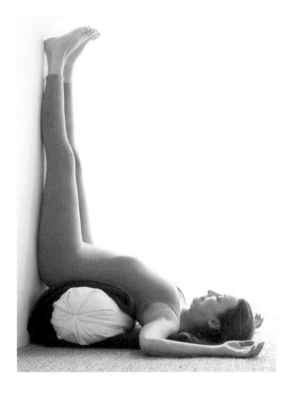

8. CORPSE POSE (Savasana) Do Corpse Pose as described on page 252. Remain in this pose for at least 5 to 10 minutes, breathing normally with a focus on your exhalations.

EFFECTS This restorative pose helps bring calm and clarity to your mind and refreshes and rejuvenates your whole body.

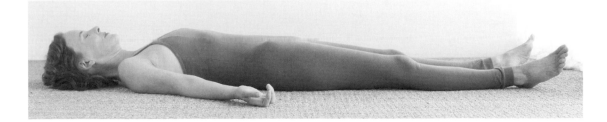

A SEQUENCE FOR FATIGUE

1. Reclining Bound Angle Pose
   (Supta Baddha Konasana)
2. Seated Forward Bend
   (Paschimottanasana)
3. Head-on-Knee Pose (Janu Sirsasana)
   or Easy Seated Forward Bend
   (Adho Mukha Sukhasana)
4. Simple Seated Twist Pose
   (Bharadvajasana)
5. Downward-Facing Dog Pose
   (Adho Mukha Svanasana)
6. Standing Forward Bend (Uttanasana)
7. Headstand (Sirsasana)
8. Inverted Staff Pose (Viparita Dandasana)
9. Shoulderstand (Sarvangasana)
10. Half-Plough Pose (Ardha Halasana)
11. Bridge Pose (Setu Bandha Sarvangasana)
12. Legs-Up-the-Wall Pose (Viparita Karani)
13. Corpse Pose (Savasana)

1. RECLINING BOUND ANGLE POSE (Supta Baddha Konasana) Do Reclining Bound Angle Pose as described on page 251. If this pose causes discomfort in your knees, simply cross your legs in front of you instead of binding them.

EFFECTS This pose should be extremely relaxing and restorative, helping to replenish your energy and improve circulation to your abdomen and heart.

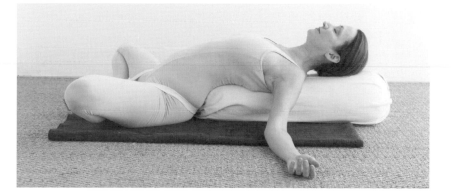

2. SEATED FORWARD BEND (Paschimottanasana)
Sit on your mat (or on one or two folded blankets) with your legs stretched out in front of you. Place a folded blanket or a bolster across your lower legs. Take a full, deep breath and lift your arms over your head, stretching up through your spine and lifting your sternum and head. Keep your back slightly concave. As you exhale, bend forward and extend your torso over your legs, cradling your head in your arms on your support. (If you feel strain in your back or in your legs, add more height to your support or rest your head on a padded chair.) Stay in the pose for 1 to 2 minutes, then slowly return to an upright position.

EFFECTS This pose helps bring a sense of safety and calm as it balances and restores your nervous system. You should feel refreshed and that your energy is more focused.

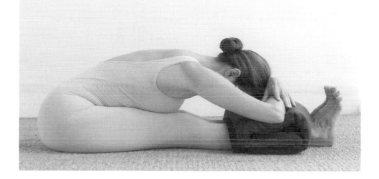

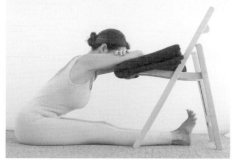

Modification

3. HEAD-ON-KNEE POSE† **(Janu Sirsasana)** Sit on the floor with your legs stretched out in front of you. Bend your right knee to the side so it is at a 45-degree angle to your left leg and your right heel is near the right side of your groin. Push your right knee as far back as you comfortably can; keep your left leg straight.

Place a folded blanket or a bolster on your outstretched leg, and turn your abdomen and chest so your sternum is in line with the center of your left leg. As you inhale, lift your trunk up from the base of your pelvis; as you exhale, reach your arms out in front of you as you lean your trunk forward. Fold your arms on your support and cradle your head on your arms. (If you feel any strain, add more height to your support or rest your head on a padded chair. If you still feel pressure or strain in your back or legs, do Easy Seated Forward Bend as described on page 262.)

Stay in this pose for at least 1 to 2 minutes, resting your head, the base of your skull, your eyes, and your brain. Inhale while coming up, straighten your right leg, and reverse sides by bending your left knee.

EFFECTS This pose helps calm your mind and your nerves.

†CAUTION Do not do this pose unsupported if you have diarrhea or feel nauseous.

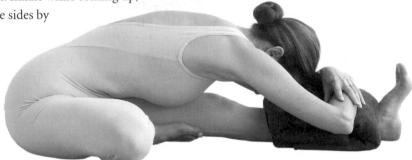

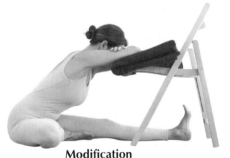

Modification

4. SIMPLE SEATED TWIST POSE† (Bharadvajasana) Sit up straight with your legs stretched out in front of you and your left hip elevated on two folded blankets. Bend both legs to the right so your feet are next to your right hip. Keeping your thighs and knees facing forward, make sure your right ankle rests on the arch of your left foot and your buttocks are not on your foot. Draw your shoulder blades into your back, broaden your chest, and extend your spine upward. On an exhalation, turn your abdomen, ribs, chest, and shoulders (in that order) to the left; place your right hand on the outside of your left thigh and your left hand on the blankets behind you. Remain in this pose for 20 to 30 seconds. Come back to the center position, straighten your legs, and change sides.

EFFECTS Gentle twists like this one replenish your adrenal glands, restore your nervous system, and bring energy and stability to your whole system.

†CAUTION Do not practice twists if you have diarrhea or feel nauseous. Do not do this pose if you have arthritis in your knees. If you suffer from sacroiliac pain, release your pelvis whenever you twist.

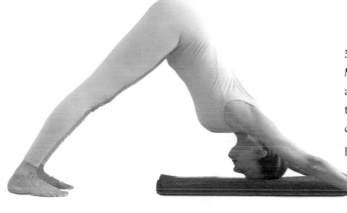

5. DOWNWARD-FACING DOG POSE (Adho Mukha Svanasana) Do Downward-Facing Dog as described on page 248. Remain in this position for 1 to 2 minutes, or as long as you are comfortable.

EFFECTS This pose helps calm jittery nerves, cool your mind, and give a sense of release and relief.

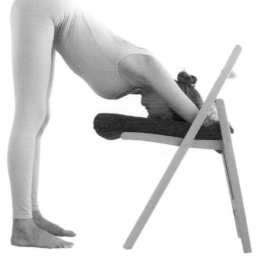

6. STANDING FORWARD BEND (Uttanasana) Do Standing Forward Bend as described on page 256. Remain in the pose for 1 or 2 minutes, or as long as you feel comfortable.

EFFECTS This variation is particularly good for calming your mind and relieving fatigue.

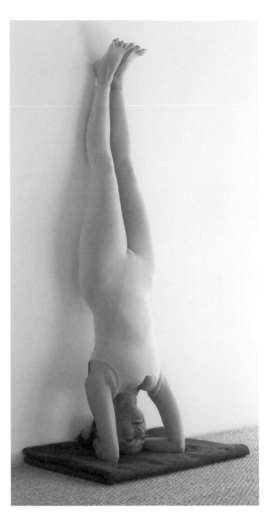

7. HEADSTAND† (Sirsasana) Do Headstand as described on page 249.

EFFECTS This pose brings fresh blood to your heart and head. Invigorating and energizing, it helps balance your endocrine system and rejuvenate your whole body.

†CAUTION Do this pose only if it is already part of your yoga practice. Do not do this pose if you have high blood pressure, have your period, or suffer from neck or back problems or migraines.

8. INVERTED STAFF POSE† (Viparita Dandasana) Do Inverted Staff Pose as described on page 257. Remain in this pose for a minute or two, depending on your comfort level.

EFFECTS This pose helps soothe agitation, calm your mind, and build self-esteem.

†CAUTION Seek the advice of an experienced teacher if you have neck problems. Do not do this pose if you have a migraine or tension headache or diarrhea.

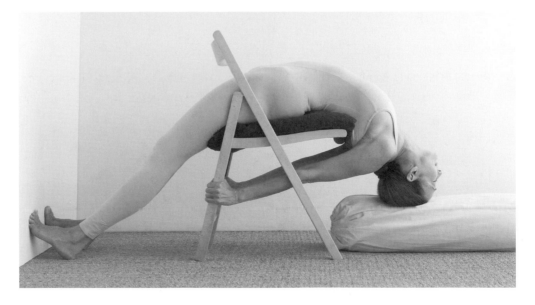

9. SHOULDERSTAND† (Sarvangasana)

Do Shoulderstand as described on page 250. Remain in the pose, breathing normally, for several minutes.

EFFECTS Try this pose to help mitigate the effects of hypertension, including anxiety-produced fatigue.

†CAUTION Do not do this pose if you suffer from neck or shoulder problems, if you have high blood pressure, if you are menstruating, or if you have a migraine or tension headache.

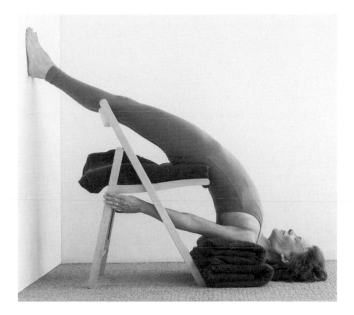

10. HALF-PLOUGH POSE† (Halasana)

Do this pose as described on page 250. Supporting your legs completely enables your whole body to rest and your mind to cool. Stay in the pose for 3 to 5 minutes, breathing normally.

EFFECTS This pose calms jittery nerves and combats fatigue.

†CAUTION Do not do this pose if you suffer from neck or shoulder problems, or if you have your period.

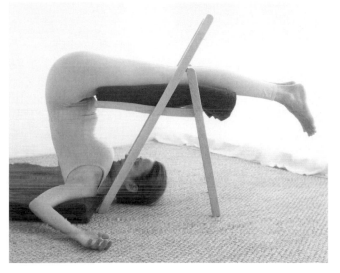

11. BRIDGE POSE (Setu Bandha Sarvangasana)
Do Bridge Pose as described on page 251.

EFFECTS This pose helps calm and restore your nervous system, rest your heart, and relieve nervous exhaustion.

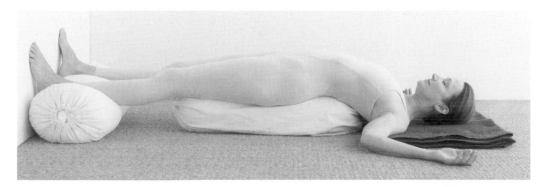

12. LEGS-UP-THE-WALL POSE† (Viparita Karani) AND CYCLE Do Legs-Up-the-Wall Pose and Cycle as described on page 258. Remain in each stage of the cycle for as long as you like, at least 3 to 5 minutes.

EFFECTS This pose can help calm and restore your body, mind, and spirit, leaving you refreshed and renewed.

†CAUTION This pose may be done during menstruation if you don't use a bolster; your pelvis should not be higher than your chest when you are menstruating.

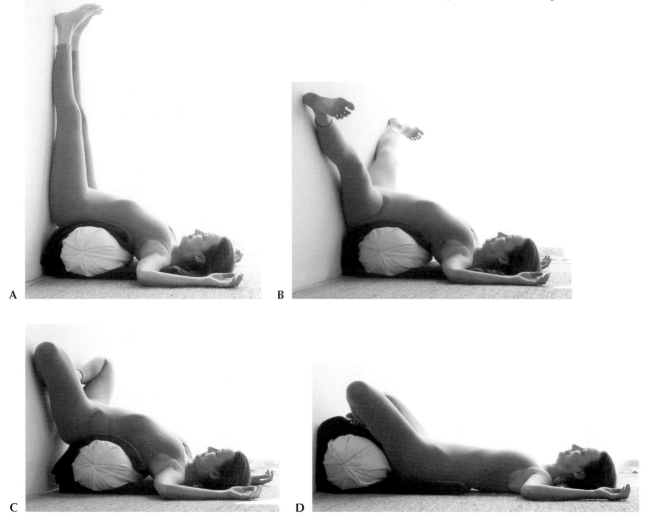

A

B

C

D

13. CORPSE POSE (Savasana) Do Corpse Pose as described on page 252. Remain in this pose for at least 5 to 10 minutes.

EFFECTS This deeply relaxing pose helps soothe and calm, as well as restore and rejuvenate. Try to end every practice with at least 5 to 10 minutes of this pose.

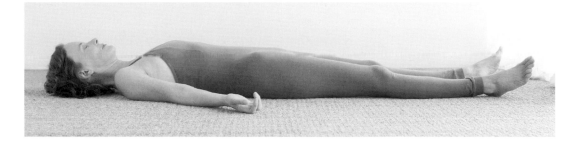

Chapter 12 *Improving Digestion*

NO ONE REALLY LIKES TO TALK ABOUT IT, BUT POOR DIGESTION plagues most women, especially as they get older. In fact, ayurvedic physicians will tell you that most diseases arise from a weak or malfunctioning digestive system. Carmen can attest to that. She says her problems started about the time she turned forty-five. Sometimes she'd eat three meals a day and feel fine; other times, by the end of the evening, her belly would blow up as if she were six months pregnant. The pain sometimes radiated down her back and into her legs, usually accompanied by gas and horrible constipation that left her both anxious and exhausted. By morning, she generally felt better. This pattern continued for more than a year and made Carmen feel like she was losing her mind. She figured it must be diet-related, but no single culprit emerged when she stopped eating various foods.

By the time she made an appointment with her doctor, she had eliminated almost everything from her diet. As a result, she had lost twelve pounds and was subsisting on oatmeal and scrambled eggs, too afraid to put anything else into her stomach. Luckily she benefited from a combination of Western and ayurvedic support and a series of yoga postures that worked not only on her gastrointestinal (GI) area, but also on her liver, pancreas, kidneys, and endocrine glands.

Carmen suffered from irritable bowel syndrome (IBS), or what some people call spastic colon. Not everyone has such severe discomfort, but constipation, occasional bouts of diarrhea, and chronic gas and indigestion are common complaints of many women as they age. Although most people hate to talk about their bowels—and their friends certainly don't like to hear about them—ignoring digestive disorders can seriously jeopardize your health and vitality. At best, these symptoms can be annoying, but at worst, they can lead to chronic fatigue syndrome, premature aging, arthritis, skin eruptions, allergies, and even autoimmune diseases.

Patricia Says

Whether we're teenagers or postmenopausal wise women, we need to make peace with and accept our abdomens if we are ever to heal our digestive complaints. A daily yoga regime allows us to practice softening our abdomen, encourages us to breathe deeply into our core, and gives us time to completely relax and replenish.

YOUR DIGESTIVE SYSTEM

Most people think of digestion as beginning in the stomach, but it actually starts in your mouth, with your first bite of food or your first sip of liquid. As you chew your food, the hypothalamus (in your

273

THE DIGESTIVE SYSTEM

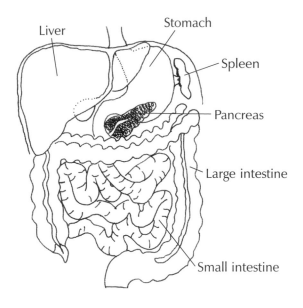

Liver

Stomach

Spleen

Pancreas

Large intestine

Small intestine

brain) signals your digestive system that food is on its way. Tiny glands in your mouth release saliva laced with special digestive enzymes that break down the food and lubricate it enough to send it through your esophagus and into your stomach. Muscle contractions in your stomach help break up the food even more. Assisted by hydrochloric acid, which destroys any bacteria associated with food, these contractions turn the food particles into a thick paste called chyme.

The chyme passes through your duodenum and, with the help of more muscle contractions, into your small intestine, which absorbs the nutrients it receives into its lining. In order to do this, the small intestine must rely on the gallbladder, liver, and pancreas to deliver bile and additional enzymes to break down the food particles into usable molecules, and to remove all toxic or useless chemicals you've ingested. From there, anything left goes to your large intestine, which takes what it needs and pushes the remains down and out through your rectum.

WHAT COULD GO WRONG?

Carmen is convinced that her digestive system has a mind of its own, that there's a reason her condition is called "irritable bowel" syndrome. Although she's been pretty successful in controlling the problem lately, when it was at its worst, she came to see her belly as a recalcitrant child who rebelled when no one was paying proper attention to it. Actually, according to Michael Gershon of Columbia-Presbyterian Medical Center in New York City, Carmen isn't so far off the mark. In a 1997 *Yoga Journal* article by Kristen Barensen, Gershon explains that your gastrono-intestinal tract has a "gut brain"—a primitive enteric (or intestinal) nervous system with its own sets of neurotransmitters (dopamine, serotonin, norepinephrine, and a blood-brain barrier), much like those found in your central brain. This gut brain communicates with your central brain via the vagus nerve. When you suffer from acute gastro-intestinal problems, it's possible that your central brain is either ignoring or overstimulating your gut brain.

THE AYURVEDIC APPROACH

It's clear your entire body works to ensure that you digest whatever you ingest. Your brain sends signals via the vagus nerve to your esophagus, stomach, and intestines; your thyroid gland regulates metabolism—the speed at which your body breaks down and uses food; and your liver and gallbladder deliver the right amount of bile and digestive enzymes to keep everything flowing.

Ayurvedic physicians will tell you that when one part of the equation breaks down, it affects the rest of the process. If your brain is preoccupied by stress, nerves, and fear, it may "forget" to send the right signals to your gut brain that food is on its way. Similarly, a sluggish thyroid can mean a sluggish digestive system. If your liver is weakened or on overload because of stress, drugs, alcohol, environmental toxins, or unhealthy foods, it may not produce enough bile to break down food particles. Undigested food particles, according to the ayurvedic system, cause myriad problems.

Digestive Disorders

• Constipation is not generally life-threatening. It usually indicates that you've changed your diet or daily routine or that you're experiencing more stress than you can handle. Avoid laxatives if at all possible. Instead, add herbs and spices that increase your digestive fire, and eat more fruits and vegetables for fiber. If your constipation lasts more than a couple of weeks, if it's accompanied by abdominal pain or severe bloating, or if you suddenly lose weight, by all means, visit your doctor.

Nancy Lonsdorf, M.D., coauthor of *A Woman's Best Medicine: Health, Happiness, and Long Life through Ayurveda*, explains that a woman ingests more than just food. Information, emotions, and visual stimulation all find their way into your mind and soul, as well as into your physical body. If you allow what you ingest to go undigested (in other words, if you're unable to process it and let it go), Lonsdorf cautions that this excess baggage can create what ayurveda calls ama, the sticky matter that accumulates in your body when something is amiss. In ayurvedic thinking, ama is the root of all disease, the undigested experience or foodstuff left in your body. It's the substance that blocks your arteries, the fog that clouds your thinking, and the resistance you feel that prevents you from being open and loving.

If ama is allowed to accumulate in your digestive tract, it impedes the muscle contractions that help food particles break down and pass through the proper channels. It clogs the vagus nerve and prevents clear communication between your brain and your enteric nervous system; it can also get in the way of liver and gallbladder function by creating excess "bad" cholesterol and gallstones. It can cause constipation or set up an inflammatory reaction such as colitis or Crohn's disease, or even show up as fibroid growths in your uterus or breasts.

The Digestive Fire

Holistic practitioners the world over agree that deep within the belly lies more than just a stomach, intestines, and bowels. Westerners might call it vital energy; for traditional Chinese doctors, it is chi; ayurvedans refer to it as agni—the great digestive fire. Agni governs metabolism, breaking down the food you eat and turning it into energy you absorb and waste products you eliminate. The thirteen types of agni loosely correspond to the Western understanding of digestive enzymes. In ayurvedic medicine, what you eat isn't nearly as important as how you eat it and how you digest it. If your vital fire or agni is weak, you will experience problems no matter what kind of food you put into your mouth. Weak digestive agni prevents food from breaking down completely, causing it to remain in your system and become ama.

"Undigested" emotions can also contribute to ill health, according to ayurveda. Repressed anger or resentment, in particular, can produce ama, upsetting the delicate balance of your gallbladder, bile duct, and small intestines.

WHY DO WOMEN HAVE MORE DIGESTIVE PROBLEMS?

According to some statistics, nearly 30 percent of the world's population suffers from irritable bowel syndrome, meaning periodic bouts of abdominal pain caused by muscle spasms that bring on diarrhea or severe constipation. And guess what? Two-and-a-half times more women suffer than men from IBS.

Helen, a yoga teacher from Nevada, says she notices that a lot of her students in their late forties or early fifties who have digestive disorders also struggle with body-image problems and even eating disorders like anorexia or bulimia. Elaine, a friend of mine in New York City, agrees. She says she's looked the same for most of her adult life. In fact, she prided herself on keeping her slim figure and flat stomach well into her late forties. But all of a sudden her body began to change, and she panicked. She stopped eating dairy products—she reasoned she might be lactose-intolerant. That didn't help. So she stopped eating wheat—no pasta, no bread. That helped a little. Before she knew it, she became obsessive about food.

While food allergies could be the culprit, chances are that something else is going on with Elaine that, according to Patricia, speaks more of Western society's view of women than of Elaine's inability to tolerate any sort of food. Our ideal of beauty that's limited to thin, young women with flat stomachs runs counter to the vision of the belly as a vessel where a woman holds her creativity, power, and intuition. A bloated belly, chronic constipation, or excessive tension in the abdomen may signal a woman's inability to assert herself, to establish her voice in the world.

From a physiological perspective, Patricia says that by repeatedly holding in her stomach and hiding it under tight jeans or tummy-trimming panty hose, Elaine runs the risk of obstructing blood flow to her digestive tract and reproductive organs, which could result in disorders within those systems.

The desire for a flat belly can also take an emotional toll. Patricia remembers a time in her life when she sought help from a hypnotherapist. At one point in the session, she recalls, "the therapist asked me to relax my abdomen. After trying for about half an hour, I was finally able to let go. As I released the grip on my abdomen, a floodgate of tears opened up. I realized then just how much I was storing there and how very attached I was to the flat abdomen image. I didn't even like myself when I could see my belly. So much of me was invested in what I looked like and not how I felt." These days, in Patricia's menopause workshops, she encourages women to let go of their abdomens, to keep their bellies soft, and many of them respond with relief, often declaring they can no longer hold it all in. They want to reconnect with their intuition, their creativity, and when they do, their belly begins to blossom, open, and soften. And they can accept it with pride.

Digestive Disorders

- Diarrhea can be a sign of anxiety. It can also be your body's way of getting rid of toxins or parasites, or a sign of a viral infection. Avoid over-the-counter treatments that stop diarrhea because they will also stop your body from eliminating the toxins. Drink lots of water and herbal teas with chamomile, nettle, and alfalfa. Ayurvedic physicians recommend nutmeg for emergencies. If you see blood in your stools or the diarrhea persists for several days, check with your doctor.

Ayurvedic physicians point to another reason women often have digestive troubles as they age. During your reproductive years, you are blessed with a built-in cleansing system—your monthly cycle. With your period, your body has an opportunity to rid itself of stored up detritus—undigested food particles, toxins, and other impurities—along with the endometrial lining. When you go through menopause, you no longer have that luxury. Ayurvedic physicians, therefore, often prescribe a gentle monthly cleanse, which can be a combination of light fasting and cleansing herbs. It's best to consult an ayurvedic physician about a program that works best for your body type.

Physiologically, as a perimenopausal woman, you'll have more trouble with your digestion than your younger sisters for two reasons. First of all, your gastrointestinal tract slows down because your body produces less estrogen—a natural GI stimulant. Second, your liver, which provides many of the building blocks for breaking down food, is much too busy recycling unused hormones to have much time for digestive work. That's because once you enter perimenopause, your pituitary gland sends large quantities of follicle-stimulating hormone (FSH) and luteinizing hormone (LH) into your system in hopes of jump-starting ovarian production of estrogen. The excess FSH and LH make their way to your liver for disposal.

Emotionally, your struggle with body image may place added stress on your digestive system. It becomes a vicious cycle—you struggle to hold your stomach in; it reacts by bloating, cramping, and distending; you punish it even more by withholding nourishment, in the form of either food or soothing, healing breath; and your stomach rebels even more, making sure it gets your attention.

Recipe for a Belly Massage

Treat yourself to a soothing belly massage to promote better digestion and ease a gaseous stomach. Warm some unfiltered, unprocessed organic sesame oil (available through ayurvedic mail order or at well-stocked natural foods stores) that has been scented with a few drops of lemon balm or lavender essential oil. Rub generously on your belly in slow, luxurious motions for at least three to five minutes. Always rub in a clockwise motion to promote better digestion.

WHAT CAN YOU DO ABOUT IT?

Is poor digestion really an inevitable part of aging, or is there something you can do to help your body process what you give it? Do you really have to contend with constipation, irritable bowels, a bloated stomach, and indigestion just because you are perimenopausal? Not necessarily. Obviously, if you go into this stage of your life with healthy eating and sleeping habits and a consistent, preventive yoga practice, you stand a better chance of staying healthy. But even if this isn't your situation, yoga and lifestyle changes offer hope.

Exercise

Most exercise helps energize a sluggish digestive system. Walking, jogging, or jumping on a trampoline can stimulate bowel muscles. Conversely, lack of exercise can lower your metabolism and weaken your body's natural cleansing systems. Yoga, as you'll see, not only helps stimulate gastrointestinal function but also helps balance your thyroid gland, calm your central nervous system, and soften and bring healing breath to your abdominal region. It can also reconnect you to your spiritual source of strength and creativity.

Diet

If you suffer from constipation, it's probably time to reevaluate your diet. Stop eating so much bread and cheese. Increase your intake of fresh fruits; green, leafy vegetables; and fiber-rich grains and cereals. Drink lots of liquids—particularly warm water—throughout the day. Ayurvedic physicians say that sips of unflavored hot water help break up ama and encourage the flow of waste products out of your body, without stimulating digestive enzymes. Avoid mucus-producing foods (fried or processed, anything containing partially hydrogenated oils, and foods made with white flour or white sugar) which can tax your liver and overload your intestines.

Essential fatty acids (EFAs), especially flaxseed, help promote bowel regularity and can benefit your entire endocrine system. For example, flaxseed calms the mucus membranes in your intestines. Buy the seeds and sprinkle them on your cereal or add them to your smoothies every morning. Alternatively, you can purchase flaxseed oil from a health food store and take a tablespoon once or twice a day. Likewise, adding seaweed to your diet gives your thyroid gland the added boost of iodine it needs to function optimally. You can buy seaweed at your health food store or, if you don't like the taste, get the capsule form.

If eating brings on embarrassing and painful bouts of gas, you need to watch your intake of breads and dairy products. Also, don't eat foods high in simple sugars or starches, which will encourage the growth of intestinal yeast (*Candida albicans*), according to K. P. Khalsa, a medical herbalist and ayurvedic specialist. To further prevent such growth, restore your body's beneficial bacteria (the normal flora residing in your bowels) with probiotics—acidophilus and bifidobacterium—available in the refrigerated section of your health food store. Probiotics are the healthy bacteria your body needs to manufacture and absorb nutrients. Such bacteria—called *Lactobacillus acidophilus*—can only be replenished through supplementation.

When I met with ayurvedic healer Maya Tiwari, she told me that a key to good digestion is consistency. She counseled that I should eat my main meal before 2:00 PM and a lighter meal between 6:00 and 8:00 PM. Eating late at night interferes with your body's nighttime ritual of cleansing and rebuilding. If you go to bed on a full stomach, Maya says, your body must work to digest the food and has no time or energy to cleanse and restore. She also advises eating only fresh foods, in season, and whenever possible choosing organic foods to minimize your exposure to environmental pollutants, food additives, and pesticides. For example, eating fresh, young salad greens in the early spring

Digestive Disorders

• Indigestion could be a sign of overeating or consuming fatty, sugary, or fried foods. Gentle herbs like chamomile and peppermint help soothe your stomach; bitters like gentian and turmeric get the digestive juices flowing properly; and licorice before a meal can be a good antacid. If indigestion keeps recurring, there's blood in your stools, or you have pain in your chest or left arm, see a physician.

is a great way to get your digestive system going. They provide the bitters you need to get the enzymes fired up. They also contain loads of vitamins and minerals, such as folic acid, vitamins C and A, potassium, iron, magnesium, calcium, and zinc. My favorites are nettles, dandelion greens, sorrel, and chickweed.

Herbs and Spices

Chris Clark, M.D., medical director of the Raj, an ayurvedic treatment center in Fairfield, Iowa, told me that a woman can more easily digest foods she thought she couldn't tolerate by adding digestive herbs and spices to them. If your abdomen is gassy and distended, use spicy, carminative herbs. Ginger, fennel, cumin, garlic, rosemary, and cardamom work well and taste good. Western herbs like chamomile, lemon balm, and hops help release tension in your lower intestines and are good for relieving a spastic colon and promoting appetite. You can combine these herbs in a delicious tea by steeping them for five to ten minutes. Sip a cup before bed to calm your stomach and help you sleep.

German researchers found that five to ten drops each of peppermint oil and caraway seed oil in an eight-ounce glass of warm water relieved IBS symptoms in 90 percent of sufferers. Siberian ginseng can also help, especially if you suffer from nervous exhaustion or stress-related digestive problems. This type of ginseng is an adaptogenic herb, which means it is both stimulating and relaxing, depending on what your body needs. It acts on your pituitary gland and replenishes your adrenals.

Digestive Disorders

• Irritable bowel syndrome is characterized by bouts of constipation and diarrhea, usually along with abdominal distention and pain. Stress and poor diet exacerbate IBS. Make an appointment with a nutritionist or naturopathic doctor for dietary suggestions if you feel you're not getting anywhere on your own. This syndrome can sometimes be the result of candidiasis, a yeast buildup in the intestines caused by antibiotics and stress, which strips the intestines of their natural bacteria-fighting flora.

• Inflammatory bowel diseases like Crohn's disease, ulcerative colitis, and diverticulitis can be serious conditions that require medical attention. A diet rich in fiber, folates, and zinc, along with a regular yoga practice and stress-relieving activities, can help your recovery process.

Supplements

As we age, our bodies produce digestive enzymes less efficiently than they did when we were younger, so the food we eat breaks down more slowly. It lingers in the intestines and kind of ferments, which causes flatulence and gastric distress. Sometimes a supplement of betaine hydrochloric acid or a daily dose of bitters (gentian, barberry, dandelion root, milk thistle, ginger) will stimulate digestion. Bear in mind that bitters are named for their taste; gentian is especially foul, but particularly effective. Fenugreek is another bitter herb that ayurvedic physicians favor, along with turmeric and lemon. A simple cup of hot water flavored with fresh lemon or chopped, fresh ginger can also help stimulate digestion.

HOW YOGA CAN HELP

A well-rounded, daily yoga practice can do wonders for digestive health. Patricia teaches that yoga has a powerful ability to squeeze stale blood out of an organ and then soak it with new, oxygenated blood, which freshens and enlivens the tissues and enhances physiological function.

Yoga provides the balance between activity and rest that your body needs to function properly. Specific poses and breathing exercises can also address specific digestive complaints. If your digestive woes accompany perimenopause or postmenopause, you'll want to pay particular attention to your adrenals, thyroid, and liver, in addition to your belly and intestinal tract.

If you suffer from too much digestive fire—characterized by bouts of indigestion, acid reflux, or burning sensations after eating—you need postures that will cool your system down. The best poses for this are supported backbends, what Patricia calls "the suptas." These poses lift your diaphragm a bit to take pressure off your stomach and get fresh blood circulating in your abdomen. You don't want to do forward bends if you have a "burning belly" or diarrhea because these poses put too much pressure on your abdomen and create heat.

Forward bends do help, however, if you are constipated or bloated or feel gassy. Besides their inherently calming effect on your central nervous system, the gentle pressure forward bends exert on your abdomen can help release trapped gas. Both standing and seated forward bends pacify your adrenals and kidneys, while simultaneously getting your digestive juices flowing again.

Standing poses, if you feel up to doing them, can improve digestion and elimination. If you need to, you may do these poses with your back against the wall for support. Much like supported backbends, these modified poses can cool your digestive system and increase circulation in your abdominal organs.

Adding some twists will help tone and energize your adrenals, liver, and intestines. Even a simple twist can relieve gastritis, according to Patricia. Your gallbladder loves the massaging, squeezing effect of twisting poses, which helps prevent the formation of gallstones and assists in the proper digestion of fat.

Inversions relieve digestive problems in a number of ways. Just by reversing gravity, you give your abdominal organs a break. This relieves congestion and, once again, increases blood flow to the area. Inversions are a great way to improve elimination and soothe a gassy stomach. They also balance your endocrine system (particularly your hypothalamus, which controls digestive function, and your thyroid and parathyroids, which govern metabolism) and your central nervous system. A cautionary note, however: Don't confuse your poor digestive system by turning upside down too soon after eating. Always wait at least one and a half or two hours before inverting. And don't practice inversions if you feel nauseous or have a headache.

Ending your practice with Corpse Pose (Savasana) brings you back to your core and enables you to soothe your abdominal organs with the healing power of your breath.

Patricia Says

• If you feel ill, do not worry about getting stronger and better in the poses you choose to practice. Your focus should be internal.

• Soften your abdomen; relax your sphincter muscles; let go of tension in your shoulders, neck, face, and fingers; and as you exhale, send the breath directly into your abdomen and pelvic area.

• Don't worry if you can't get through the sequences we've provided. I know it sounds obvious, but choose only the poses that make you feel better and stay away from any that make you feel worse.

• Consistency of practice is essential in preventing any digestive problems.

• Learning to be sensitive to your inner body takes practice, but the more inner sensitivity you gain, the more you'll be able to use yoga practice to help yourself.

Patricia Says

Do not do inversions if you feel nauseous. Turning upside down can increase acid reflux. Instead, do any of the "suptas"—supported reclining poses— we show here. They will calm your stomach.

A SEQUENCE FOR IMPROVING DIGESTION

1. Reclining Hero Pose (Supta Virasana)
2. Reclining Bound Angle Pose (Supta Baddha Konasana)
3. Downward-Facing Dog Pose (Adho Mukha Svanasana)
4. Head-on-Knee Pose (Janu Sirsasana)
5. Seated Forward Bend (Paschimottanasana)
6. Head-on-Knee Pose (Janu Sirsasana)
7. Headstand (Sirsasana)
8. Child's Pose (Adho Mukha Virasana)
9. Inverted Staff Pose (Viparita Dandasana)
10. Shoulderstand (Sarvangasana)
11. Bridge Pose (Setu Bandha Sarvangasana)
12. Legs-Up-the-Wall Pose (Viparita Karani)
13. Corpse Pose (Savasana)

1. RECLINING HERO POSE (Supta Virasana) Kneel on the floor with your knees together and your feet pointing straight back, slightly wider than your hips. Place a bolster vertically behind you with a blanket on the far end for your head. Sit between your feet on the floor or on a block. Lean back onto your forearms, and gently bring your trunk to rest on the bolster and your head on the blanket. Place your arms over your head or in a relaxed position at your sides. If you feel discomfort in your lower back, add another bolster or blanket for support. Close your eyes, and concentrate on breathing deeply into your abdomen, with a slight emphasis on the exhalations. Remain in this pose for at least 1 to 2 minutes.

To come out, press up to a seated position using your hands. Release your legs one at a time and stretch them out in front of you.

EFFECTS This pose creates space in your abdomen by lifting your diaphragm. It also increases blood flow to the area and cools a "burning belly."

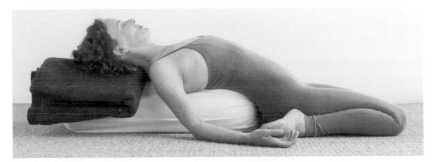

2. RECLINING BOUND ANGLE POSE (Supta Baddha Konasana) Place a bolster vertically behind you and sit just in front of it with your knees bent and your sacrum touching the bolster's edge. Place a strap behind your back, at your sacrum; draw it forward over your hips, across your shins, and under your feet (see page xv). Put the soles of your feet together and let your knees and thighs fall to the sides. Cinch the strap securely under your feet. Lie back so your head and torso rest comfortably on the bolster and your buttocks and legs are on the floor. (If you feel any discomfort in your lower back, add some height to your support with a folded blanket or

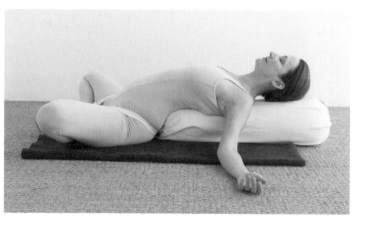

two. If you feel any strain in your neck, place a folded blanket under your head and neck. If you feel any muscle tension in your legs, roll two blankets vertically and place one under the top of each thigh.) Rest in this pose for as long as you like, breathing deeply.

To come out, draw your knees together, slip the strap off, and slowly roll to one side. Use your hands to push yourself up to a seated position.

EFFECTS This pose cools digestive fire and calms your belly by lifting your diaphragm off your stomach and liver. It also increases blood flow to your abdomen and intestines.

3. DOWNWARD-FACING DOG POSE† (**Adho Mukha Svanasana**) Lie facedown on your sticky mat. Place your palms on the floor by each side of your chest with your fingers well spread and pointing straight ahead. Come up on your hands and knees. That's your position. Now place a bolster or one or two folded blankets so your support is in line with your sternum. Your support should be high enough to support your head, but low enough to lengthen your neck. Return to your hands-and-knees position, and turn your toes under.

Exhale, press your hands firmly into the mat and extend up through your inner arms. As you exhale, raise your buttocks high into the air and move your thighs up and back. Keep stretching through your legs and bring your heels toward the floor. Keep your legs firm and your elbows straight as you lift your buttocks upward and release your head onto your support. The action of the arms and legs serves to elongate your spine and release your head. Remain in this pose for 30 seconds to 1 minute.

Come back to your hands-and-knees position. Bring your feet together, keep your knees slightly spread, and sit back on your heels. Bend down and rest your forehead on your support. Release your arms down by your sides with your palms up, and relax completely. Stay like this for 1 to 2 minutes, breathing deeply.

EFFECTS This gentle inversion helps balance your hypothalamus, which controls digestion, and relieves constipation and indigestion.

†CAUTION Do not do this pose if you are nauseous or vomiting.

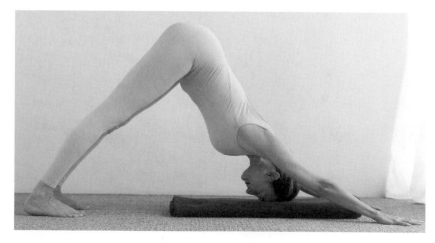

4. HEAD-ON-KNEE POSE† (**Janu Sirsasana**) Sit on your sticky mat with your legs stretched out in front of you. Bend your right knee to the side so your right heel is near the right side of your groin. Push your right knee as far back as you comfortably can; keep your left leg straight. Turn your abdomen and chest to the left so your sternum is in line with the center of your left leg. Bend your left knee and loop a strap around the ball of your foot. Straighten your left leg. With an exhalation, bend forward from your hips while pulling on the strap. Inhale and lift your trunk up from the base of your pelvic area. Look forward, over your outstretched leg, and keep your back slightly concave. Stay in this position for 20 to 30 seconds, breathing normally. Release the pose and switch legs.

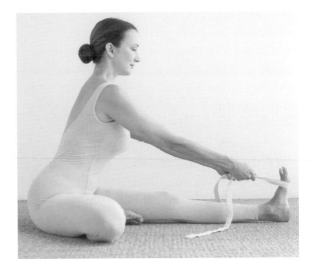

EFFECTS This twisting pose is helpful for toning and improving circulation to your kidneys and abdominal organs. It may also relieve hemorrhoid pain.

†CAUTION Do not do this pose if you have diarrhea or feel nauseous.

5. SEATED FORWARD BEND† (**Paschimottanasana**)
Sit on your mat (or on one or two folded blankets) with your legs stretched out in front of you. Place a folded blanket or a bolster across your lower legs. Take a full, deep breath and lift your arms over your head, stretching up through your spine and lifting your sternum and head. Keep your back slightly concave. As you exhale, bend forward and extend your torso over your legs, cradling your head in your arms on your support. (If you feel strain in your back or in your legs, add more height to your support or rest your head on a padded chair.) Stay in the pose for up to 5 minutes, then slowly return to an upright position.

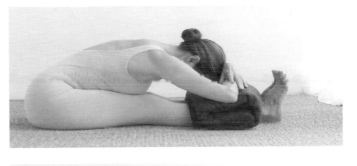

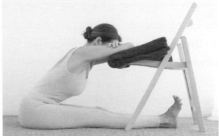

Modification

EFFECTS This pose warms your belly and calms your nerves. It's also good for relieving constipation and flatulence.

†CAUTION Do not do this pose if you have acid indigestion or diarrhea.

6. HEAD-ON-KNEE POSE† (Janu Sirsasana) Sit on the floor with your legs stretched out in front of you. Bend your right knee to the side so it is at a 45-degree angle to your left leg and your right heel is near the right side of your groin. Push your right knee as far back as you comfortably can; keep your left leg straight.

Place a folded blanket or a bolster on your outstretched leg, and turn your abdomen and chest so your sternum is in line with the center of your left leg. As you inhale, lift your trunk up from the base of your pelvis; as you exhale, reach your arms out in front of you as you lean your trunk forward. Fold your arms on your support and cradle your head on your arms. (If you feel any strain in your neck, add more height to your support or rest your head on a padded chair. If you feel any pressure or strain in your back or legs, simply cross your legs in front of you.)

Stay in this pose for at least 1 to 2 minutes, resting your head, the base of your skull, your eyes, and your brain. Inhale while coming up, straighten your right leg, and reverse sides by bending your left knee.

EFFECTS This pose helps soothe your sympathetic nervous system, and its twisting action tones your kidneys and helps improve bladder function.

†CAUTION Do not do this pose if you have diarrhea or feel nauseous.

Modification

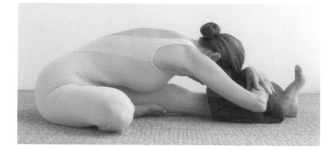

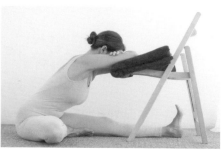

7. HEADSTAND† (Sirsasana) (Before beginning, see pages 16–17.) Place a folded blanket against the wall. Kneel in front of it with your feet and knees together. Interlace your fingers firmly, thumbs touching and your hands cupped. Position your hands no more than 3 inches from the wall with your elbows shoulder-width apart and wrists perpendicular to the floor. Your wrists, forearms, and elbows form the foundation for this pose.

Lengthen your neck and place the crown of your head on the blanket. The back of your head should be in contact with your hands. Press your forearms into the floor and lift your shoulders away from the floor. Maintain this action throughout the pose. Straighten your legs, raise your hips, and walk your feet in until your spine is almost perpendicular to the floor. Exhale, raise your legs up one at a time, and bring your heels to the wall.

Keep your heels and buttocks against the wall. Roll your thighs in, lift your tailbone, lengthen your legs upward, and keep your feet together. Balance on the crown of your head, press your forearms into the floor, and continue to lift your shoulders away from your ears. Keep your breathing even, your eyes and throat soft, and your abdomen relaxed. With regular practice, you can learn to bring your buttocks and heels away from the wall. Hold the pose as long as you can, up to 5 minutes.

To come out, exhale and bring your legs down to the floor one at a time. Bend your knees, sit back on your heels, and rest for a few breaths before raising your head.

EFFECTS This posture helps stabilize your digestive tract and ease spastic colon, particularly when practiced with Shoulderstand (Sarvangasana).

CAUTION Do this pose only if it is already part of your yoga practice. Do not do this pose if you have acid indigestion, high blood pressure, a headache, or your period.

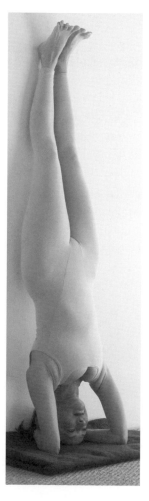

8. CHILD'S POSE† (Adho Mukha Virasana) Kneel on the floor with a vertical bolster directly in front of you, the short end between your knees. Spread your knees wide and straddle the bolster, bringing your toes together. Bend forward and stretch your arms and trunk up and over the bolster, pressing it into your abdomen. Rest your head on the bolster and relax completely for a minute or two, breathing steadily. Push yourself up with your hands to release the pose.

EFFECTS This pose helps relieve constipation, bloating, and flatulence.

†CAUTION Do not do forward-bending poses if you suffer from acid indigestion.

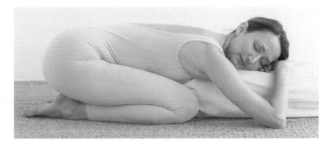

9. INVERTED STAFF POSE† (Viparita Dandasana) (Before beginning, see pages 34–35.) Place a folded blanket on a chair that has been placed about 2 feet from the wall—far enough away so your feet can touch the wall when your legs are outstretched. Place a bolster (or two, depending on your flexibility) in front of the chair to support your head. Sit backward on the chair, facing the wall, with your feet through the chair back. Letting your hands slide down the sides of the chair and supporting yourself on your elbows, lean back slowly until your head and neck extend past the front of the chair seat.

Still holding the sides of the chair, arch back so your shoulder blades are at the front edge of the seat. (You may need to scoot your buttocks farther toward the back of the seat.) Take your feet to the wall, legs slightly bent, and move your hands to the back legs of the chair (your arms should be between the front legs). Rest your head on your support. Lengthen your legs, pressing the chair away from the wall, and roll your thighs in toward each other. (If you feel strain in your lower back, elevate your feet on a block or low stool.) Breathe quietly for 1 to 2 minutes. If you can't maintain the pose that long, do it for 30 seconds, sit up, and repeat a couple of times.

To come out, bend your knees and place your feet flat on the floor. Hold on to the sides of the chair back and carefully come up, lifting from your sternum. Lean over the chair back for a few breaths to release your back.

EFFECTS This is an excellent pose to help relieve an acidic stomach, abdominal cramping, and flatulence.

†CAUTION Seek the advice of an experienced teacher if you have neck problems. Do not do this pose if you have a migraine or tension headache or diarrhea.

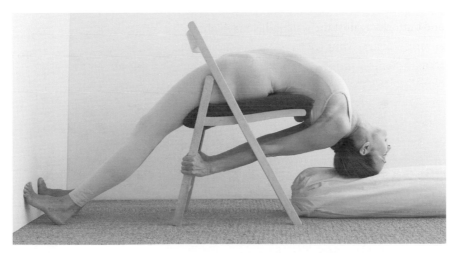

10. SHOULDERSTAND† **(Sarvangasana)** (Before beginning, see page 50.) Place a chair with its back about 8 to 10 inches away from the wall. Put a folded sticky mat or blanket on the chair seat, and two or three folded blankets in front of the chair. Sit backward on the chair with your legs bent over the top of the back; move your buttocks into the center of the chair seat.

Holding the sides and then the front legs of the chair, slowly lower your torso so your shoulders are on the blankets and your head is on the floor. You must extend your spine and open your chest to get the proper position. Move your hands, one at a time, to hold the back legs of the chair; your arms should be between the front legs. Stretch your legs, rotate your thighs in, rest your heels against the wall, or lift your legs straight up. Keep your legs together and extended from your groin to your heels. Close your eyes, breathe normally, and bring your chest toward your chin. Hold this pose for 3 to 5 minutes, or as long as you're comfortable.

To release from the pose, bend your knees, place your feet on the chair back, release your hands, and slide down until your sacrum rests on

the blankets and your calves are on the chair seat. Rest here a moment, then roll to your side and sit up slowly.

EFFECTS This is an excellent restorative pose if you have colitis, chronic constipation, or hemorrhoids.

†CAUTION Do not do this pose if you suffer from neck or shoulder problems, if you have high blood pressure, if you are menstruating, or if you have a migraine or tension headache.

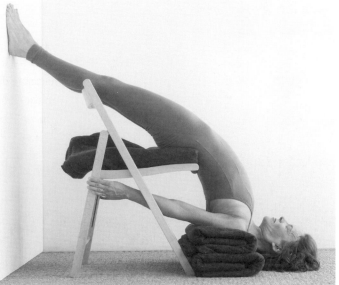

11. BRIDGE POSE (Setu Bandha Sarvangasana) Place a bolster horizontally against the wall and another vertically, forming a T shape. Spread a folded blanket on the floor at the end of the vertical bolster that is farthest from the wall (for your head). Sit on the end of the vertical bolster that is closest to the wall. Keeping your knees bent, lie back over the bolster. Slide down until the end of the bolster is in the middle of your back and your shoulders just reach the floor. Rest your shoulders and head on the blanket. Stretch your legs toward the wall and put your heels on the horizontal bolster so your feet touch the wall. Your legs should be straight out in front

of you, hip-width apart. Rest your arms in any comfortable position—over your head or out by your sides. Close your eyes and relax completely, breathing deeply. Stay in this position for 5 to 10 minutes, or as long as you like.

To come out, bend your knees and slowly roll to one side. Using your hands, push yourself up to a seated position.

EFFECTS This gentle backbend helps calm your digestive system and relieve a bloated, crampy stomach. It will also increase the blood supply to your abdominal organs and improve overall digestion.

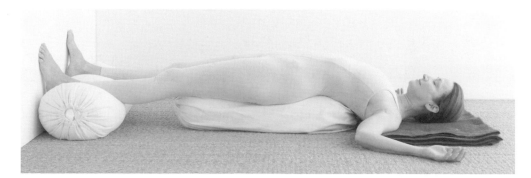

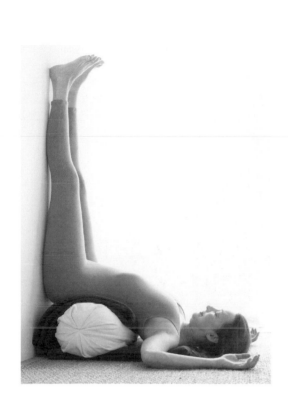

12. LEGS-UP-THE-WALL POSE† (Viparita Karani) Place a bolster about 3 inches from the wall. (If you are tall, you may need a higher support, such as a folded blanket on top of the bolster.) Sit on the bolster so your right hip and side are touching the wall. Using your hands to support you, lean back and swivel your body around, taking your right leg and then your left leg up the wall. Keep your buttocks close to or against the wall; if they moved away from the wall as you lifted your legs, place your feet on the wall and use your hands for support to lift your hips and move your buttocks back into position. (If you feel discomfort in your legs, push your buttocks slightly away from the wall.) Lie down so your lower back and ribs are supported by the bolster, your tailbone is releasing down toward the floor, and your shoulders and head are on the floor. (If your neck is uncomfortable, put a folded towel or blanket under it.) Extend through your legs and place your arms out at your sides, elbows bent and palms up. Remain in this position, breathing normally, for 5 minutes or longer. (If you wish, you can drape an eyebag over your eyes to help remove all distractions.)

To come out, place your feet on the wall and gently push yourself off the bolster. Slowly roll to one side and push up to a seated position.

EFFECTS This is an excellent pose for relieving diarrhea and nausea.

†CAUTION Do not do this pose when you are menstruating.

13. CORPSE POSE (Savasana) Lie on your back with your legs stretched out in front of you. Place your arms comfortably at your sides, slightly away from your torso, with your palms facing upward. Actively stretch your arms and legs away from you, then allow them to release completely. Close your eyes and let everything relax. Remain in this pose, breathing normally, for 10 minutes.

EFFECTS This position offers complete repose. It is excellent for helping to alleviate stress-related symptoms, such as stomach pain, diarrhea, or nausea, by balancing your central nervous system.

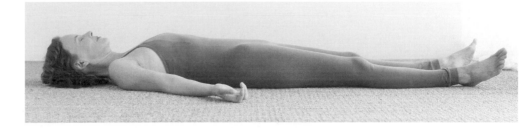

A SEQUENCE FOR RELIEVING DIARRHEA

1. Cross Bolsters Pose
2. Reclining Bound Angle Pose (Supta Baddha Konasana)
3. Bridge Pose (Setu Bandha Sarvangasana)
4. Legs-Up-the-Wall Pose (Viparita Karani)
5. Corpse Pose (Savasana)

1. CROSS BOLSTERS POSE Place a bolster on your mat and lay another one across the center of the first to form a cross. Sit on the middle of the top bolster and carefully lie back so your spine is supported on the bolster and the back of your head touches the floor. (If that is too much of a stretch or puts strain on your neck, place a folded blanket underneath your head.) Place your arms on either side of your head, palms up, elbows bent, and relax completely. (If you feel any strain in your lower back, raise your feet on a block.) Relax in this pose for several minutes, softening your belly and breathing healing energy into it. To come out of the pose, bend your knees and roll to one side. Help yourself up using your hands.

EFFECTS This pose helps relieve indigestion, flatulence, and diarrhea.

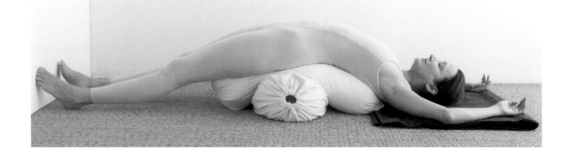

2. RECLINING BOUND ANGLE POSE (Supta Baddha Konasana) Do Reclining Bound Angle Pose as described on page 282.

EFFECTS Try this posture to help ease indigestion and flatulence, as well as diarrhea.

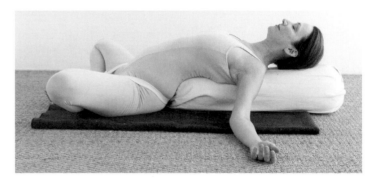

3. BRIDGE POSE (Setu Bandha Sarvangasana) Do Bridge Pose as described on page 286. Remain in this pose for 3 to 5 minutes.

EFFECTS Try this pose to help improve your overall digestion, tone your abdominal region, and relieve diarrhea.

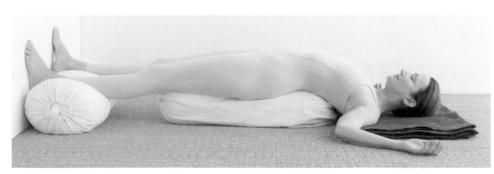

4. LEGS-UP-THE-WALL POSE† (Viparita Karani)

Do Legs-Up-the-Wall Pose as described on page 287. Stay in this pose for at least 5 minutes.

EFFECTS This pose helps relieve diarrhea, indigestion, and nausea.

†CAUTION Do not do this pose when you are menstruating.

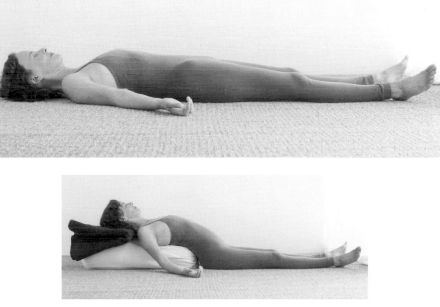

5. CORPSE POSE (Savasana)

Do Corpse Pose as described on page 287. Remain in the pose for 10 minutes. (If it is more comfortable, you can open your chest by lying back on a vertical bolster and supporting your head with a folded blanket.)

EFFECTS This position offers complete repose. It is excellent for helping to alleviate stress-related symptoms, including diarrhea and abdominal cramps.

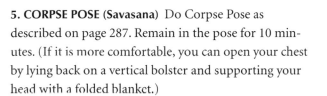

Modification

A SEQUENCE FOR IRRITABLE BOWEL SYNDROME

1. Corpse Pose (Savasana)
2. Reclining Bound Angle Pose (Supta Baddha Konasana)
3. Reclining Hero Pose (Supta Virasana)
4. Reclining Easy Seated Pose (Supta Sukhasana)
5. Inverted Staff Pose (Viparita Dandasana)
6. Bound Angle Pose (Baddha Konasana)
7. Wide-Angle Seated Pose I (Upavistha Konasana I)
8. Downward-Facing Dog Pose (Adho Mukha Svanasana)
9. Headstand (Sirsasana)
10. Shoulderstand (Sarvangasana)
11. Half-Plough Pose (Ardha Halasana)
12. Bridge Pose (Setu Bandha Sarvangasana)
13. Legs-Up-the-Wall Pose (Viparita Karani)

1. CORPSE POSE (Savasana) Do Corpse Pose as described on page 287. Open your chest by lying back on a vertical bolster and supporting your head with a folded blanket. Remain in the pose, breathing normally, for 10 minutes.

EFFECTS This position offers complete repose. It is excellent for helping to alleviate stress-related symptoms, including diarrhea and abdominal cramps.

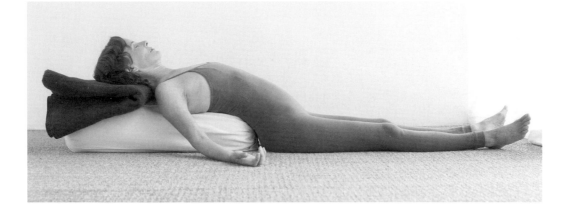

2. RECLINING BOUND ANGLE POSE (Supta Baddha Konasana) Do Reclining Bound Angle Pose as described on page 282.

EFFECTS Try this pose to help relieve indigestion, flatulence, and diarrhea.

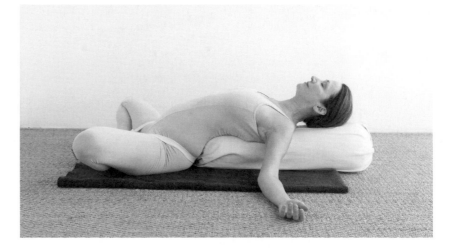

3. RECLINING HERO POSE (Supta Virasana) Do Reclining Hero Pose as described on page 281.

EFFECTS This pose helps ease stomach acidity, abdominal cramping, and flatulence.

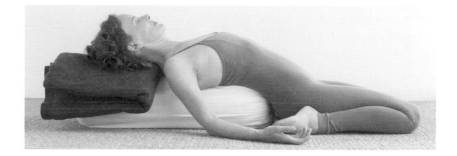

4. RECLINING EASY SEATED POSE (Supta Sukhasana)
Place a bolster vertically on the floor behind you and sit just in front of it with your knees bent and your sacrum touching the bolster's edge (just like in Reclining Bound Angle Pose). You may put a folded blanket on the bolster to support your head. Cross your legs comfortably at your shins and extend up through your spine. Using your hands to support you, lie back on the bolster. Rest your arms out to the sides, bring your shoulder blades into your back ribs, and lift your chest. This should be a restful pose and you should feel no discomfort anywhere.

(If you feel any strain in your back, add more height to your support.) Remain in the pose for at least 1 to 2 minutes. To come out, uncross your legs, place your feet flat on the floor, and roll slowly to one side. Use your hands to push yourself up to a sitting position.

EFFECTS This pose can help ease abdominal cramping, indigestion, and flatulence.

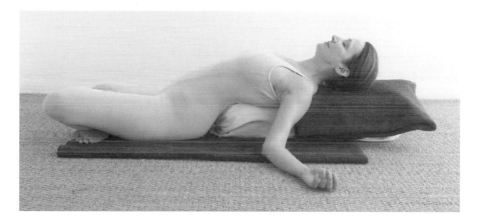

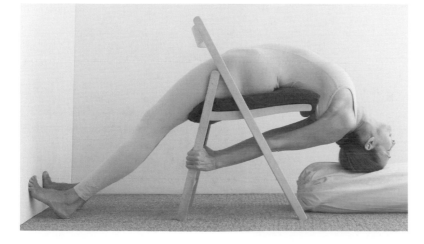

5. INVERTED STAFF POSE† (Viparita Dandasana) Do Inverted Staff Pose as described on page 285.

EFFECTS Try doing this pose to help relieve diarrhea, abdominal cramping, flatulence, and indigestion.

†CAUTION Seek the advice of an experienced teacher if you have neck problems. Do not do this pose if you have a migraine or tension headache or diarrhea.

6. BOUND ANGLE POSE (Baddha Konasana) Sit against the wall on a block or folded blanket (about 4 inches thick) with your back straight and your abdomen lifted. Bending your legs, open your knees out and bring the soles of your feet together. Hold the tops of your feet and draw your heels in toward your perineum or pubic bone. The outer edges of your feet should remain on the floor. Lengthen your spine upward, leading with the crown of your head. Stretching your inner thighs from the groin to the knee, gently lower your knees as far as possible. Place your hands behind you to sit up straighter, and lift your abdomen. Stay in this position for 1 minute or more, breathing normally. To come out, relax your arms by your sides and bring your knees up one at a time. Stretch your legs out in front of you.

EFFECTS This pose increases circulation to your abdomen and pelvis, improving digestive function.

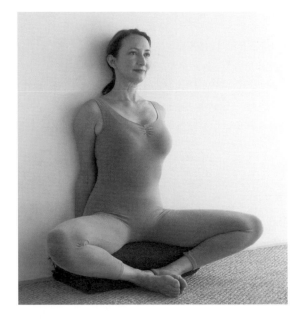

7. WIDE-ANGLE SEATED POSE I (Upavistha Konasana I) Sit against the wall on a block or a folded blanket (about 4 inches thick). Spread your legs wide apart and flex your feet. Adjust the flesh of your buttocks by drawing it behind you and out to the sides. Place your hands on the floor behind you, draw your abdomen and floating ribs up toward your chest, and pull your shoulder blades into your back. Sit up tall, stretching through your legs. Stay in this pose for at least 1 minute. To come out, relax your arms and bring your legs together.

EFFECTS This pose increases circulation to your abdomen and pelvis, improving digestive function.

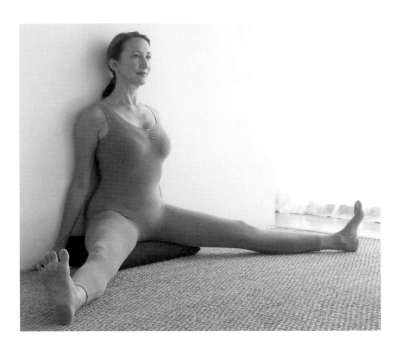

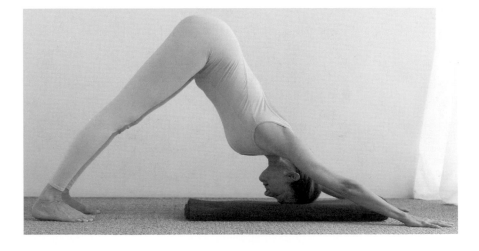

8. DOWNWARD-FACING DOG POSE (Adho Mukha Svanasana) Do Downward-Facing Dog as described on page 282.

EFFECTS This pose helps calm your nervous system and relieve constipation and indigestion.

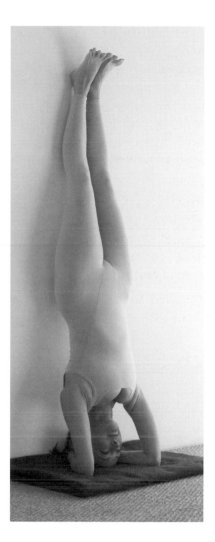

9. HEADSTAND† (**Sirsasana**) Do Headstand as described on page 284.

EFFECTS This posture helps stabilize your digestive tract and ease spastic colon, particularly when practiced with Shoulderstand (Sarvangasana).

†CAUTION Do this pose only if it is already part of your yoga practice. Do not do this pose if you have high blood pressure, have your period, or suffer from neck or back problems or migraines.

10. SHOULDERSTAND† (**Sarvangasana**)
Do Shoulderstand as described on page 286, remaining in the pose for several minutes or as long as you're comfortable.

EFFECTS This is an excellent restorative pose if you have irritable bowel syndrome, colitis, chronic constipation, or hemorrhoids.

†CAUTION Do not do this pose if you suffer from neck or shoulder problems, if you have high blood pressure, if you are menstruating, or if you have a migraine or tension headache.

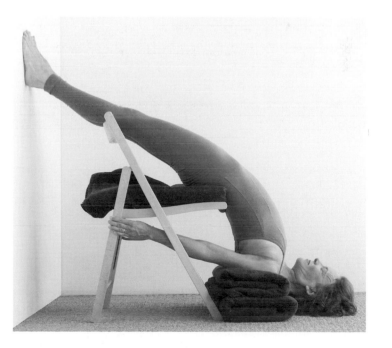

11. HALF-PLOUGH POSE† (**Ardha Halasana**) Lie on your back with your legs outstretched, your shoulders on a folded blanket, and your head beneath the chair seat. As you exhale, bend your knees and swing or lift your buttocks and legs, so your thighs rest completely on the chair seat. (Pad the seat with blankets if you need more height for your legs to be parallel to the floor.) Move your chest in toward your chin. Rest here, with your palms up and your eyes closed, for at least 3 to 5 minutes, breathing deeply. To come out, place your hands on your back and slowly roll down.

EFFECTS Try this pose to help soothe your nerves and relax your mind. It's good for relieving stomach disorders and digestive complaints associated with anxiety.

†CAUTION Do not do this pose if you suffer from neck or shoulder problems, or if you have your period.

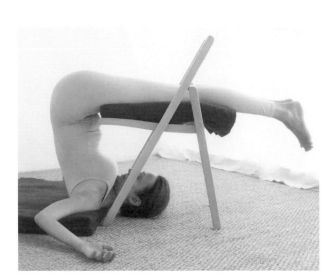

12. BRIDGE POSE (Setu Bandha Sarvangasana) Do Bridge Pose as described on page 286. Remain in this pose for 3 to 5 minutes.

EFFECTS This posture helps improve your overall digestion, tone your abdominal region, and relieve diarrhea and abdominal cramping.

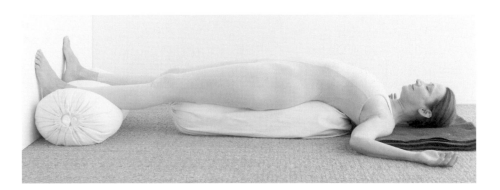

13. LEGS-UP-THE-WALL POSE† (**Viparita Karani**) Do Legs-Up-the-Wall Pose as described on page 287. Stay in this pose for at least 5 minutes.

EFFECTS This is a wonderful pose to soothe your sympathetic nervous system and relieve anxiety-related digestive orders such as diarrhea, indigestion, and nausea.

†CAUTION Do not do this pose when you are menstruating.

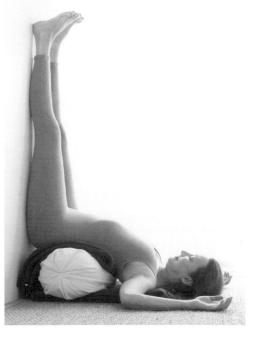

PART FIVE

Wisdom from the Heart

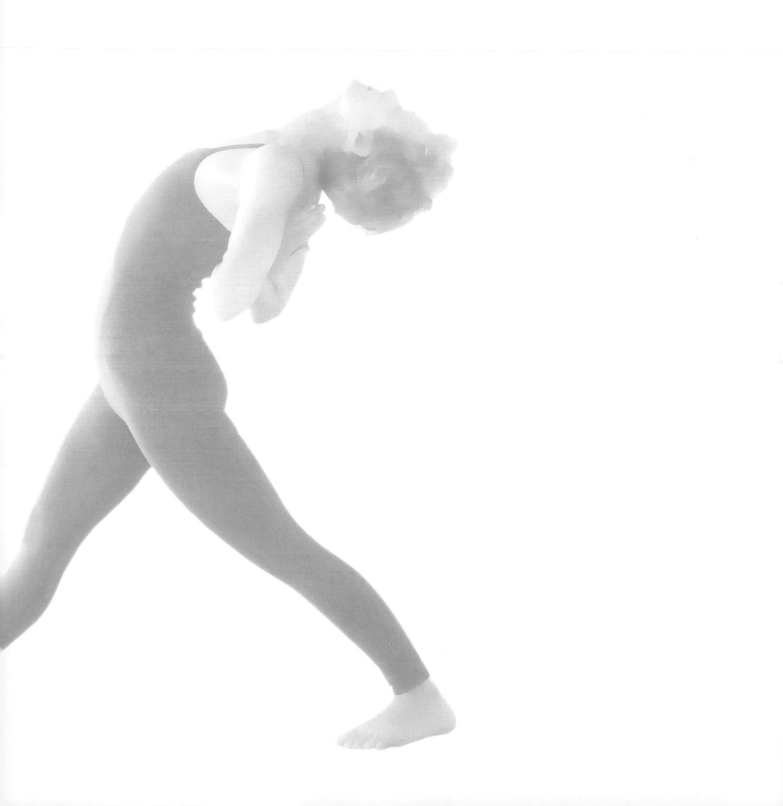

Introduction

About ten years ago, I went to an herb conference in Massachusetts, where I met three incredible women. Juliette de Bairacli Levy, then in her late seventies, spun tales of her life as a healer among the gypsies in Greece and as a champion for animals throughout the world. Adele Dawson, eighty-five, delighted everyone with her self-effacing humor; rich stories of her life as an herbalist and a gardener; and infectious passion for the trees, flowers, and forest creatures that lived near her home. Hortense Robinson, seventy, spoke shyly and hesitantly of her life and teaching as a Mayan healer in Belize, which had begun a decade earlier and continued to flourish as word of her ability to heal and give counsel spread throughout the country. That night in Massachusetts, as I (and two hundred others) sat at their feet, these women told their tales—not from the distant past of their youth, but as part of their present, active lives. Being among them, I felt nurtured, healed, invigorated, and inspired. They became my role models and my teachers.

Every woman needs role models as she moves through the stages of her life. Who better to turn to than women who have already experienced what she's going through? Patricia says older women have always motivated her. Even when she was in her twenties, she revered women whose wisdom is born of and ripened by their experiences, their work in the world. All of these women clearly have what Margaret Mead called postmenopausal zest. I much prefer this image to that of a barren old crone whose youthfulness and usefulness are part of her past.

The wisewoman years share much with early girlhood. Before puberty stifles a young girl's voice, she speaks up with refreshing (and sometimes alarming) candor and present-moment innocence. This honesty and directness return as you age, enriched by a lifetime of relationships and experiences. As an older woman no longer plagued by the unpredictability of perimenopausal hormones, you may find your energy and spirit soaring to prepubescent levels. Patricia says many women at this stage turn to a strong yoga practice, particularly if they have been physically active throughout their lives.

If you've succeeded in reaching sixty-five in good health, gerontologists say you have a good chance of living another fifteen to eighteen years. Your challenges at this stage—and how you choose to face them—will determine the richness of those additional years. Physically, the postmenopausal years bring the threat of osteoporosis, heart disease, and a variety of other illnesses. Mentally, you may fear losing your memory and slipping into dementia. Interestingly enough, the very things that help prevent (or manage) the physical symptoms can also reduce the likelihood of mental deterioration. Your body and mind need stimulation in order to stay strong and alert. Staying active in your community, doing a daily yoga class, reading, writing, keeping in touch with friends—all these activities bring a sense of well-being, usefulness, and joy that increase your ability to keep growing and age gracefully.

Supporting one another is critical at this stage of our lives. Many women outlive their husbands by a decade or more and fear growing old alone. Patricia repeatedly reminds her students that supporting each other at all stages of life is essential to their physical, mental, and spiritual health. Learning from one another, spending time together, and sharing information—as well as joys and sorrows—are the greatest gifts we can give ourselves and each other.

Physically, yoga is an ideal companion at this stage of your life. No matter what shape your body or mind is in, you can always do some kind of yoga. Some days you may feel like doing a vigorous practice; other days your body needs a restorative, gentle practice; and still other times you may only have the energy to do deep breathing exercises. No matter what type of yoga you choose on any particular day, Patricia says your body and your mind reap profound benefits.

Mentally and emotionally, yoga brings stability and calm, strengthening your immune system and pacifying your nervous system. Hannah, a seventy-six-year-old who has done yoga since she was sixty-eight, says the most important gift yoga has given her is awareness of her own body's abilities. Learning to stand tall in Mountain Pose (Tadasana), balance in Half-Moon Pose (Ardha Chandrasana), and stretch through Extended Triangle Pose (Utthita Trikonasana) have made her feel stronger. She's no longer afraid of falling. She trusts her balance and that gives her the sense of independence and freedom she felt she had lost.

On a very deep level, yoga shows you the inherent wisdom of your body as you move in, through, and out of each pose. And it allows you the quiet time and space to get reacquainted with the intuitive side of your mind and the teachings of your heart so that you can share those gifts with the rest of the world.

Try the yoga poses and lifestyle suggestions Patricia and I have provided to address the most common complaints of postmenopause. Of course, if you suffer from heart disease or osteoporosis, have your doctor evaluate your yoga routine to make sure it's safe and effective for you, especially if you are a beginning student.

Chapter 13 *Minimizing Postmenopausal Symptoms*

Your postmenopausal years bring with them a new array of physical and emotional challenges. You'll need to find ways to address annoying symptoms like vaginal dryness and atrophy, urinary incontinence, and decreased mobility in your joints. Stimulating these areas through a consistent yoga practice can help counteract the worst of these problems.

VAGINAL DRYNESS AND DECREASED LIBIDO

Although not every postmenopausal woman suffers from decreased libido (a lack of interest in sex), most will admit that their vaginal lubrication has changed. And, for some, that symptom alone reinforces the stereotype of the sexless, dried-up crone and has them reaching, however reluctantly, for hormone replacement therapy (HRT).

Of course, the fact that the medical profession believes "vaginal atrophy" is an inevitable condition of menopause (indeed, just the idea that physicians call it that) is enough to make any woman fear this stage of her life. While decreased levels of progesterone and estrogen can certainly cause thinning of the vaginal tissue and a decrease in its natural, protective lubrication, you don't have to give up sex unless you choose to. Having a dry, irritated vagina can make intercourse uncomfortable for some and downright painful for others, but it's not an irreversible problem. Lubricants, estrogen creams, diet, and certain yoga postures can help minimize the effects of declining hormone levels. Many postmenopausal women are able to enjoy sexual relations just as much as they did when they were younger (and sometimes more).

Most women will say they feel sexiest when they feel good about themselves—when they're well rested, thinking clearly, feeling beautiful. It's hard to feel all those things when you've got insomnia, fuzzy thinking, low self-esteem, and periodic hot flashes. Other women admit that menopause has become a good excuse for not making love with someone who doesn't make them feel desirable and happy. Physiologically, you'll probably need to address a few things that conspire against pleasurable lovemaking. First of all, your vaginal opening is smaller, thinner, smoother, and dryer than before. This lack of mucus makes lubrication more difficult, and you may not be able to achieve orgasm as quickly as you used to. In addition, your breasts may not be as sensitive as they once were. Martine, a yoga teacher, says that lack of lubrication has been the number-one challenge for her as she grows older. At fifty-seven, she feels as sexually alive as ever, but even during arousal her vagina doesn't lubricate as quickly as it did only a few years ago. Having a sensitive lover helps a lot, she points out.

The most common way to treat vaginal dryness is with estrogen, but many women are reluctant to sign up for HRT because of its side effects, especially if this is their only postmenopausal complaint. Hormone creams present a safer option, though they still have side effects for some women. Martine says she was initially pleased with the combination testosterone-estriol-progesterone cream she received from her doctor. But her breasts became sore after using it for only three months, which she felt negated the early success of the medication. According to Susan Love, M.D., author of *Dr. Susan Love's Hormone Book: Making Informed Choices About Menopause*, you need only a small amount (often much less than the recommended dosage) of a very-low-dose cream to get results, which may help some women avoid the side effects Martine experienced. Dr. Love also points out that some of these creams are made from estriol, a much less potent type of estrogen, and have been beneficial for those suffering from urinary incontinence.

Even if you are not sexually active, it's still important to maintain a healthy level of vaginal lubrication to guard against vaginal, uterine, urinary, and bladder infections. But before you choose hormonal therapy (even in cream form), try a few natural remedies.

Use It or Lose It

The more you make love, the more toned and lubricated your vagina will stay. All the activity increases blood flow to the vagina and stimulates the mucous membranes. And even though sex also strengthens the surrounding muscles, do Kegel exercises religiously. Most women have known about these exercises since they were teenagers. The squeeze-and-release movements strengthen your pelvic floor muscles, increase circulation, and have the added benefit of improving orgasms and vaginal tone. To do Kegel, simply tighten the muscles you use when you want to stop urinating, hold for five seconds, and release completely. Repeat several times in a row, several times a day. Do this when you're working, talking on the phone, sitting at a stop light, even during intercourse.

Diet

Drink loads of water, at least eight to ten glasses a day (herbal tea included). Avoid beverages that contain caffeine or alcohol. And cut out white sugar (especially if you're prone to vaginal yeast infections), processed foods, and red meat. All of them place additional stress on your adrenal glands. Instead eat foods high in phytoestrogens like green leafy vegetables (kale, mustard greens, dandelions), soy, and flaxseed and drink cranberry juice (sweetened with white grape juice, not corn syrup).

Supplements

Increase your intake of vitamin E (up to 600 IU/day for two months or more), zinc, and essential fatty acids (like flaxseed or borage oil). Susun Weed, author of *Menopausal Years: The Wise Woman Way*, suggests motherwort tincture (ten to twenty drops several times a day) if your vaginal dryness has escalated to the burning, itchy stage. Plantain ointment brings instant relief for many women. Aloe vera gel (2 tablespoons mixed in a ¼-cup of water) is herbalist Amanda McQuade Crawford's recipe to soothe a raw, irritated vagina.

Lubricants

Astroglide and K-Y jelly work wonders. Don't think you have to use them because you've failed as a lover; treat them as a sexual enhancement aid and have some fun with them! Experiment with more sensual lubricants like aloe vera gel, olive oil, or vitamin E oil. Ayurvedic healers swear by gently heated sesame oil. Don't use estrogen creams as lubricants for making love, otherwise your partner could end up with excess estrogen in his system.

Attitude

It's not easy to break through the stereotype of older women as dried-up crones, but plenty of women have. I was inspired several years ago when I heard herbalist Rosemary Gladstar give a lecture on herbal support for the menopausal years. She talked about approaching the transition with such anticipation and excitement that one woman in the audience asked whether Rosemary was nervous about getting older. Rosemary looked at her, beamed, and announced, "Oh no, I feel terrific; so moist and juicy!"

Rosemary's attitude is far from unusual. Lots of women report that their libidos took an upswing at menopause, since it was the first time in their lives they didn't have to worry about getting pregnant. One California yoga practitioner said that, at fifty-five, she feels as sexy and desirable as ever. Other women are content without a lot of sexual contact. Another yoga teacher says she doesn't feel any less passionate than when she was younger; it's just that her passion is directed more inward, toward her spiritual practice, and that feels good to her.

Christiane Northrup, M.D., suspects that fallen libido for some women means they've simply exhausted their life energy (or chi) through years of stress, and they have nothing left over for sexual intimacy. Which is all the more reason to replenish your adrenals through yoga and lifestyle changes.

Women who have turned away from sexual contact by choice must still honor their pelvic organs. As the lining of your cervix thins and your vaginal lining becomes drier, both of these organs are prone to diseases and infections, not to mention itchy, burning discomfort. An active yoga practice, coupled with some of the suggestions we've outlined here, will help keep your creative juices flowing whether you channel them into your work, your love life, or your spiritual journey.

How Yoga Can Help

Although no one can promise that practicing yoga will enhance your sex drive and keep you lubricated, it certainly can't hurt. Exhausted adrenal glands exacerbate the problem because your body can't depend on them to deliver the estrogen it needs. To keep your adrenals active and healthy, Patricia says you must first pacify them with forward bends, then practice yogic twists to activate them.

Patricia suggests backbends to tone and strengthen your nervous system. Most women know the benefits of Kegel exercises, but several yoga poses will also tone and strengthen the pelvic floor and enhance circulation to the area. Standing and seated forward bends done with a slightly concave back and inversions help strengthen your pelvic wall, tone and lift your uterus, and reinforce your perineal and anal muscles. Combined with Kegel exercises that work the voluntary muscles, yoga can enhance the inner supporting ligaments of your uterus. The poses Patricia suggests in this chapter can tone your reproductive organs and increase circulation to them.

URINARY INCONTINENCE

Valerie, a yoga teacher from Los Angeles, can't get many of the women in her classes to talk about it, but she suspects bladder and urethral problems are more common after menopause than women like to admit. She suffers occasionally herself.

Two types of incontinence can plague you at this stage of life: stress incontinence or urge incontinence. You know you have stress incontinence if small amounts of urine leak out when you laugh too hard, sneeze, cough, run, or move in any way that increases abdominal pressure or tugs at the opening of the urethra. Weakened pelvic floor muscles (which support your bladder, rectum, uterus, and vagina) are generally responsible.

Urge incontinence occurs when involuntary bladder contractions cause bladder pressure to exceed the urethra's ability to hold the urine back. You can tell you have this type of incontinence when you have to urinate suddenly and can barely get to a bathroom in time. Just like the vaginal lining, the mucous of the bladder and urethra depends on estrogen to stay supple and strong. Once estrogen declines, the lower urinary tract loses elasticity and the ability to function optimally. Hormonal fluctuations can cause excitability in the sacral nerves surrounding the pelvic organs, which can make you feel like you have to go more often. If you've had a hysterectomy, you may have more problems with this type of incontinence than if you went through menopause naturally.

The Medical Question

Before you try anything drastic to help your condition, rule out the possibility of a bladder or urethral infection, which can cause temporary stress or urge incontinence. Hormonal therapy—natural or otherwise—generally has little effect one way or the other, although studies show that small amounts of intravaginal hormone creams made of estriol (the weakest of the estrogen hormones) can help. The good news about estriol, according to Susan Love, is that "much less [of it] is absorbed from the vagina into the rest of the body, making [it] a good choice for women whose only problem is urinary tract infections." Some women get good results with natural progesterone cream (from wild yams), which helps tone the bladder tissue. Every doctor and herbalist I talked to recommended Kegel exercises. Yoga teachers encourage you to do standing and seated forward extensions, which can lift and tone your uterus.

Diet

Stay away from caffeine and alcohol, which can make incontinence worse. Ayurvedic physicians recommend an adrenal-pacifying diet that excludes hot, spicy, and acidic foods. Ironically enough, drinking lots of water can actually help urinary tract problems, especially if you are prone to infections. Eat foods rich in phytoestrogens, and follow the dietary suggestions for vaginal dryness and decreased libido. Possible herbal support includes black cohosh, nettles, and catnip.

How Yoga Can Help

Focus on yoga poses that strengthen your pelvic floor muscles and increase circulation to the pelvic area, especially if you've had a cesarean section or a hysterectomy or suffer from a prolapsed uterus. According to Geeta Iyengar, bending forward with a slightly concave back can help lift a prolapsed bladder or urethra and soften your vaginal walls and vulva. It also strengthens your pelvic muscles. All the forward bends we've provided in this chapter should be practiced with a slightly concave back. Inversions will drain venous blood from your pelvic organs and increase circulation to keep them supple.

If you have a more advanced practice, adding a rotation to your Headstand (Sirsasana) or Shoulderstand (Sarvangasana) will further stimulate your adrenals. Placing your legs with the soles of your feet together (Baddha Konasana) or with your legs wide apart (Upavistha Konasana) in Headstand or Shoulderstand can give you immediate relief from any pressure you feel in the pelvis. Bridge Pose (Setu Bandha Sarvangasana) also helps tone the lateral muscles supporting your uterus.

Bending back, either unsupported or over a chair or bolster, allows your perineal and anal muscles to work hard and maintain their tone and elasticity. Even a restorative pose like Reclining Bound Angle Pose

(Supta Baddha Konasana) over a bolster can be invaluable for lifting and strengthening the urethra. Coming in and out of twisting poses alternately squeezes venous blood from your pelvis and soaks it with fresh, oxygenated blood to stimulate your pelvic organs. Patricia teaches Great Seal Pose (Maha Mudra) with concave back to tone your uterus and help lift it.

STIFF, ACHY JOINTS

Lynn, a fifty-six-year-old writer and editor, couldn't figure out what was wrong with her shoulders and elbows. They often felt stiff and sore; sometimes when she grabbed a jar or heavy can, she experienced pain in her elbow, much like she would imagine athletes do when they suffer from tennis elbow. She acknowledges that her work keeps her chained to her computer, often for long stretches of time, but it had never been a problem before. She was relieved to hear Susan Love speak at a conference and mention, almost in passing, that many women complain about joint pain during menopause. The most common sites are shoulders, elbows, and knees. Lynn was also relieved that she didn't suffer from stiffness in her lower back, hips, or wrists—often a sign of osteoporosis or weak kidneys.

Should swelling and redness accompany your joint stiffness, seek medical advice to rule out osteoarthritis or rheumatoid arthritis. Don't ignore the pain or stiffness; the earlier you treat it, the easier it will be to work through. (For additional yoga poses, diet, and other lifestyle changes that can help joint pain as well as more serious arthritic conditions, see chapter 8).

How Yoga Can Help

For problem joints associated with menopause and postmenopause, the poses in the Sequence for Joint Stiffness should help. Lynn found it most beneficial to move in and out of the poses, a suggestion Patricia gives all her postmenopausal students. For example, she has them practice Reclining Big Toe Pose I (Supta Padangusthasana I) with a strap, gently moving each leg back and forth in its socket to keep the joint mobile.

A SEQUENCE FOR VAGINAL HEALTH

1. Mountain Pose (Tadasana)
2. Standing Forward Bend (Uttanasana)
3. Downward-Facing Dog Pose (Adho Mukha Svanasana)
4. Spinal Twist Pose (Marichyasana III)
5. Inverted Staff Pose (Viparita Dandasana)
6. Great Seal Pose (Maha Mudra)
7. Upward-Facing Bow Pose (Urdhva Dhanurasana)
8. Shoulderstand (Sarvangasana)
9. Half-Plough Pose (Ardha Halasana)
10. Bridge Pose (Setu Bandha Sarvangasana)
11. Legs-Up-the-Wall Pose (Viparita Karani)
12. Corpse Pose (Savasana)

1. MOUNTAIN POSE (Tadasana) Stand up straight legs together (with big toes touching, if that's comfortable). Distribute your weight evenly between the front of your feet and your heels. Place a block between your upper thighs and press firmly against it, without gripping or clenching your vaginal or anal muscles. Tighten your knees by pulling up with your quadriceps (front thigh muscles). Raise your sternum (breastbone) and broaden your chest by rolling your shoulders back and drawing your shoulder blades in. Lift your abdomen and draw your tailbone in without pushing your thighs forward. Extend your arms downward with palms facing your thighs and fingers together. Keep your shoulders moving away from your ears. Remain in this pose for 30 to 60 seconds, breathing normally.

EFFECTS This posture helps lift and tone your uterus and improve circulation to your pelvis.

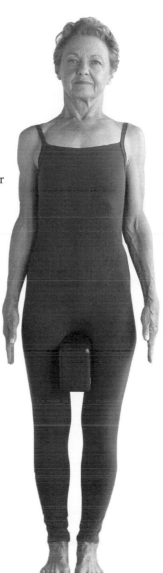

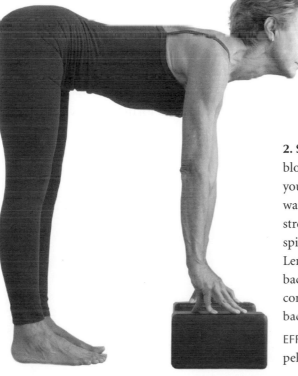

2. STANDING FORWARD BEND (Uttanasana) Place two blocks about shoulder-width apart on the floor in front of you. Stand with your feet together. Turn your palms outward and lift your arms to the side and over your head, stretching your whole body. As you exhale, extend your spine and bend forward, resting your hands on the blocks. Lengthen your spine, lifting your head up and keeping your back concave. Breathe normally for 30 to 60 seconds. To come out, place your hands on your hips and lift your torso back to a standing position.

EFFECTS This posture helps lift your uterus and tone your pelvic floor.

3. DOWNWARD-FACING DOG POSE (Adho Mukha Svanasana) Put two blocks against the wall. Lie facedown with your feet in front of the blocks. Place your palms on the floor by your sides with your fingers well spread and pointing toward your head. Turn your toes inward. Come up on your hands and knees. Step your feet onto the blocks.

Exhale and press your hands into the floor and your toes onto the blocks. Raise your buttocks high into the air. Move your thighs up and back, keep stretching through your legs and bring your heels toward the blocks as you lift your buttocks higher. The action of the arms and legs serves to elongate the spine and release your head. Stay in this pose for 30 seconds to 1 minute, breathing deeply.

To come out, step off the blocks and return to your hands and knees. Keep your knees spread slightly and sit back on your heels.

EFFECTS Use this pose to help lift and tone your uterus, improve circulation to your pelvis, and strengthen your pelvic floor.

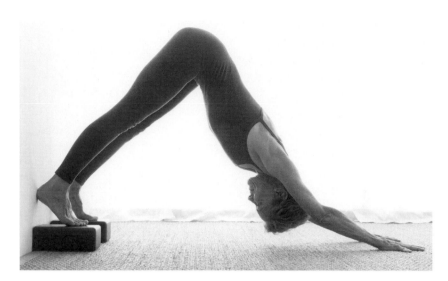

4. SPINAL TWIST POSE (Marichyasana III) Sit with your legs stretched out in front of you. Bend your left leg up, with your foot resting flat on the floor near your pubic bone and your calf against your thigh. Keep your right leg outstretched and active. Take a deep breath. As you exhale, extend your spine and rotate your torso toward your left leg, so that your abdomen is close to your thigh. Place your left hand on the floor (or a block) behind you, several inches away from your buttocks; open your chest. Raise your right arm and bend your elbow, placing the outside of the elbow on the outside of your left knee. Your fingertips should point toward the ceiling. Turn your head to look over your left shoulder. Hold the pose, breathing normally, for 10 to 15 seconds. Release your head, arms, and legs, and sit with your legs outstretched before repeating on the other side.

EFFECTS This is a good pose for toning and massaging your reproductive organs, liver, and kidneys.

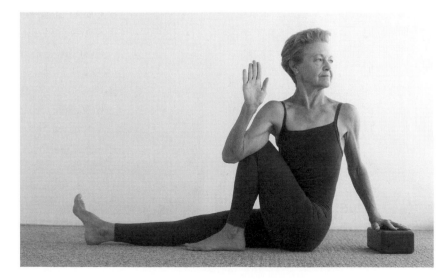

5. INVERTED STAFF POSE† (Viparita Dandasana) (Before beginning, see pages 34–35.) Place a folded blanket on a chair that's about 2 feet from the wall—far enough away so your feet can press into the wall when your legs are outstretched. Sit facing the wall, with your feet through the chair back. Hold on to the sides of the chair and support yourself on your elbows as you arch back slowly. Your head, neck, and shoulders should extend past the chair seat, and your shoulder blades should touch the front edge of the seat. (You may need to scoot toward the back edge of the seat to do this.) Take your feet to the wall and move your hands (one at a time) to the back legs of the chair. Lengthen your legs and roll your thighs in. (If you have neck problems, rest your head on a bolster or two. If you feel any pain in your lower back, elevate your feet on a block or bolsters placed against the wall.) Breathe quietly for 30 to 60 seconds.

To come out, bend your knees and place your feet flat on the floor. Grasp the sides of the chair back and lift from your sternum. Lean over the chair back for a few breaths to release your back.

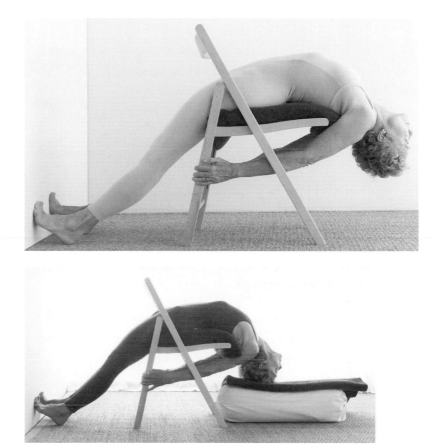

Modification

EFFECTS This pose stimulates your adrenals and can help correct a displaced bladder or prolapsed uterus.

†CAUTION Seek the advice of an experienced teacher if you have neck problems. Do not do this pose if you have a migraine or tension headache or diarrhea.

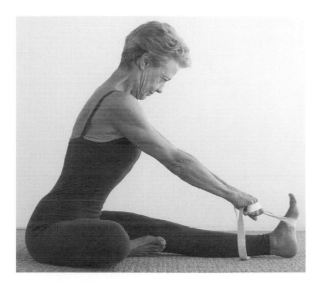

6. GREAT SEAL POSE (Maha Mudra) Sit up tall with your legs stretched out in front of you. Place your right heel close to your groin so your right leg is perpendicular to your left. Extend your arms and wrap a strap around the ball of your foot. Pressing your thighs into the floor, raise your torso, and straighten your arms. Your back should be slightly concave and your sternum lifted. Lower your chin toward your chest and exhale completely. Inhale fully and lift from your pubic bone, drawing your abdominals up and back toward your chest as you elongate your spine. Hold the breath for 3 to 5 seconds, expanding your chest further. Exhale and repeat before switching sides.

EFFECTS This pose helps balance your endocrine system, realign your uterus, and tone your pelvic floor muscles.

7. UPWARD-FACING BOW POSE† (Urdhva Dhanurasana) Lie on your back with your knees bent, your feet hip-width apart, and your heels close to your buttocks. Bend your elbows and place your hands alongside your head with your fingers pointing toward your feet. As you exhale, raise your hips and chest, straighten your arms, and stretch your legs. Lift your tailbone and move the backs of your thighs toward your buttocks. To come out of the pose, bend your knees and elbows, and slowly lower your body to the floor. Hold this pose for 5 to 10 seconds, if you can. If not, come in and out of the pose two or three times.

If you have trouble pushing up into a backbend, try the modification on page 37.

EFFECTS You can use this pose to help strengthen your pelvic and abdominal muscles and stimulate your endocrine glands. It also helps correct a prolapsed uterus.

†CAUTION Do the unsupported version of this pose only if it is already part of your yoga practice. Seek the advice of an experienced teacher if you have neck problems. Do not do this pose if you have a migraine or tension headache or suffer from any serious illness.

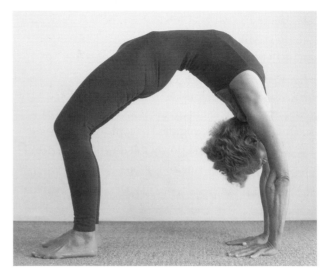

8. SHOULDERSTAND† (Sarvangasana) (Before beginning, see page 50.) Place a chair with its back about 8 to 10 inches away from the wall. Put a folded blanket on the chair seat, and two or three folded blankets in front of the chair. Sit backward on the chair with your legs bent over the top of the back; move your buttocks into the center of the chair seat.

Holding the sides and then the front legs of the chair, slowly lower your torso so your shoulders are on the blankets and your head is on the floor. You must extend your spine and open your chest while doing this to get the proper position. Move your hands, one at a time, to hold the back legs of the chair; your arms should be between the front legs. Stretch your legs, rotate your thighs in, rest your heels against the wall or lift your legs straight up. Keep your legs together and extend from groin to heels. Close your eyes, breathe normally, and bring your chest toward your chin. Hold for 3 to 5 minutes.

To release from the pose, bend your knees, place your feet on the chair back, release your hands, and slide down until your sacrum rests on the blankets and your calves are on the chair seat. Rest here a moment, then roll to your side and sit up slowly.

EFFECTS This posture helps improve thyroid and parathyroid function and soothe your nerves, and it may help to correct a displaced uterus.

†CAUTION Do not do this pose if you suffer from neck or shoulder problems, if you have high blood pressure, or if you have a migraine or tension headache.

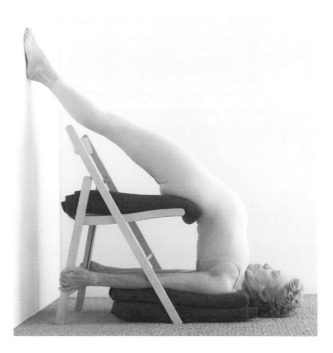

9. HALF-PLOUGH POSE† (**Ardha Halasana**) Place a folded blanket on your sticky mat with the rounded edge near the legs of a chair. Lie on your back with your legs outstretched, your shoulders on the blanket, and your head beneath the chair seat. As you exhale, bend your knees and swing or lift your buttocks and legs, so your thighs rest completely on the chair seat. (Pad the seat with blankets if you need more height for your legs to be parallel to the floor.) Move your chest in toward your chin (not your chin toward your chest). Relax with your palms up and your eyes closed. Remain in this position for at least 5 minutes. To come out, place your hands on your back and slowly roll down, one vertebra at a time. Roll to one side and sit up.

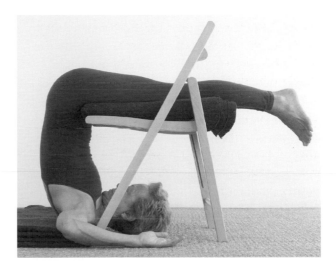

EFFECTS This pose helps relieve pain and heaviness in your uterus. It also may help relieve symptoms from urinary disorders.

†CAUTION Do not do this pose if you suffer from neck or shoulder problems.

10. BRIDGE POSE (**Setu Bandha Sarvangasana**) Place a bolster horizontally against the wall and another vertically, forming a T shape. Fold a blanket on the floor for your head. Sit on the end of the vertical bolster that is closest to the wall. Keeping your knees bent, lie back over the bolster. Slide down until the end of the bolster is in the middle of your back and your shoulders just reach the floor. Rest your shoulders and head on the blanket. Keeping your feet and heels together, stretch your legs toward the wall and put your heels on the horizontal bolster so your feet touch the wall. Your legs should be straight out in front of you. Rest your arms in any comfortable position. Close your eyes and relax completely, softening your abdomen, and breathing deeply. Stay in this position for 5 to 10 minutes.

To come out, bend your knees and slowly roll to one side. Push yourself up to a seated position.

EFFECTS This pose strengthens and tones your pelvic organs and brings a sense of calm to your body and mind.

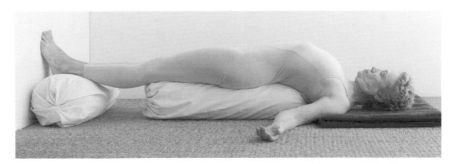

11. LEGS-UP-THE-WALL POSE (Viparita Karani) Place a bolster about 3 inches from the wall. (If you are tall, you may need a higher support, such as a folded blanket on top of the bolster.) Sit on the bolster so your right hip and side are touching the wall. Using your hands to support you, lean back and swivel your body around, taking your right leg and then your left leg up the wall. Keep your buttocks close to or against the wall. (If you feel stiffness or discomfort in your legs, push your buttocks slightly away from the wall.) Lie down so your lower back and ribs are supported by the bolster and your shoulders and head are on the floor. (If your neck is uncomfortable, put a folded towel or blanket under it.) Extend through your legs and place your arms out at your sides, elbows bent and palms up. Rest in this position, eyes closed, for at least 5 to 10 minutes.

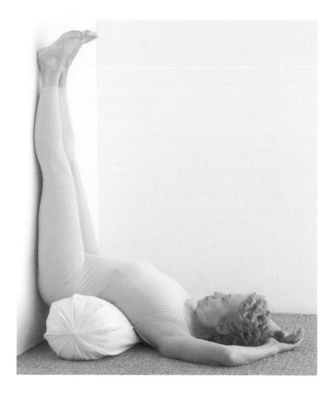

To come out, gently push away from the wall until your buttocks are off the bolster and resting on the floor. Roll to one side. Breathe quietly for a few breaths, then use your arms to help you to a seated position.

EFFECTS This pose lifts and tones your pelvic organs and relieves nervous exhaustion.

12. CORPSE POSE (Savasana) Lie on your back with your legs stretched out in front of you. Place your arms comfortably at your sides, slightly away from your torso, with your palms facing upward. Actively stretch your arms and legs away from you, then allow them to release completely. Close your eyes and let everything relax. Take a few deep breaths, inhaling into your chest without tensing your throat, neck, or diaphragm. Exhale your body into the floor, releasing your shoulders, neck, and facial muscles. Relax your pelvic floor muscle (the muscle you use to stop urinating) and the muscles in your buttocks and abdomen; release your lower back. As you relax, breathe normally for at least 10 minutes. To come out of the pose, bend your knees, roll slowly to one side, and after a few breaths, gently push yourself to a seated position.

EFFECTS This is a very restful pose that can help you build confidence, relieve fatigue and depression, and rejuvenate your whole body. By helping to balance your sympathetic nervous system, it soothes your reproductive organs as well.

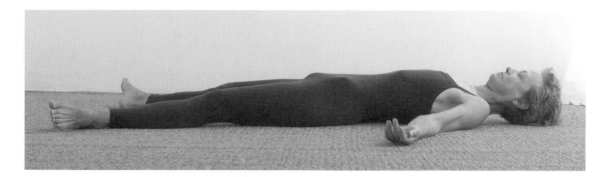

A SEQUENCE FOR URINARY INCONTINENCE

1. Standing Forward Bend (Uttanasana)
2. Wide-Angle Standing Forward Bend (Prasarita Padottanasana)
3. Great Seal Pose (Maha Mudra)
4. Bound Angle Pose (Baddha Konasana)
5. Wide-Angle Seated Pose I (Upavistha Konasana I)
6. Reclining Bound Angle Pose (Supta Baddha Konasana)
7. Shoulderstand (Sarvangasana)
8. Plough Pose (Halasana)
9. Bridge Pose (Setu Bandha Sarvangasana)
10. Legs-Up-the-Wall Pose (Viparita Karani)
11. Corpse Pose (Savasana)

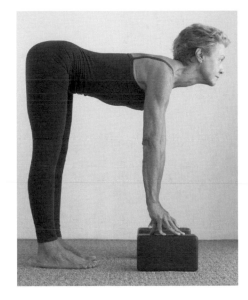

1. STANDING FORWARD BEND (Uttanasana) Do Standing Forward Bend as described on page 305. Remain in the pose for 30 to 60 seconds.

EFFECTS This pose helps lift your uterus and tone your pelvic floor.

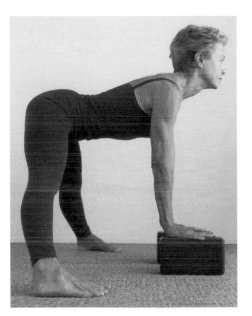

2. WIDE-ANGLE STANDING FORWARD BEND (Prasarita Padottanasana)
Place two blocks, shoulder-width apart, in front of you on the floor. Step your feet apart about 4 feet (or as wide as possible), keeping the outer edges of your feet parallel. Tighten your quadriceps to draw your kneecaps up and keep your thighs well lifted. On an exhalation, bend forward from your hips and place your hands on the blocks—in line with your shoulders—between your feet. Lift your hips toward the ceiling, draw your shoulder blades into your back, and extend your chest forward. Look up and extend your trunk forward, keeping your entire spine concave. Stay in this pose for 1 minute, if possible. To come out, bring your hands to your hips, and raise your trunk. Step your feet together.

EFFECTS This position helps lift and tone your uterus and improves circulation to your pelvis.

3. GREAT SEAL POSE (Maha Mudra)
Do Great Seal Pose as described on page 307.

EFFECTS Use this pose to help balance your endocrine system, realign your uterus, and tone your pelvic floor muscles.

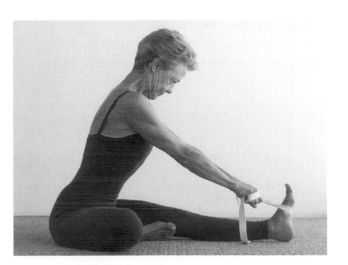

4. BOUND ANGLE POSE (Baddha Konasana) Sit on a block with your back against the wall and your abdomen lifted. Bending your legs, open your knees out and bring the soles of your feet together. Hold the tops of your feet and draw your heels in toward your pubic bone. The outer edges of your feet should remain on the floor. Place your hands on the block behind you. Lengthen your spine upward, leading with the crown of your head. (If you have trouble with this, try the modification on page 316.) Stretching your inner thighs from groin to knee, gently lower your knees as far as possible. Stay in this position for 30 seconds or more, breathing normally. To come out, relax your arms and bring your knees up one at a time.

EFFECTS This pose helps tone and massage your kidneys, strengthen your bladder, and lift your uterus.

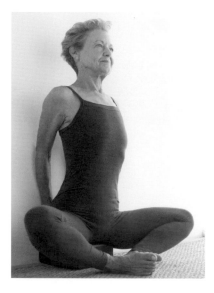

5. WIDE-ANGLE SEATED POSE I (Upavistha Konasana I) Sit on a block with your back against the wall and spread your legs wide apart; flex your feet. Adjust the flesh of your buttocks by drawing it behind you and out to the sides. Place your hands behind you on the block to help draw your abdomen in, open up your chest more, and draw your shoulder blades into your back. Sit up tall, stretching from groin to heels and keeping your knees straight. Stay in this pose for 30 seconds or more, breathing normally.

EFFECTS This pose helps increase circulation to your pelvic region, tones your uterus, and strengthens your bladder.

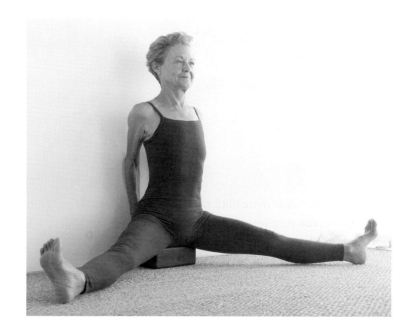

6. RECLINING BOUND ANGLE POSE (Supta Baddha Konasana) Place a bolster vertically on the floor behind you with a blanket on the far end for your head and neck. Sit just in front of the bolster with your knees bent and your sacrum touching the bolster's edge. Place a strap behind your back, at your sacrum; draw it forward over your hips, across your shins, and under your feet (see page xv). Put the soles of your feet together and let your knees and thighs fall to the sides. Cinch the strap securely under your feet. Lie back so your head and torso rest comfortably on the bolster and your buttocks and legs are on the floor. (If you feel any discomfort in your lower back, add some height to your support with a folded blanket or two. If you feel any muscle tension in your legs, roll two blankets vertically and place one under the top of each thigh.) Rest in this pose for at least 5 to 10 minutes, breathing deeply.

To come out, draw your knees together, slip the strap off, and slowly roll to one side. Use your hands to push yourself up to a seated position.

EFFECTS This posture helps calm your nervous system and take pressure off your pelvic area.

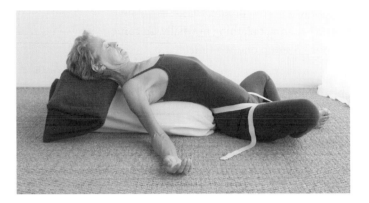

7. SHOULDERSTAND† (Sarvangasana) (Before beginning, see pages 18–19.) Lie on your back with two folded blankets supporting your shoulders and your arms stretched out beside you. On an exhalation, bend your knees and raise your legs toward your chest. Pressing your hands into the floor, swing your bent legs over your head; support your back with your hands and press your elbows firmly into the blankets. Raise your torso up until it is perpendicular to the floor and your knees are close to your chest. Supporting your back, raise your legs until your thighs are parallel to the floor; raise them some more until your knees point toward the ceiling. Now raise your legs completely and extend up through your heels until your whole body is perpendicular to the floor. Use your hands to lift your back ribs.

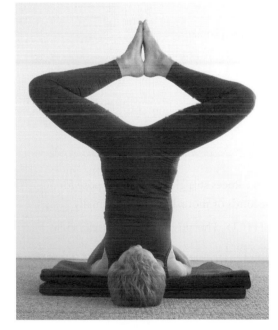

Bend your legs, spread your knees outward, and press the soles of your feet firmly together. Remain in this pose for several breaths, working up to 1 to 2 minutes. Return to Shoulderstand by straightening your legs. Keeping your hands on your back for support, roll down slowly. Rest here for a few breaths.

EFFECTS This pose can help correct urinary disorders and is very soothing for your entire nervous system.

†CAUTION Do not do this pose if you suffer from neck or shoulder problems, if you have high blood pressure, or if you have a migraine or tension headache.

8. PLOUGH POSE† **(Halasana)** Lie on your back with two folded blankets supporting your neck and shoulders; your head is on the floor. Bend your knees and bring your thighs in to your chest. On an exhalation, swing or lift your buttocks and legs up, supporting your back with your hands, and extend your legs over your head, placing your toes on the floor behind you. Keep your thighs active by tightening your knees to create space between your face and your legs. Stay in this pose, breathing deeply and slowly, for 30 seconds; work up to 3 minutes. To come out, slowly roll down one vertebra at a time. Rest with your back flat on the floor, breathing deeply, for several breaths.

EFFECTS This pose helps soothe your nerves and relieve urinary problems.

†CAUTION Do not do this pose if you have neck problems.

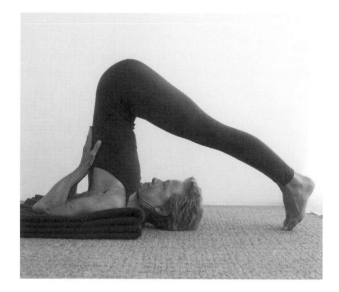

9. BRIDGE POSE (Setu Bandha Sarvangasana) Place a block vertically against the wall and have another at your side. Lie on your back with your arms at your sides and your knees bent. Raise your hips and chest as high as possible and support your back with your hands, fingers pointing in toward your spine. Keeping your head and shoulders flat on the floor, lift your spine even farther, increasing the arch, and place the other vertical block under the fleshy part of your buttocks. Stretch out one leg at a time, resting each heel on the vertical block against the wall. Release your arms so that your hands reach just beyond the block under your sacrum. Hold the pose for at least 30 seconds, breathing normally.

To come out, bend your knees and place your feet on the floor. Then release the block under your sacrum and slowly roll down one vertebra at a time. Hug both knees to your chest and rest for several breaths.

If this pose is too difficult, you can substitute the version described in the Woman's Restorative Sequence (see page 51).

EFFECTS Use this posture to help tone your kidneys and relieve anxiety.

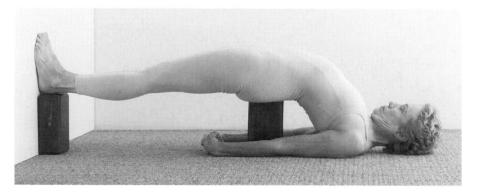

10. LEGS-UP-THE-WALL POSE (Viparita Karani) Do this pose as described on page 310. Remain in the pose for 5 minutes or more.

EFFECTS This pose helps soothe your nerves, ease symptoms from kidney disorders, and calm your digestive system.

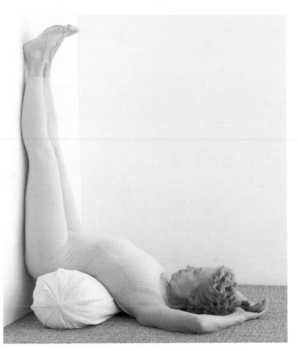

11. CORPSE POSE (Savasana) Do this pose as described on page 310. Remain in the pose for at least 5 to 10 minutes.

EFFECTS This will soothe and reenergize your whole body.

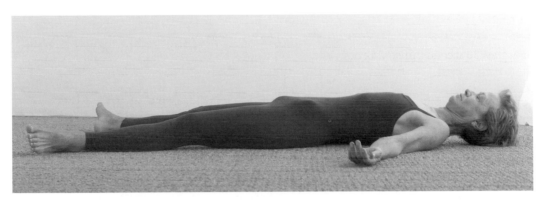

1. Bound Angle Pose (Baddha Konasana)
2. Wide-Angle Seated Pose I
   (Upavistha Konasana I)
3. Reclining Big Toe Pose I
   (Supta Padangusthasana I)
4. Downward-Facing Dog Pose
   (Adho Mukha Svanasana)
5. Downward-Facing Dog Pose
   (Adho Mukha Svanasana)
6. Upward-Facing Dog Pose
   (Urdhva Mukha Svanasana)
7. Mountain Pose with Arms Overhead
   (Urdhva Hastasana in Tadasana)
8. Standing Forward Bend (Uttanasana)
9. Extended Triangle Pose
   (Utthita Trikonasana)
10. Extended Side-Angle Pose
    (Utthita Parsvakonasana)
11. Wide-Angle Standing Forward Bend
    (Prasarita Padottanasana)
12. Child's Pose (Adho Mukha Virasana)
13. Reclining Bound Angle Pose
    (Supta Baddha Konasana)
14. Corpse Pose (Savasana)

1. BOUND ANGLE POSE (Baddha Konasana) Do this pose as described on page 312, or place your hands on a chair in front of you for support. Remain in this pose for 30 seconds or more, breathing normally.

EFFECTS This pose helps tone and strengthen your spine and increase flexibility.

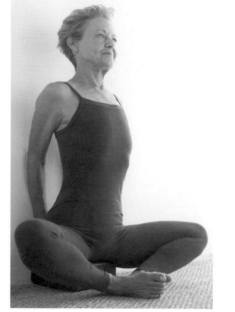

Modification

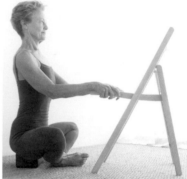

2. WIDE-ANGLE SEATED POSE I (Upavistha Konasana I) Do Wide-Angle Seated Pose I as described on page 312. Remain in this pose for 30 seconds or more, breathing normally.

EFFECTS You can use this pose to help alleviate arthritis pain in your hips and to release a tight groin. It elongates and strengthens your spine, bringing flexibility to your back muscles.

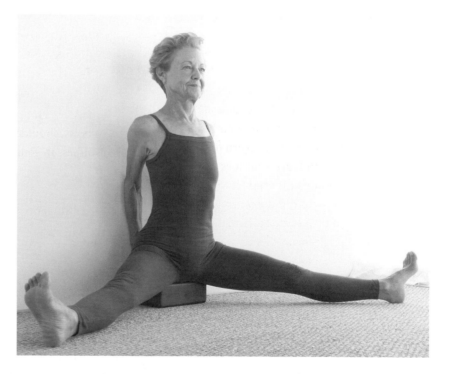

3. RECLINING BIG TOE POSE I (Supta Padangusthasana I) Lie flat on the floor with your legs outstretched and together. As you inhale, draw your left knee up to your chest and place a strap around the ball of your foot. Exhale as you extend your leg straight up to the ceiling (A). With both hands pulling the strap, ease your leg closer to your head (if possible), keeping your left buttock firmly on the floor (B). Keep your right leg on the floor, actively pressing it into the ground, with your toes toward the ceiling. For additional support, press your foot into the wall. Move your leg gently back and forth in its socket to increase mobility and to keep the joints fluid. Release the strap slowly and change legs.

EFFECTS This active pose helps create more flexibility in your hip joints and groin, release stiffness in your lower back, stretch your hamstrings and calf muscles, and strengthen your knees.

A

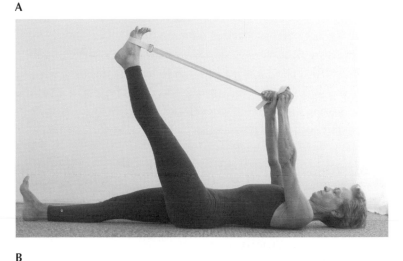

B

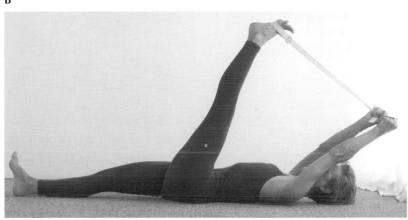

4. DOWNWARD-FACING DOG POSE (Adho Mukha Svanasana) Lie facedown on your sticky mat. Place your palms on the floor by each side of your chest with your fingers well spread and pointing straight ahead. Come up on your hands and knees. That's your position. Now place a bolster or one or two folded blankets vertically so your support is in line with your sternum. Your support should be high enough to support your head, but low enough to lengthen your neck. Return to your hands-and-knees position, and turn your toes under.

Exhale, press your hands firmly into the mat and extend up through your inner arms. As you exhale again, raise your buttocks high into the air and move your thighs up and back. Keep stretching through your legs and bring your heels toward the floor. Keep your legs firm and your elbows straight as you lift your buttocks upward and release your head onto your support. The action of the arms and legs serves to elongate your spine and release your head. Hold this pose for 30 seconds to 1 minute, breathing deeply.

Come back to the hands-and-knees position. Bring your feet together, keep your knees slightly spread, and sit back on your heels. Bend down and rest your forehead on your support. Let your arms lie by your sides with your palms up, and relax completely. Stay like this for a minute or so, breathing deeply.

EFFECTS This pose can help ease arthritic pain in your elbows, shoulders, wrists, and hands. It also helps release stiffness in your back and hamstrings.

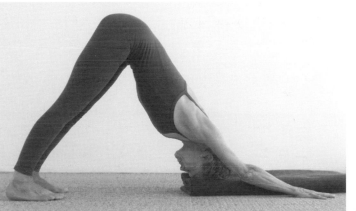

5. DOWNWARD-FACING DOG POSE (Adho Mukha Svanasana)
Place two blocks against the wall, shoulder-width apart. Kneel in front of the wall and place your palms on the blocks. Curl your toes under and walk your feet back, keeping them hip-width apart, so they are about 4 feet away from and in line with your hands. As you exhale, press your feet into the floor and your hands into the blocks and continue the pose as described on page 317.

6. UPWARD-FACING DOG POSE (Urdhva Mukha Svanasana) Lie facedown with your feet hip-width apart, your toes pointing back and legs active. Bend your elbows and place your hands next to your floating ribs, fingers pointing toward your head. Roll your inner thighs toward each other and, leading with your sternum and the crown of your head, raise the upper part of your body off the mat. Press your hands firmly into the mat and raise your sternum as high as you can, while bringing the pelvis toward the hands. Lift your hips off the mat, keep your thighs strong and your knees pulled up so they don't rest on the floor. Move your shoulder blades into your back ribs, expand your chest, and take your head back, looking up at the ceiling. (If you have neck trouble, look straight ahead.) Remain in this position for 15 to 20 seconds. (Put your hands on blocks if you can't lift your thighs off the floor or open your chest.) To come out, exhale as you bend your elbow, resting the hips, thighs, and chest on the mat.
Lower your head down and relax.

EFFECTS This pose alleviates stiffness in your shoulders and upper back, and lower back tension. Opening your chest can lift your spirits when you are depressed and helps calm agitated or nervous energy.

Modification

7. MOUNTAIN POSE WITH ARMS OVERHEAD (Urdhva Hastasana in Tadasana) Stand in Mountain Pose (see page 305; omit the block). Turn your palms outward and slowly lift your arms out to the side and over your head, keeping your shoulders down and away from your ears. Lift your chest and draw your shoulder blades deep into your back. Breathe normally and stay in this position for 20 to 30 seconds, if possible. Otherwise, come in and out of the pose two to three times, breathing evenly. To come out, release your arms down to your sides.

EFFECTS This pose can help ease arthritic pain in your shoulders, arms, and spine; strengthen your knees, legs, and ankles; and stretch your hamstrings.

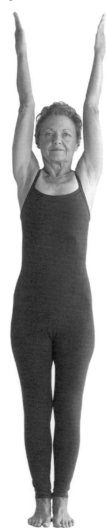

WISDOM FROM THE HEART

8. STANDING FORWARD BEND

(Uttanasana) Stand in Mountain Pose (Tadasana). Balance the weight evenly between your feet, lengthen up through your inner thighs, and roll your thighs in. Keep your legs and knees firm as you lift your arms overhead, stretching up through your waist and ribs. As you exhale, bend forward from your hips and release your side body down toward your knees. Press your hands into the floor next to your feet (A). (If you can't touch the floor, rest your hands on blocks or hold your shins.) Come back to Mountain Pose, clasp your hands behind your back, and as you exhale, bend forward, gently extend through your arms and bring your hands overhead toward the floor (B). Keep your shoulder blades moving into your back, away from your neck.

EFFECTS Use this posture to strengthen and stretch your hamstrings and knees, as well as to increase flexibility in your hip joints and shoulders.

9. EXTENDED TRIANGLE POSE (Utthita Trikonasana)

Stand in Mountain Pose (Tadasana). Step your feet about 3½ feet apart; turn your right foot out 90 degrees and your left foot slightly inward. The heel of your right foot should line up with the arch of your left. (Place a block beside the outside edge of your right foot if you need to.) Stretch your arms out to the sides, draw up through your quadriceps, and lift your abdomen and chest. On an exhalation, keeping your back straight, extend your trunk to the right and bring your right hand down to the floor or the block. Press your hand into the floor or block, stretch across your chest and up through your left arm. Draw your shoulder blades in, turn your chest toward the ceiling, and look straight ahead or up at your left hand. Turn your abdomen to the left. Breathe normally and hold this pose for 20 to 30 seconds. On an inhalation, lift up and straighten your torso. Repeat the pose on your left side, then turn your toes forward and step your feet together.

EFFECTS This is a good pose to strengthen your legs, knees, and ankles, and to relieve stiffness in your elbows, shoulders, neck, and wrists.

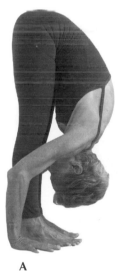

A

B

Modification

10. EXTENDED SIDE-ANGLE POSE (Utthita Parsvakonasana) Stand in Mountain Pose (Tadasana). Step your feet out as wide as possible (about 4½ feet apart, if you can); turn your left foot out 90 degrees and your right foot slightly inward. The heel of your left foot should line up with the arch of your right. Stretch your arms out to the sides. As you exhale, bend your left knee so your thigh is parallel and your shin is perpendicular to the floor. (If your knee extends beyond your ankle, widen your stance.) Keeping your back straight, exhale and extend your trunk to the left, bring your left hand down to the floor (or a block), and stretch your right arm up over your right ear. Draw your shoulder blades in, turn your chest toward the ceiling, and look straight ahead or up toward the ceiling. Turn your abdomen to the right. Breathe normally and hold this pose for 20 to 30 seconds, if possible. Inhale as you lift up and straighten your torso. Repeat the pose on your right side, then turn your toes forward and step your feet back to Mountain Pose.

EFFECTS This pose helps open your hip joints and elongate your spine. It also helps strengthen your legs, knees, and ankles and relieve stiffness in your elbows, neck, and shoulders.

Modification

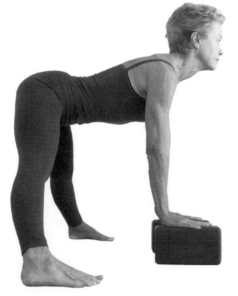

11. WIDE-ANGLE STANDING FORWARD BEND (Prasarita Padottanasana) Do Wide-Angle Standing Forward Bend as described on page 311, continuing in the pose for 20 to 30 seconds. If you have trouble holding this pose, move in and out of it a few times.

EFFECTS This pose helps release tension in your back, shoulders, and legs.

12. CHILD'S POSE (Adho Mukha Virasana) Kneel on the floor with your knees slightly wider than your hips and bring your big toes together. Bend forward and stretch your arms and trunk forward. Rest your head on the floor or a blanket.

EFFECTS This pose stretches and tones your entire spine while releasing the muscles in your neck and upper back.

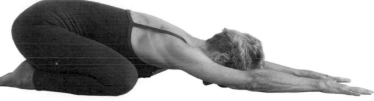

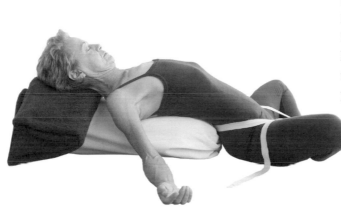

13. RECLINING BOUND ANGLE POSE (Supta Baddha Konasana) Do Reclining Bound Angle Pose as described on page 313. Extend from your groin to your knees and release any tension in your thighs, knees, and ankles. Remain in the pose up to 5 to 10 minutes.

EFFECTS This pose helps you gently open your chest, hips, and groin area, improving circulation.

14. CORPSE POSE (Savasana) Do Corpse Pose as described on page 310. (If your lower back hurts or feels tight, put a bolster under your knees.) Remain in this pose, breathing normally, for at least 5 to 10 minutes.

EFFECTS This posture allows your whole body to relax.

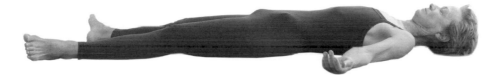

Chapter 14   *Relieving Osteoporosis*

THE THOUGHT OF OSTEOPOROSIS, EVEN MORE THAN HOT FLASHES and seemingly unending perimenopausal PMS, can engender fear in most women—even those who have sailed through menopause relatively unscathed—and have them clambering to fill prescriptions for hormone replacement therapy (HRT). One friend of mine, who has had no problems so far in her menopausal journey, actually began HRT recently because she's terrified of developing osteoporosis. Like me, Freida is a very thin Caucasian woman with a small frame—a body profile that's at high risk for the disease. What scares her most, she says, is that she could have osteoporosis right now and not even know it.

Adding to Freida's fear is the definition of osteoporosis itself. I always thought osteoporosis (literally, "soft bones") meant bone fractures associated with an abnormal loss of bone mineral density—a disease characterized by broken bones, the telltale dowager's hump, and shrinking stature. I associated it with my ninety-two-year-old Aunt Emma who, when asked how she's doing, always replies, "Just fine, dear, only shorter." Calling it an inescapable condition of aging, doctors now define osteoporosis simply as loss of bone mass, which means the body loses more bone cells than it can create, causing the bones to grow weak and unstable and increasing the risk of fractures. The problem with this definition, of course, is that every woman loses more bone than she builds by the time she reaches her late thirties.

The statistics are frightening. According to the U.S. National Osteoporosis Foundation, this silent disease affects 28 million Americans, 80 percent of them women, and does damage long before you even know you have it. By the time the baby boomers have finished menopause, an alarming 41 million women will be considered at high risk for the disease. Articles by the mainstream press abound with such startling statistics as one out of every two women in America over the age of fifty will suffer an osteoporotic fracture; 37,500 Americans die from complications of such fractures; 90 percent of all women over seventy-five have osteoporosis; and ten years after menopause, women have lost over 30 percent of their bone mass.

With statistics like these, doctors understandably want to prescribe something that will prevent or at least delay the effects of bone loss. And women understandably want to fill those prescriptions to prevent the "inevitable"—an osteoporotic fracture in their later years.

However, many women have begun to question the assertion that osteoporosis is a foregone conclusion. Freida, in fact, asked her doctor why she should spend the majority of her postmenopausal years on medication for something that may or may not affect her by the time she reaches seventy-five or eighty. She wondered whether there wasn't something she could do that didn't require taking hormones. Her doctor encouraged her to get a bone density scan to assess her bone mineral density (BMD), begin taking calcium/magnesium supplements, continue exercising every day, and reassess her diet. She reminded Freida that the healthier she is going into menopause—that is, the more bone mass she builds now—the less likely it is that she will have osteoporotic problems.

WHAT CAUSES OSTEOPOROSIS?

Holistic health care providers remind us that osteoporosis is a disease created largely by our Western lifestyle. No one can think that nature would create a woman's body to self-destruct after menopause, inadvertently allowing her ovaries to stop producing the estrogen and progesterone she needs to live a healthy life. According to Susan Love, M.D., author of *Dr. Susan Love's Hormone Book: Making Informed Choices About Menopause*, osteoporosis is not as common as the mainstream medical press wants you to believe. She says only about 25 percent of women will ever develop osteoporosis. Dr. Love also reminds women that a low BMD reading does not automatically mean you have osteoporosis; it is, however, an indication of a higher risk factor and a wake-up call to reassess your lifestyle. Although it's true that estrogen and progesterone contribute to bone stabilization, it's also true that nature gives you what you need through other hormones and organs. It's up to you, however, to keep your body healthy. If you get very little exercise; smoke; eat too much protein, sugar, and processed foods; and drink too much alcohol and caffeine, you run the risk of depleting the hormonal resources you do have and setting yourself up for osteoporosis later on.

Risk Factors for Osteoporosis

- Caucasian ancestry
- Family history of osteoporosis
- Consistent program of excessive exercise or no exercise
- Amenorrhea (delayed menses)
- Thin, small-boned frame
- Poor calcium absorption (determined by blood tests and bone scans)
- Hyperthyroidism
- Smoking
- Excessive intake of alcohol, red meat, and caffeine
- Exposure to environmental toxins
- Premature menopause or removal of ovaries before natural menopause
- Use of prescription drugs such as anti-epileptic medicine, steroids, and blood thinners

How Your Body Makes Bone

Beginning in puberty, the correct balance of estrogen and progesterone ensures that your menstrual cycle is well regulated and that you can experience a healthy, trouble-free pregnancy. Estrogen predominates during the first half of your cycle, preparing your uterus for implantation of a fertilized egg and simultaneously stimulating your bones to retain calcium. By slowing the action of osteoclasts (the cells that break down bone), estrogen exerts some control over how much bone you lose. Progesterone, on the other hand, stimulates osteoblasts (the cells that build new bone). Because progesterone is manufactured in your ovaries during the second phase of your cycle, if you don't ovulate, you don't build new bone efficiently and you'll lose bone mass faster. Too much stress, excessive exercise, rapid weight loss, vitamin and mineral deficiency, and certain prescription drugs can all contribute to anovulatory periods and, as a result, lost bone mass.

Estrogen and progesterone are not the only hormones your endocrine system manufactures that play a part in maintaining healthy bone mass. According to Susan Love, hormones from your parathyroid and thyroid glands work to regulate your metabolism and ensure that your body gets the calcium it needs. If there's not enough calcium to go around, the parathyroid gland instructs your kidneys to hold on to their reserve and tells the osteoclasts to break down more bone and release the calcium into your bloodstream. Your adrenal steroid glands (the ones that respond to physical stress) help your bones give up calcium in an emergency (called bone resorption); and testosterone and other androgens (which your adrenals manufacture after menopause) promote bone growth to balance the bone-resorbing action of the steroids.

Osteoclast cells search for old or damaged bone matter, breaking it down and removing it. Osteoblast cells move in and create new bone matter. To stimulate new growth, bone cells rely on vitamins such as A, C, and K, and minerals like calcium, magnesium, phosphorous, manganese, zinc, copper, and silicon. Vitamin D helps your bones absorb and use the calcium they need. Before you are thirty-five years old, the action of the osteoblasts and osteoclasts is balanced—old bone dissolves, new bone forms. By thirty-five, however, you've reached your peak bone mass, the osteoblasts break down more than the osteoclasts can build, and your body doesn't make much new bone after that.

All this bone making and breaking has an important goal: to ensure that your body has adequate levels of calcium to function properly. Without enough calcium, your body can't regulate its heartbeat, the flow of its nerve impulses, or critical blood-clotting functions. The strength of your muscles and bones, and even your teeth and gums, depend on calcium. In fact, calcium is so critical that one of the endocrine glands—the parathyroid—is designated as your body's calcium regulator. If you have enough calcium, the parathyroid instructs your bones to store the excess (which strengthens them); if you're lacking calcium, the parathyroid demands that your bones give some back (which results in softer, more porous bones).

Of course, if all you needed to prevent osteoporosis were plenty of calcium and additional estrogen, American women—who drink more milk and take more hormone therapy than any other women in the world—would have the lowest rate of osteoporosis. We don't; we have the highest. The fact is, your body has to be able to use the calcium it receives, and your lifestyle can interfere with that.

FIGHTING BACK

Even if you do everything right, your body will lose bone mass at an accelerated rate as soon as you go through menopause, and as far as researchers know now, hormone replacement therapy won't stop that from happening. Scientists do know, however, that this rapid bone loss continues to some extent for at least five to ten years after menopause and then levels off. So, again, the more bone mass you have going into menopause, the better off you'll be ten, twenty, or even thirty years down the line. Even women in countries where osteoporosis is not a problem experience a certain degree of bone mass loss. The key to maintaining healthy bones and preventing the crippling effects of osteoporosis lies in a balanced diet with adequate calcium, a good weight-bearing exercise program, and a lifestyle that allows you time and space to deal with the stresses that come your way.

• To work with osteoporosis, it's important to incorporate inversions and weight-bearing asanas in your daily practice. Downward-Facing Dog Pose (Adho Mukha Svanasana), Headstand (Sirsasana), and Upward-Facing Bow Pose (Urdhva Dhanurasana) are all beneficial. If you are an advanced practitioner, standing on your hands or doing an elbow balance (such as Pincha Mayura-sana) works well, too. These poses, as well as Upward-Facing Bow Pose, enable you to lift your own weight, which is very important for building bone mass.

Unfortunately, no one has control over some of the risk factors for the disease. For example, Freida, being a woman, has less bone mass than a man; there's nothing she can do about that. She is also thin, small-boned, and Caucasian, and both her grandmother and her mother have suffered stress fractures of the vertebrae in their later years. There's nothing she can do about those factors, either. What she can do, however, is create a lifestyle that promotes preventive care for her bones. These lifestyle choices should ideally happen long before a woman enters perimenopause, preferably in her twenties and thirties, but it's never too late to start.

Exercise

Even the most conservative doctor believes exercise increases bone mass in postmenopausal women. The key, according to Kendra Kaye Zuckerman, M.D., director of the osteoporosis program at Allegheny University Hospitals in Philadelphia, is that you must exercise consistently—at least thirty minutes a day, five days a week. Exercise works, according to Krishna Raman, M.D., author of *A Matter of Health,* because it stimulates bone remodeling and "improves the absorption of calcium from the intestine and promotes its deposition on the bones." Not just any kind of exercise will do, however. Weight-bearing exercise and movements that exert pressure on your bones stimulate bones to retain calcium. Health care providers recommend walking or running because they stimulate the bones in your feet, legs, pelvis, and spine by combining the effects of gravity and muscle contraction. In contrast, swimming (which can help joint pain and limited mobility) does nothing to increase bone density.

If you have already begun to lose bone mass—and may therefore be susceptible to vertebral stress fractures—running can put too much stress on your knees, ankles, and lumbar spine. The other problem with confining weight-bearing exercise to walking or running is that these activities only benefit your lower limbs and do nothing to strengthen your wrists, shoulders, upper back, or elbows.

One additional caveat about aerobic exercise: Be careful not to overdo it. Excessive exercising, and a corresponding drop in body fat, can actually increase your chances of osteoporosis, according to the National Osteoporosis Foundation.

Good Posture

As we have discussed throughout this book, correct posture is critical to keeping your spine healthy. If you have poor posture on top of a weakened spine, it can increase your likelihood of vertebral fracture. If your head sits in front of your shoulders, the weight is not evenly distributed along your spine. Instead, the front part of the thoracic vertebrae receive the majority of the weight and are prone to stress fractures.

Standing postures like Mountain Pose (Tadasana) help strengthen your back muscles and improve your posture. Including forward and backward bends in your daily yoga practice can strengthen the front and back of your spinal column, and help increase overall flexibility. Modified backbends can passively lengthen your thoracic spine and help prevent stress fractures. (See additional poses in chapter 8.)

Patricia Says

• Maintain good posture, with your head over your shoulders and your shoulders in line with your hips, to prevent pressure on your spine. Practice sitting, standing, and walking with the same posture you use in Mountain Pose (Tadasana).

• Put your body through its full range of motion—from standing to sitting, right side up and upside down, back and forth, and twisting side to side—to increase and maintain mobility and flexibility.

• Incorporate restorative poses that allow your body and your muscles to relax completely.

Diet

The food you eat has an important effect on maintaining bone mass. Even if you've been less than diligent in the past, it's never too late to improve your diet. Evaluate your present intake against the following suggested guidelines.

Eat Less Animal-Derived Protein Research shows that vegetarian women lose far less bone mass than their meat-eating sisters. In fact, one study conducted in southwestern Michigan reported that women who were vegetarians for twenty years had only 18 percent bone mass loss, while their carnivorous counterparts suffered 35 percent loss. One reason for that, according to Dr. Dean Ornish, director of the Preventive Medicine Research Institute in Sausalito, California, is that a diet high in animal protein can cause your body to excrete too much calcium through urine. That means your body actually gets rid of the calcium before you can benefit. Vegetarians, on the other hand, excrete far less calcium and therefore profit from its bone-strengthening capabilities.

Supplement Your Diet with Calcium Adequate amounts of calcium (1,000 mg/day before and during menopause, 1,500 mg/day after menopause) are critical to healthy bones and a healthy heart. Remember, however, no amount of calcium supplementation will do you any good if your diet prevents your body from absorbing it. Whether you ingest too little calcium or your body excretes too much, your bones will suffer. According to a 1998 article in *Internal Medicine News*, taking calcium (1,200 to 1,500 mg/day) and vitamin D (700 to 800 IU/day) supplements reduces fractures in postmenopausal women by 50 percent. If you don't drink much milk or you suffer from lactose intolerance, don't despair. You can get adequate calcium from a variety of sources—dark green leafy vegetables, almonds, tofu, soy products, miso, seaweed, and salmon. Drink calcium-enriched orange juice—one glass delivers as much calcium as a glass of milk. Good calcium-providing herbs include nettles, horsetail, sage, oatstraw, borage, raspberry leaf, and alfalfa.

If you use calcium supplements, be sure to take them according to the directions on the label for maximum absorption. (Note: Don't try to get your calcium from antacids that contain aluminum, which causes the calcium to be excreted.) Some calcium, like calcium carbonate, gets absorbed better with food; other types, like calcium citrate, work better on an empty stomach. To use the calcium you do take in, your body needs adequate amounts of not only vitamin D, but also magnesium, trace minerals, and hydrochloric (or stomach) acid—which postmenopausal women often lack. Women need approximately 2.0 mg of copper, 3.0 mg of manganese, and 12 mg of zinc every day. Nuts, berries, tofu, and tomatoes give you enough manganese and copper; seafood and peas are good sources of zinc. Trace minerals enhance calcium's ability to increase bone density as well. You can purchase betaine hydrochloric acid at your local health food store if you need it.

You also need to beware of calcium robbers. Too much salt can leach calcium from your bones, just as protein can. Watch out for hidden salt in processed foods, soft drinks, and canned goods. Phosphates in carbonated soft drinks can also steal from your body's calcium supply; so can caffeine, alcohol, and nicotine. Some researchers warn that consuming more than three or four cups of caffeinated coffee a day can increase your risk factor for bone loss by 80 percent. Cigarette smoking and even moderate alcohol consumption can double your risk.

Patricia Says

• To keep joints mobile and flexible, move in and out of standing poses several times before holding the position. Do not hold a pose too long or lock your joints, but focus on creating freedom in your joints.

• Don't practice poses that compress your spine—keep it elongated.

• If you already have osteoporotic fractures, avoid sudden or jerking movements. Do not do Headstand (Sirsasana) or other unsupported inversions that could bring weight to bear on your spine.

Sunbathe Everyone knows the dangers of getting too much sun. However, twenty-five to thirty minutes three or four times a week give you all the vitamin D your body needs to absorb and use calcium effectively. So, slather on plenty of sunblock and head outside.

Additional Supplements Besides taking enough calcium, magnesium, and trace minerals, increasing your vitamin K intake may help your bones stay less breakable, according to researchers at Tufts University. If you're not on blood-thinning medication, you may want to ask your doctor whether increasing your daily intake of vitamin K makes sense. It's actually pretty easy to get all you need from the food you eat. Just one-half cup of collard greens, for example, can give you over 400 mcg of vitamin K; the same amount of spinach yields 360 mcg; and broccoli packs 113 mcg into that little half cup. Essential fatty acids, vitamins B_6 and C, and folic acid also contribute to good, healthy bone structure.

Adequate Estrogen

Your body must have an adequate supply of estrogen to keep your bones strong and healthy and to minimize bone mass loss. Once you go through menopause, your ovaries no longer make the amount of estrogen your body's used to, so it must look for another supplier. Be patient. Remember, each time you enter a new phase of life, your body needs time to adjust. You've been through periods of raging hormones at least twice in you life (and more if you've had babies) and you've lived to tell about it. Now your body needs time to figure out this phase.

While it's working things out, your bones will lose density, and there's not a lot you can do about it. Your body will turn primarily to the adrenals to get its hormones; body fat and muscles also manufacture (and even the ovaries continue to provide) some estrogen. If your adrenal glands are depleted through stress, poor diet, or illness, they can't do their job. If you have dieted excessively and don't have much body fat, your body won't find adequate estrogen there, either.

Hormone Replacement Therapy In a lecture she gave at Kripalu Yoga Center in May 1999, Susan Love posed an interesting question. If, as studies show, a woman will lose significant bone mass twice in her life—during the five to ten years after menopause and then again in her seventies—but bone fractures, especially in the hips, generally don't occur until a woman is in her seventies and eighties, should she take HRT from perimenopause on to prevent fractures that most probably will occur when she's quite old (if at all)? Is it possible to wait until a woman reaches seventy or seventy-five and then give her the smallest amount of estrogen possible to prevent such breakage? The most dangerous side effects of hormone therapy—increased risks for breast and endometrium cancer—appear to be the result of long-term use (more than five years). If women have to go on hormones at forty-five or fifty years old to prevent a potential hip fracture thirty years from now, Dr. Love warns, they may be setting themselves up to die of breast or uterine cancer long before they're old enough to break a bone. Unfortunately, there are no clear-cut answers to these questions yet.

John Lee, M.D., coauthor of the well-known and somewhat controversial book *What Your Doctor May Not Tell You About Menopause: The Breakthrough Book on Natural Progesterone,* prescribes natural progesterone cream to his female patients suffering from osteoporosis, with what he says are often outstanding results. His theory is that estrogen, while increasing bone mass in existing bones, does nothing to create new bone. But progesterone does, as long as the progesterone you take is not synthetic. Dr. Lee recommends using a progesterone cream, because he has encountered very few, if any, side effects this way. Dr. Love recommends using micronized progesterone, which has been shown in studies to build bone as well as prevent resorption. Unfortunately,

---

HRT and Osteoporosis

A study cited in the April 15, 2001, issue of the *American Journal of Medicine* appears to indicate that hormone replacement therapy does not prevent or help reverse osteoporosis. This study is part of the Heart and Estrogen/Progestin Replacement Study (HERS), which tracked 2,700 postmenopausal women for four years to determine (in part) the effect HRT had on bone fractures. According to the results, HRT was no more effective than a placebo in protecting women from broken bones.

the micronized progesterone used in the clinical trials she describes is not available in this country; other brands can be ordered (with a doctor's prescription) from alternative compounding pharmacies such as the Women's International Pharmacy in Madison, Wisconsin. Again, there aren't enough studies yet to prove the progesterone theory or to categorically show that taking estrogen or a combination of estrogen and progesterone will prevent age-related bone fractures.

Other promising medical alternatives to hormones include bisphosphonates like Fosamax. Bisphosphonates work by preventing osteoclasts from reabsorbing bone. Unfortunately, there are not enough long-term studies yet to determine how well they work. Two other treatments that show promise are calcitonins, which are hormones from the thyroid, and a bioflavonoid called ipriflavone, which may increase bone density. Recent studies show the parathyroid hormone (PTH) as a promising therapy for actually stimulating bone growth with few side effects. The bad news on PTH so far is that it can only be administered through daily injection; the good news is that women need take it for only a year or two.

Even if you do decide to take hormones or some other form of treatment—either now or when you get older—remember that pharmaceutical therapy (or herbal alternatives) alone will not help you prevent osteoporosis. You still need to pay attention to your diet; you still need daily exercise, preferably including a well-rounded yoga practice with weight-bearing poses; and you still need to honor your body's signals to rest and renew. Osteoporosis is a crippling, painful disease; but with proper attention to all aspects of your health, it needn't be an inevitable consequence of aging.

HOW YOGA CAN HELP

Yoga helps your body in several ways. Many health practitioners see its usefulness in combating the stress that can compromise your neuroendocrine and immune systems. But yoga does more than that. In a 1988 article in *Yoga Journal*, author Mary Schatz, M.D., says yoga can stimulate your bones to retain calcium, provided your body gets enough calcium in the first place. The secret? Yoga emphasizes weight-bearing poses (like arm balances, inversions, and standing poses) that affect your whole spine, arms, shoulders, elbows, legs, knees, ankles, and feet, while encouraging full range of motion. In a small, as yet unpublished study conducted at California State University at Los Angeles in 2000, researchers discovered what therapeutic yoga teachers have known all along: Yoga actually increases bone density. Nine female subjects practiced yoga, and the other nine did not. Bone density tests were given at the beginning of the study and again after six months. The yoga practitioners saw an increase in bone density in their vertebrae, but the nonpractitioners saw no change at all. Interestingly enough, the yoga practitioners also had a decrease in density of the hip bone. Ironically, doctors believe this decrease actually signals a subsequent rise in bone density.

B. K. S. Iyengar contends that through the process of squeezing out the old, stale blood or lymphatic fluids, and soaking the area with freshly oxygenated blood or fluids, yoga helps your body use the nutrients it needs. Inversions, particularly Shoulderstand (Sarvangasana) and Plough Pose (Halasana), work particularly well. These poses, according to Iyengar, regulate your thyroid and parathyroid glands (critical for metabolism) by creating a chin lock that squeezes stale blood from the area. As you come out of the pose, and release the lock, the neck region is bathed in fresh blood. In other words, inversions aid circulation in and around your head and neck, which can rejuvenate the glands.

In Patricia's practice, she teaches forward bends to quiet the adrenal glands, mitigating the effects of the fight-or-flight response, and backbends to energize them. She says twists are equally effective for regulating the adrenals, which provide adequate amounts of estrogen and androgen for healthy bones.

Many older people fall because they lose confidence in their ability to move properly; others suffer from poor eyesight, weakened muscles (often from lack of use), poor posture, or arthritis. Yoga can help improve your posture and coordination, strengthen your muscles, increase your flexibility, and promote better balance.

You may do the yoga poses in the following sequence supported as we show here, or if you have a daily practice and are symptom-free, do the full pose (as shown in chapters 1 and 2). If you already suffer from the effects of osteoporosis or you're at high risk for the disease, check with your health practitioner before you begin. You'll find a few asanas that are good if you have limited mobility, but talk with your doctor first. It's clear that osteoporosis presents a real catch-22 for those who suffer. If you do too much—or the wrong kind of exercise—not only do you experience more pain, you run the risk of breaking more bones. If you don't exercise, your muscles will grow stiffer and weaker and you'll lose the vital calcium you need to prevent additional fractures. So it's imperative that you seek advice from a therapeutic yoga teacher and a knowledgeable health practitioner.

A SEQUENCE FOR OSTEOPOROSIS

1. Mountain Pose (Tadasana) with different arm positions
2. Standing Forward Bend (Uttanasana)
3. Downward-Facing Dog Pose (Adho Mukha Svanasana)
4. Warrior I Pose (Virabhadrasana I)
5. Warrior II Pose (Virabhadrasana II)
6. Extended Triangle Pose (Utthita Trikonasana)
7. Revolved Triangle Pose (Parivrtta Trikonasana)
8. Standing Spinal Twist Pose (Utthita Marichyasana)
9. Camel Pose (Ustrasana)
10. Upward-Facing Bow Pose (Urdhva Dhanurasana)
11. Child's Pose (Adho Mukha Virasana)
12. Legs-Up-the-Wall Pose† (Viparita Karani) and Cycle
13. Corpse Pose (Savasana)

1. MOUNTAIN POSE (Tadasana) Stand up straight, your legs together (with big toes touching, if that's comfortable). Distribute your weight evenly between the front of your feet and your heels. Tighten your knees by pulling up with your quadriceps (front thigh muscles). Raise your sternum (breastbone) and broaden your chest by rolling your shoulders back and drawing your shoulder blades in. Lift your abdomen up and draw your tailbone in without pushing your thighs forward. Extend your arms downward with palms facing your thighs and fingers together (A). Keep your shoulders moving away from your ears. Visualize your spine elongating, rising out of your center, as you plant your feet firmly on the ground. Breathe normally, relax your pelvic floor muscles (the ones you contract to stop urinating), your shoulders, and your neck. Remain in the pose for 30 to 60 seconds.

ARMS OVERHEAD (Urdhva Hastasana) Standing in Mountain Pose (Tadasana), turn your palms outward and slowly lift your arms to the side and over your head, keeping your shoulders down and away from your ears (B). Lift your chest and draw your shoulder blades deep into your back. (If you have trouble with balance, you may step your feet apart a little or practice with your back against a wall.) Stay in this pose for 20 to 30 seconds, if possible. Otherwise, come in and out two or three times.

ARMS IN PRAYER POSITION (Namaskar Arms) To further open your chest and shoulder area, continue standing in Mountain Pose (Tadasana), put your hands together in prayer position behind your back (C). Be careful not to arch your back. (If that's too much of a stretch, cross your arms behind you, holding your elbows.) Your posture should remain in alignment, just as it does when you have your arms by your sides.

EFFECTS The different arm positions help alleviate stiffness in your shoulders, arms, and upper and lower back; improve circulation throughout your body; and correct postural problems.

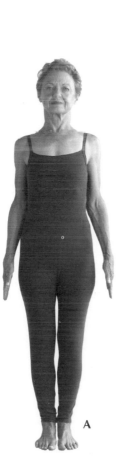

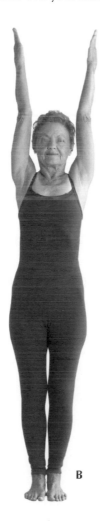

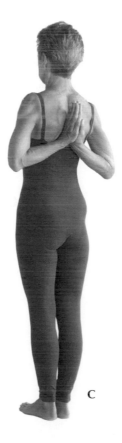

A

B

C

Modification

2. STANDING FORWARD BEND (Uttanasana)

Stand with your feet slightly apart. Clasp your hands behind your back and, as you exhale, lengthen your waist and side ribs toward the floor. Bend forward, extend through your arms, and bring your hands overhead toward the floor. Keep your shoulder blades moving away from your neck. Remain in this position for 10 to 15 seconds, slowly coming back to a standing position, and rest for a few breaths.

EFFECTS By clasping your hands behind your back, you open your chest more and release tension and stiffness in your shoulders, elbows, wrists, and fingers.

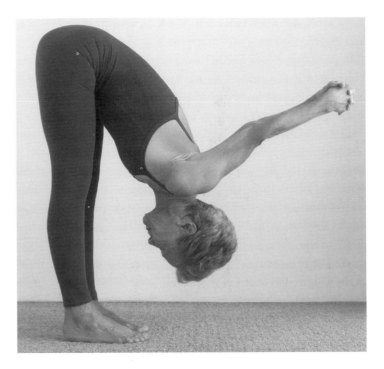

3. DOWNWARD-FACING DOG POSE (Adho Mukha Svanasana)

To find the correct distance between your hands and feet for this pose, lie facedown. Place your palms on the floor by each side of your chest with your fingers well spread and pointing toward your head. Turn your toes inward. Come up on your hands and knees. (If you are flexible enough, keep your feet close together.)

Exhale, press your hands into the mat and extend up through your inner arms. Exhale again and raise your buttocks high into the air. Move your thighs up and back, keep stretching through your legs, and bring your heels toward the floor as you lift your buttocks higher. The action of the arms and legs serves to elongate the spine and release your head. Stay in this pose for 30 seconds to 1 minute, breathing deeply. Let your head rest completely and release the base of your neck. To come out, return to your hands and knees, sit back on your heels, and lift your head up.

EFFECTS This weight-bearing exercise strengthens your arms, legs, and spine; helps elongate your spine; and eases tension and stiffness in your shoulders, neck, and arms.

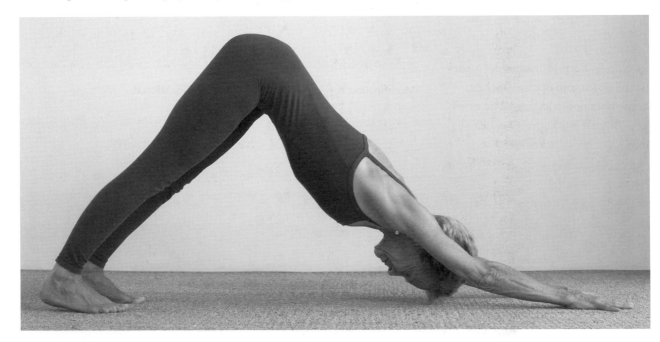

4. WARRIOR I POSE (Virabhadrasana I) Stand in Mountain Pose (Tadasana). Step your feet as far apart as is comfortable (about 4½ feet) with your toes pointing forward. Stretch your arms out to the sides at shoulder level, parallel to the floor, with palms down. Turn your palms up and raise both arms until they are in line with your ears and parallel to each other; your elbows should be straight. Draw up through your quadriceps and lift your abdomen and chest. As you exhale, simultaneously turn your torso and right leg 90 degrees to the right and your left foot about 60 degrees to the right. Inhale and stretch through your upper arms; exhale and bend your right knee so your thigh and shin form a right angle. (If your knee extends beyond your ankle, you need to widen your stance.) Stretch your torso up toward the ceiling as you take your head back as far as it is comfortable and look up at your thumbs. (If this is too hard on your neck, keep your head straight and your gaze forward.) Move in and out of the pose several times to create mobility in your hips and knees.

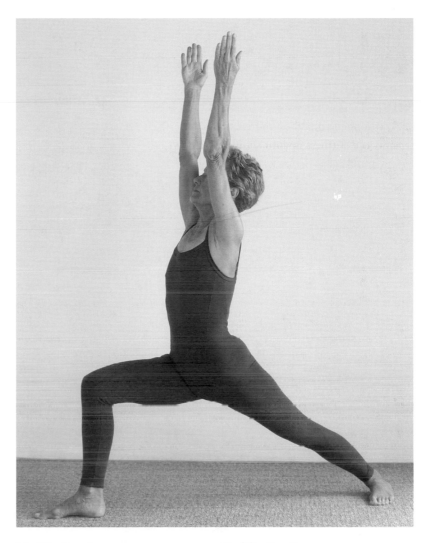

MODIFICATION If you need additional support or stability, press the toes of your front foot into the wall and place your hands on the wall in front of you. Look straight ahead. Move in and out of the pose with each exhalation, bending and straightening your front leg three or four times. As you bend your knee the last time, release your hands from the wall, and stretch your arms over your head with your palms facing each other. Keep your shoulder blades in and down, and open your chest. Remember not to let your knee extend beyond your ankle. Breathe normally for several breaths. Return to Mountain Pose (Tadasana) and switch legs.

EFFECTS This weight-bearing pose helps increase mobility in your hips and lower back. Moving in and out of the pose helps keep your joints flexible.

Modification A

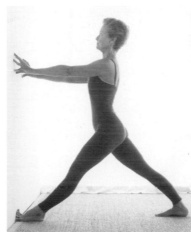

Modification B

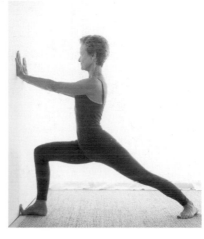

5. WARRIOR II POSE (Virabhadrasana II) Stand in Mountain Pose (Tadasana). Step your feet out as wide as possible (about 4½ feet apart, if you can); turn your left foot out 90 degrees and your right foot slightly inward. The heel of your left foot should line up with the arch of your right. Stretch your arms out to the sides so they're parallel to the floor. As you exhale, bend your left knee so your thigh is parallel and your shin is perpendicular to the floor. (If your knee extends beyond your ankle, you need to widen your stance.) Turn your head to look over your left arm just past your fingertips. Imagine both arms are engaged in a tug-of-war. Move in and out of the pose several times to increase mobility in your joints.

MODIFICATION If you need support, practice with one foot pressed up against and your hand resting on the wall. Move in and out of the pose by straightening as you inhale and bending the knee of the leg closest to the wall as you exhale, releasing your arms slightly, if necessary. As you come into the pose for the last time, remove your hand from the wall, and remain in the pose for several breaths. Step your feet together and change sides.

EFFECTS This pose is great for improving posture; elongating and strengthening your spine; and increasing flexibility in your hips, back, and legs. Because it is a weight-bearing exercise for your feet, ankles, and legs, it stimulates the bones in those areas to retain calcium.

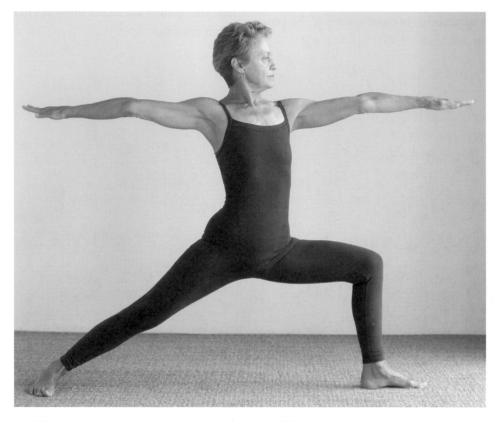

Modification A

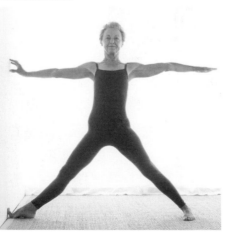

Modification B

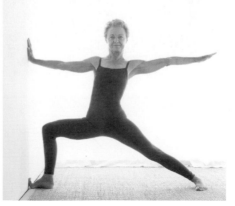

6. EXTENDED TRIANGLE POSE (Utthita Trikonasana)

Stand in Mountain Pose (Tadasana). Step your feet about 3½ feet apart; turn your right foot out 90 degrees and your left foot slightly inward. The heel of your right foot should line up with the arch of your left. Place a block beside the outside edge of your right foot. Stretch your arms out to the sides, draw up through your quadriceps, and lift your abdomen and chest. On an exhalation, keeping your back straight, extend your trunk to the right and bring your right hand down to the block. Press your hand into the block, stretch across your chest and up through your left arm. Draw your shoulder blades in, turn your chest toward the ceiling, and look straight ahead or up at your left hand. Turn your abdomen to the left. Breathe normally and hold this pose for 20 to 30 seconds. On an inhalation, lift up and straighten your torso. Repeat the pose on your left side, then turn your toes forward and step your feet back toward each other, returning to Mountain Pose.

MODIFICATION If this pose proves too challenging or if you feel unsteady, substitute a low stool or chair for the block. Place one hand on the chair and another on your hip. Keep your arms and legs active and strong. Relax your shoulders, neck, and facial muscles, and breathe normally for several breaths.

EFFECTS This pose elongates and strengthens your spine and increases circulation to your pelvic region. It is excellent for helping increase flexibility and stability. Because it is a weight-bearing exercise for your arms, legs, and spine, it stimulates the bones in those areas to retain calcium.

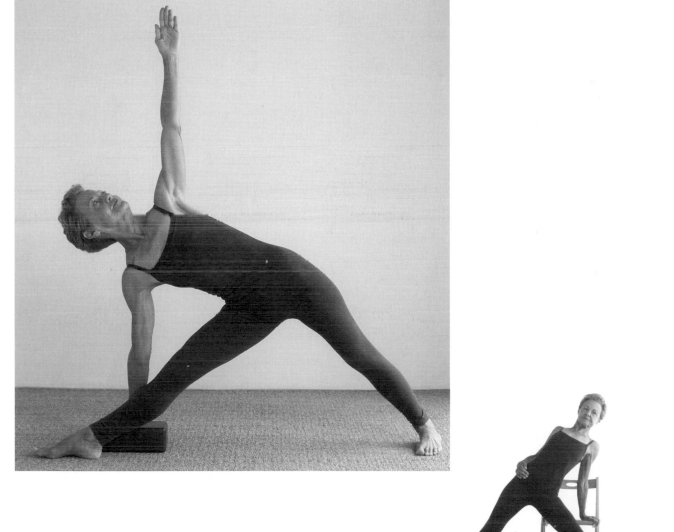

Modification

7. REVOLVED TRIANGLE POSE (Parivrtta Trikonasana) Stand in Mountain Pose (Tadasana). Step your feet about 3 to 3½ feet apart; turn your left foot out 90 degrees and your right foot slightly inward. The heel of your right foot should line up with the arch of your left. Place a block parallel to the outside edge of your left foot. As you exhale, rotate your torso so you are facing left; your right leg and knee should turn inward. Place the fingertips of your right hand on the block. Tighten both legs and keep your chest expanded by drawing your right shoulder blade into your back. Breathe normally for 15 to 20 seconds. Come up on an inhalation, turn, and repeat the pose on the other side.

If this pose is too difficult, place your hand on a chair instead of a block. Add blankets and bolsters to the chair to raise the height. Come in and out of the pose several times to keep your joints fluid and flexible. Hold the final pose for several breaths, if possible.

EFFECTS This pose stimulates the bones in your legs, arms, and spine to retain calcium. It also elongates and strengthens your thoracic spine; increases flexibility and mobility in your shoulders, hips, and back; and improves your posture.

8. STANDING SPINAL TWIST POSE (Utthita Marichyasana) Place a chair with one side against the wall and put a block on the seat area closest to the wall. (If the block slips, place a sticky mat on the chair seat first.) Stand facing the chair with the left side of your body next to the wall. Keeping your right leg firm, put your left foot up on the block. Inhale and stretch up, exhale and turn your torso toward the wall, using your right hand on your left knee and your left hand on the wall. Move in and out of this pose several times, each time taking a deeper inhalation to stretch up taller and exhaling more completely to turn your torso a little more. Turn the chair and repeat with your right foot.

EFFECTS This pose helps elongate and strengthen your spine and release stiffness in your upper and middle back.

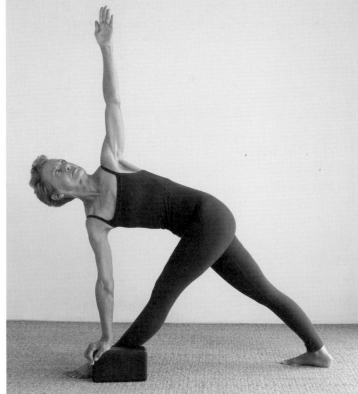

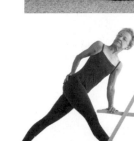

Modification

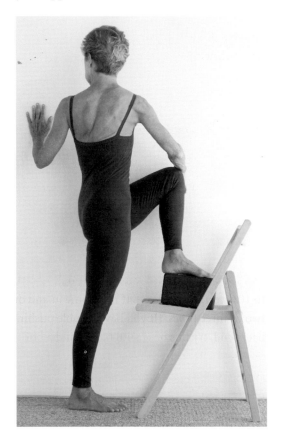

9. CAMEL POSE† (Ustrasana) Kneel on the floor with your knees and feet hip-width apart. Place your palms on your buttocks and as you exhale, move your thighs forward slightly and raise your side ribs. Gradually bend back as far as possible, lift your chest, and broaden your shoulders. Move your hands from your buttocks to your feet, and take hold of your heels. (If you can't reach your heels, place your hands on blocks positioned next to each ankle with your fingers pointing in the same direction as your feet.) Your thighs should be perpendicular to the floor. Take your head back, if that's comfortable, and breathe steadily for 10 to 15 seconds. If that's too difficult at first, come in to and out of the pose a couple of times.

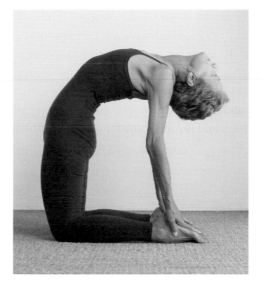

To come out, release your hands one at a time. As you exhale, slowly lift up from your sternum, using your thigh muscles. Your head should come up last.

EFFECTS This pose helps stimulate your vertebrae to retain calcium and strengthen your spine and upper back muscles.

†CAUTION Do not do this pose if you have a migraine or tension headache, or if you suffer from hypertension.

10. UPWARD-FACING BOW POSE† (Urdhva Dhanurasana) Lie on your back with your knees bent, your feet hip-width apart, and your heels close to your buttocks. Bend your elbows and place your hands alongside your head with your fingers pointing toward your feet. As you exhale, raise your hips and chest, straighten your arms, and stretch your legs. Lift your tailbone and move the backs of your thighs toward your buttocks. To come out, bend your knees and elbows, and slowly lower your body to the floor. Hold this pose for 5 to 10 seconds, if you can. If not, come in and out of the pose two or three times. (If you have trouble pushing up into a backbend, try this pose with blocks and a bolster as shown on page 37.)

EFFECTS This weight-bearing pose is extremely beneficial because it allows you to lift your own weight, stimulating the bones in your back, arms, shoulders, legs, and feet to retain calcium. It also helps increase flexibility in your chest and spine.

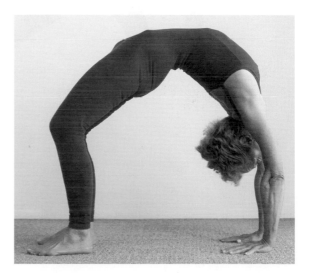

†CAUTION Do the unsupported version of this pose only if it is already part of your yoga practice. Seek the advice of an experienced teacher if you have neck problems. Do not do this pose if you have a migraine or tension headache, or suffer from heart trouble or any serious illness.

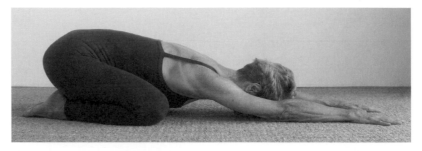

11. CHILD'S POSE (Adho Mukha Virasana) Kneel on the floor with your knees slightly wider than your hips and bring your big toes together. Bend forward and stretch your arms and trunk forward. Rest your head on the floor or a blanket. Remain in this position for 20 to 30 seconds, stretching out your back.

EFFECTS This is a restful counterpose to practice after backbends. It stretches and tones your spine and helps release tension in your back, neck, shoulders, and arms.

12. LEGS-UP-THE-WALL POSE† (Viparita Karani) AND CYCLE Place a bolster about 3 inches from the wall. Sit on the bolster so your right hip and side are touching the wall. Using your hands to support you, lean back and swivel your body around, taking your right leg and then your left leg up the wall. Keep your buttocks close to or against the wall; if they moved away from the wall as you lifted your legs, place your feet on the wall and use your hands for support to lift your hips and move your buttocks back into position. (If you feel discomfort in your legs, push your buttocks slightly away from the wall.) Lie down so your lower back and ribs are supported by the bolster, your tailbone is descending toward the floor, and your shoulders and head are on the floor (A). (If your neck is uncomfortable, put a folded towel or blanket under it.) Extend through your legs and place your arms out at your sides, elbows bent and palms up. Rest in this position, eyes closed, for 5 minutes.

CYCLE Without moving your torso, allow your legs to open out to the sides (B). Remain in this position, breathing normally, for 3 to 5 minutes.

A

B

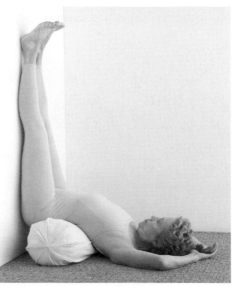

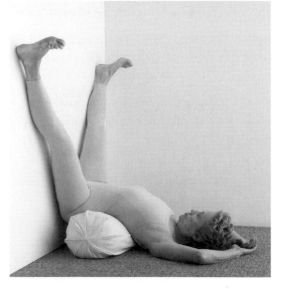

Again keeping your torso in the same position, bend your knees, cross your legs at the ankles, and continue in the pose for another 3 to 5 minutes (C).

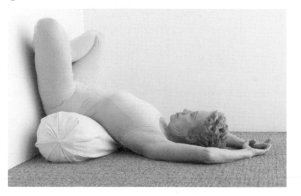

C

Gently push away from the wall until your buttocks are just off the bolster and resting on the floor; the backs of your thighs and legs rest on the bolster. Stay in this position for 5 minutes, or as long as you like (D).

To come out of the pose, uncross your legs, push gently away from the bolster, and roll to one side. Breathe quietly for a few breaths, then use your arms to help you to a seated position.

EFFECTS This restorative pose allows you to relax deeply while releasing your lower back.

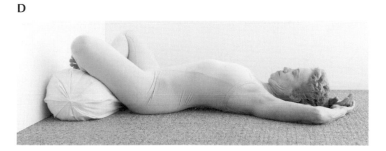

D

13. CORPSE POSE (Savasana) Lie on your back with your legs stretched out in front of you. Place your arms comfortably at your sides, slightly away from your torso, with your palms facing upward. Actively stretch your arms and legs away from you, then allow them to release completely. Close your eyes and let everything relax. Take a few deep breaths, inhaling into your chest without tensing your throat, neck, or diaphragm. Exhale your body into the floor, releasing your shoulders, neck, and facial muscles. Keep your abdomen soft and relaxed, and release your lower back. (If you feel strain in your neck, place a folded blanket under your neck and head.) Breathe normally for at least 5 to 10 minutes. To come out of the pose, bend your knees, roll slowly to one side, and after a few breaths, gently push yourself to a seated position.

EFFECTS This pose brings a sense of complete relaxation, lightness of being, and serenity.

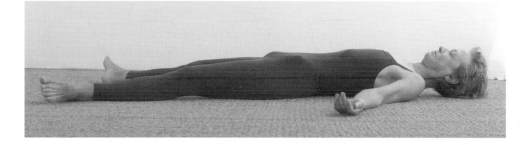

Chapter 15 Strengthening Your Heart

I ONCE ASKED MY EIGHTY-EIGHT-YEAR-OLD GRANDMOTHER WHAT she feared most about growing old. Did she worry about osteoporosis? "A little bit," she admitted, even as she stood straight and tall. "The thought of breaking my hip or my leg scares me, because then someone would have to take care of me. I couldn't stand that."

"What else?" I prodded.

"Losing my mind before my body is ready to give up," she answered.

"What about your heart, Gram? Do you ever worry about having a heart attack?" I persisted.

"Oh, no dear," she replied, "That's a man's disease. My only concern is that I have enough room in my heart to hold all my grandchildren and great-grandchildren."

Unfortunately for women, cardiovascular disease is no longer solely a man's health problem. In fact, the popular press, medical texts, family physicians, and gynecologists alike warn that after age sixty-five a woman's chances of dying from a heart attack increase dramatically. Studies show that only one in ten women between forty-five and sixty-four have some form of cardiovascular disease, but as many as one in four over the age of sixty-five are affected. In fact, more women will die from a heart attack than from all types of cancers combined.

These statistics certainly make it hard for us to ignore the risk of postmenopausal heart disease. Luckily, even high-risk women can reduce their chance of an untimely demise with lifestyle changes, which may include taking hormone replacement therapy (HRT), changing their diet, adding vitamin supplements, doing yoga, meditating, participating in support groups, and/or doing service in their communities. Yoga works particularly well in caring for an ailing heart because it addresses the problem holistically and gives women a way to manage their disease physically, emotionally, and spiritually.

YOUR HEART

The heart itself is made up of two pumps with two chambers each, an atrium on top and a ventricle on the bottom. Oxygenated blood from your lungs flows into the left atrium, travels through the left ventricle, and goes out through the aorta to the rest of your body. Once your body has finished with it, oxygen-depleted blood comes back to the heart via the right atrium, where it flows into the right ventricle, which pumps it into the lungs by way of the pulmonary artery.

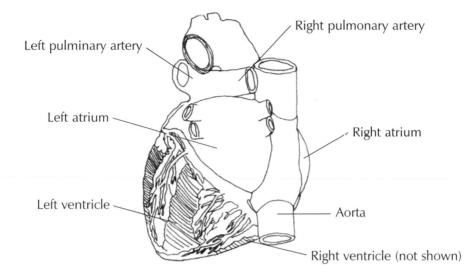

Left pulminary artery

Right pulmonary artery

Left atrium

Right atrium

Left ventricle

Aorta

Right ventricle (not shown)

The action of moving blood in and out of the heart and through the rest of your body depends on a strong heartbeat. A strong, steady beat requires a strong heart muscle that can contract rhythmically, sending rich, oxygenated blood to your body's tissues and then pumping blood back into the lungs for reoxygenation. When your body is at rest, your heart beats an average of 60 to 100 beats per minute. As the heart rests between strong contractions, it receives blood back into its upper chambers—oxygenated blood fills the left atrium and oxygen-depleted blood floods the right atrium.

When the heart pumps blood throughout your body via the arteries, it creates a certain amount of pressure against the artery walls. Health care professionals evaluate this blood pressure in your arm. When your heart contracts, your blood pressure rises, and the highest number of beats perceived (typically between 100 and 140) represents your systolic, or top-number, blood pressure. When your heart relaxes briefly between beats, the pressure drops slightly. This lower reading (usually between 60 and 85) represents your diastolic, or bottom-number, blood pressure. Your central nervous system regulates the rhythm of your heartbeat, which explains why your heart pounds so hard when you're anxious or frightened.

WHAT GOES WRONG

Physiologically, heart disease—or more accurately, cardiovascular disease (CVD)—encompasses all problems pertaining to the heart and blood vessels. One category of heart disease relates to hardening of the arteries, a process known as arteriosclerosis. This category includes coronary heart disease (CHD), characterized by decreased blood flow to the heart muscle; angina (chest pains), which reflects worsening CHD; and myocardial infarction (MI), in which a blood vessel supplying the heart becomes completely blocked. Problems with the heart's electrical wiring can result in irregular heartbeats known as arrhythmias. Structural problems also can develop, often as a result of infections, as in rheumatic heart disease, or as hereditary defects in the walls between the chambers of the heart, such as ventricular septal defects (VSD).

High blood pressure or hypertension is not solely a problem of the heart muscle itself, but can certainly contribute to CHD. High blood pressure, if left untreated, can be a factor in other heart conditions as well, in which the heart muscle simply wears out from years of struggling against the high blood pressure.

Strokes, although not directly related to a problem with the heart, can occur because of arteriosclerosis of the carotid artery (the big artery leading to the brain), among other reasons.

High Cholesterol

No doubt you have heard that cholesterol is a major risk factor for heart disease. Actually, cholesterol itself is not the problem. In fact, cholesterol—a fatty substance made by your liver—plays a central role in the creation of cell membranes. It makes bile salts to absorb fat-soluble vitamins and repairs cell damage; it is an important building block for essential hormones such as estrogen, progesterone, testosterone, and cortisol. Problems can occur when your body, accustomed to manufacturing all the cholesterol it needs, receives many times more from the foods you eat, particularly animal products, partially hydrogenated fats (used to prolong a product's shelflife), and saturated fats. Alas, no matter what they eat or how much they exercise, some women have a genetic predisposition to high cholesterol.

The cholesterol debate gets even more complex. For years, the prevailing medical wisdom has said that a high level of cholesterol causes heart disease. Now research on women's heart problems tends to distinguish between the bad kind of cholesterol (low-density lipoproteins, or LDL) and the good kind (high-density lipoproteins, or HDL). Researchers speculate that LDL—and only a certain type of LDL, mind you—causes problems in the coronary arteries.

Just like high blood pressure, LDL can damage the coronary artery walls, leading to blockages and decreased blood flow to the heart (and legs and brain). Excess LDL accumulates in the middle layer of the coronary artery. The artery attempts to get rid of the LDL by secreting chemicals to oxidize it. Once oxidized, the LDL becomes even more dangerous, forming fatty streaks within the artery. If present at a high enough level, HDL can often sweep away the oxidized LDL before it does too much damage. If there isn't enough HDL, your body's immune system sends white blood cells to the area. Unfortunately, these cells can get trapped there, too, causing plaque to form. The resultant plaque (sometimes calcified) narrows

Dietary Supplement Suggestions

Make sure your vitamin supplement contains adequate amounts of copper, chromium, and selenium, as well as the antioxidant vitamins A, C, and E. Copper, chromium, and selenium may help lower cholesterol and reduce the risk of heart attacks; the antioxidants work together to prevent LDL from oxidizing. Broccoli, green peppers, tomatoes, cabbage, green leafy vegetables, strawberries, and grapefruit contain vitamin C; carrots and other green and yellow vegetables contain plenty of vitamin A; and almonds, hazelnuts, peanuts, and sunflower seeds, as well as olive, safflower, and wheat germ oils, are good sources of vitamin E.

Patricia Says

• Do not practice unsupported inversions or full backbends if you suffer from high blood pressure, even if it is controlled by medicine. However, supported backbends like Cross Bolsters or Reclining Bound Angle Pose (Supta Baddha Konasana) are fine. They serve the dual purpose of increasing circulation to the heart and lungs and restoring balance to the nervous system.

• Do inversions if your blood pressure is normal. These poses will enhance circulation and encourage blood and lymphatic fluids to travel from your pelvis and legs up to your heart.

the artery and slows the blood flow to your heart. If your heart can't get the blood it needs to feed itself, agonizing chest pain results. This pain, called angina, is an important warning sign that your heart is in trouble. It occurs most frequently during physical exertion when your heart is pumping faster and harder; it usually disappears when your heart is at rest. If you ignore angina and make no changes in your lifestyle, you could very well be setting yourself up for a heart attack, as the artery becomes completely blocked and your heart muscle starves.

What you eat can indeed help control excess cholesterol and keep your arteries free and clear. But genetics often determines how you metabolize fat. Some women have naturally high cholesterol; others can eat anything they want, seemingly with no adverse effects. Menopause may increase LDLs in some women while lowering HDLs, particularly in sedentary women who have gained weight with the cessation of their periods.

Other Physical Indicators

Elevated triglyceride and homocysteine levels often indicate the existence of heart problems. In fact, some doctors believe an increase in either of these substances poses a greater risk to artery health than high blood pressure or high cholesterol. Triglycerides are a category of lipids, like HDL, LDL, and cholesterol. And like LDL, the lower their levels, the less likely you are to suffer from heart disease. Homocysteine is a by-product created when your body metabolizes the amino acid methionine. High levels of homocysteine and lower-than-normal levels of folic acid appear to increase the risk of coronary heart disease dramatically, particularly in women. Simply increasing your intake of B vitamins (particularly folic acid, B_{12}, and B_6) appears to lower homocysteine levels significantly.

Smoking cigarettes is as detrimental to your heart as it is to your lungs. Nicotine can oxidize LDL, damaging your arterial lining, and can even make the arteries spasm, which prevents them from moving blood efficiently. Obesity is another heart enemy, causing blood pressure to rise, especially if your waist-to-hip ratio is low; women with a small waist and big hips fare better for some reason. In other words, a pear shape is healthier than an apple shape. Fortunately, many women experience a drop in blood pressure almost immediately when they lose weight.

EMOTIONAL AND SPIRITUAL CAUSES OF HEART DISEASE

The physiology of the human cardiovascular system doesn't tell the whole story about heart disease. It's impossible to talk about good heart health without examining your emotional and spiritual status, too. You may learn from a physical that your arteries have some blockage, or that your blood pressure is high for the first time in your life, or that your LDL level is up and your HDL level is down. Even if you and your physician decide to try bringing things back into balance with exercise and diet, you won't be truly successful until you examine what else is going on in your life. Obviously your blood pressure didn't rise by itself and your arteries didn't clog for no reason.

More than ten years ago, Dean Ornish, M.D., and his team of researchers began a study that would demonstrate the effects of emotional stress, isolation, hostility, cynicism, and low self-esteem on heart disease. Believing that high levels of cholesterol, oxidized LDL, triglycerides, nicotine, and homocysteine were only part of the equation, Ornish created the Opening Your Heart program to give heart patients a chance to reverse their disease through diet, yoga, visualization, meditation, group support, and other lifestyle changes. And it worked famously. Although the results came as a surprise to the Western medical establishment, many of the women I spoke with felt it was a no-brainer. "After all," one woman commented, "how many times in my life have I felt brokenhearted, disheartened, hard-hearted, or filled with heartache? Conversely," she said, "when I'm happy, my heart leaps with joy, I feel openhearted, or my heart beats rapidly with excitement."

A Heart-Healthy Diet Program

Dr. Dean Ornish's Opening Your Heart program has successfully tested the efficacy of a very low-fat, vegetarian diet in reversing heart disease. In his book *Dr. Dean Ornish's Program for Reversing Heart Disease: The Only System Scientifically Proven to Reverse Heart Disease*, he recommends the following breakdown for your daily food intake:

• No more than 10 percent fat, using monounsaturates whenever possible

• 70 to 75 percent carbohydrates, particularly complex carbs, which are more difficult for your body to convert into fat than simple carbs.

• 15 to 20 percent protein primarily from nonanimal sources (the diet allows egg whites and nonfat milk or yogurt)

• 5 mg of cholesterol

Nischala Devi, author of *The Healing Path of Yoga: Time-Honored Wisdom and Scientifically Proven Methods That Alleviate Stress, Open Your Heart, and Enrich Your Life*, helped create the yoga program for Dean Ornish's Preventive Medicine Research Institute in Sausalito, California. She says heart function is a wonderful metaphor for the need to balance giving and receiving. Many women are so busy caring for others, they have trouble taking care of themselves. Putting themselves first makes them feel selfish, but the heart teaches that putting yourself first is self-full, not self-ish. The heart, while providing sustenance in the form of oxygenated blood to the rest of your body, never forgets to feed itself first; if it did, it would die. Just as an unhealthy heart is no good to your body, you cannot effectively nourish those around you if you're unhealthy.

My grandmother was on to something when she declared her intention to keep her heart open enough to hold the love of all her grandchildren and great-grandchildren. Her vibrancy and longevity were deeply connected to her ability to embrace and grow with each new generation, as well as to the love and respect she received from her family and friends.

Joan Borysenko, in *A Woman's Book of Life: The Biology, Psychology, and Spirituality of the Feminine Life Cycle*, says something simultaneously simple and profound: We age as we've lived. If we've grown up pushing people away, suspicious and angry over the lot we've been dealt, we'll live out our elderly years angry, embittered, and alone. On the other hand, she says, if "our focus has been on love, learning, and service, we will progressively develop our oracular wisdom and a compassion that is a natural outgrowth of empathy and interrelational thinking." Dr. Ornish's research shows that women (and men) who have maintained their social connections in their later years have fewer incidences of heart disease and immune dysfunctions.

Nischala Devi, in her heart and yoga workshops, says that women who are in emotional or psychic pain tend to shut down, closing their hearts. This in turn makes the emotional body contract, which causes even more distress. Her prescription? Yoga and positive imagery. Visualizations, affirmations, and silent recitation of mantras while doing yoga poses all allow your body to mobilize its healing forces and bring them to bear on your suffering. She also offers a simple reminder in her book: Always speak the truth "so the heart is not blocked by confusing contradictions." As the old saying goes, say what you mean and mean what you say.

Women in the throes of child-rearing and career-building can feel empty and out of the loop once their children have grown and they have retired. My friend Johanna became quite depressed after her three boys left home. She had spent her whole life as a mother and wife, nurturing and emotionally supporting her family. As she told me, "I felt worthless after they left. I always saw myself as irreplaceable in their lives and now that they had other relationships, lives of their own—which I really wanted them to have, incidentally—I felt left out. I saw myself as too old to get involved in new things, and I wasn't even sure what those new things would be. What if all I was capable of doing was cleaning toilets and picking up the dry cleaning?" When Johanna's doctor said she had high blood pressure, the news shocked her. After all, she had always enjoyed good health. Her physician, a stern but compassionate osteopath, told her he would put off prescribing antihypertensive drugs in exchange for a promise from Johanna. She needed to agree to pay more attention to her life. Learn yoga or "some stress-reducing exercises," as he called them, to quell the anxieties she felt and lift her spirits. Get out of the house and join a club, take a class, volunteer her services, anything, he said, to help her feel less isolated and depressed, and more connected and needed.

So she did. She started volunteering at her local hospice organization. There she found

Herbal Support

Master herbalist and clinical nutritionist Donald Yance, Jr., lectures extensively on heart disease. In a workshop he gave at the June 1998 International Herbalists Symposium in Massachusetts, he recommended the following herbs to his heart patients:

• Hawthorn (*Crataegus oxyacantha*) for arterial hypertension, coronary artery damage, angina pectoris, valvular deficiency, and what Dr. Yance calls a geriatric or stressed heart.

• Night-blooming cereus (*Cactus graniflorus*) for mitral or aortic regurgitation, heart palpitations, and poor cerebral blood flow. This must be taken for several months before you notice any improvement.

• Motherwort (*Leonurus cardiaca*) for nervous excitability with or without heart palpitations, hyperthyroidism, and hypertension. This is most beneficial when combined with skullcap, black cohosh, reishi mushrooms, and magnesium.

• Black cohosh (*Cimicifuga racemosa*) as an antispasmodic.

• Coleus (*Coleus forskolii*) for hypertension; it relaxes smooth muscle and works as a vasodilator.

• Broom (*Sarothamnus scoparis*) for cardiac arrhythmia and to improve venous return.

• Ginger, garlic, gingko biloba, turmeric, cayenne, and prickly ash bark to inhibit platelet aggregation and regulate blood circulation.

she could put her caregiving and organizational skills to good use. She didn't have her own kids to take care of anymore, but she found a whole new community that needed her. After six months, she says she feels happier than she's felt in years—and her lowered blood pressure readings reflect that.

Herbert Benson, M.D., a cardiologist at Harvard Medical School, is well-known for his studies showing that meditation and progressive relaxation can lower blood pressure and stabilize erratic heartbeats. More recently, researchers have expressed interest in how seeing how serving others (what ancient yogis call karma yoga) can affect heart disease. Karma yoga is not as esoteric as it sounds. Johanna's work at the hospice is a perfect example. Volunteering to serve meals at your local soup kitchen, being a Big Sister or mentor to a young girl, and organizing a food drive in your community are all examples of karma yoga—or selfless service.

THE DEBATE OVER HORMONE REPLACEMENT THERAPY

Statistics indicate that the incidence of heart disease increases significantly after a woman has gone through menopause. One of the biggest unanswered questions, however, is whether hormone replacement therapy can reverse that trend. For years, physicians—even those who did not routinely prescribe HRT or estrogen replacement therapy (ERT)—believed that women at high risk for heart disease should take estrogen alone (if they have had a hysterectomy) or a combination of estrogen and progestin if their uterus was still intact. Several studies seem to corroborate that thinking, including the Nurses Health Study, which tracked 122,000 women for twenty years and demonstrated that the women who took estrogen postmenopausally were half as likely to develop heart disease as those who didn't. Unfortunately, none of the studies was double-blind or placebo-controlled, and they all failed to study women over the age of sixty-five.

The most recent information from the Heart and Estrogen Replacement Study (HERS), a clinical trial of 2,763 postmenopausal women with heart disease, contradicts those findings and postulates that HRT does nothing to reduce the incidence of heart disease. In fact, the study suggests that the risk of heart attack may actually increase the first year of HRT therapy and then decrease again the following year. Although HRT does seem to lower LDL levels and raise HDL levels, we clearly need more studies to determine the real pros and cons. The Women's Health Initiative clinical trials, sponsored by the National Institutes for Health, has several ongoing studies for women with heart disease and without, but the results won't be published until 2008.

Patricia Says

• Do supine poses to relax the brain and abdomen and open your chest. Remember the image of an open heart. If your heart can open to receive love, happiness, and the possibilities the world has to give, it will have a harder time constricting out of fear, anger, bitterness, and loneliness. Chest openers, like those suggested in this chapter, can help regulate your breathing and open your rib cage to improve heart and lung function. Just the act of elevating your chest and releasing your shoulders can lift your spirits. By creating more space around your heart, you bring a sense of lightness to your mind.

• Do standing poses to help stretch and strengthen your whole body and to improve posture by opening your shoulders, chest, and rib cage. These poses also promote recirculation from your lower extremities. If you suffer from high blood pressure, practice standing poses without raising your arms over your head.

Patricia Says

• Include Corpse Pose (Savasana), the ultimate relaxation posture, in your daily practice. This pose restores and refreshes your mind, brings a sense of tranquillity and repose to your body and emotions, and gives you a chance to spend time reflecting and regrouping.

• Check with a doctor (preferably one well-versed in yoga), if you suffer from high blood pressure or other heart problems, before beginning the sequence that we provide.

If heart disease is a discordant symphony among multiple partners—physical indicators, negative emotions, and a lack of spiritual connection—what better conductor than yoga to bring all the players together? All the elements of a yoga practice—the physical poses, the meditative breathing, compassionate community service—work in concert to provide a healthful environment for your heart.

On a physical level, yoga asanas and the breathing technique called pranayama help to bring your autonomic nervous system into balance, which has a beneficial effect on blood pressure. Ancient yogis and modern-day teachers know intuitively what other researchers have proven in their clinical trials: Yoga helps release your body from the adverse affects of stress on the heart, immune system, and endocrine system. As Patricia teaches, creating peace, strength, and flexibility within your body translates into a sense of calm, groundedness, and flexibility in your mind. Going out into the world from this state of awareness allows you to feel more in control of your life and to notice potential problems before they turn into full-blown illnesses.

Yoga poses also enhance circulation. For your body to have good circulation, you need a strong heart, healthy muscles, and good lungs. Remember, your heart supplies oxygenated blood to the rest of your body; your muscles and lungs pump blood back into your heart. When you inhale, as your diaphragm moves down, not only does air come into your lungs, but blood and lymphatic fluid rise from your abdomen into your chest. Yoga, which translates to "union" or "joining together," works by bringing opposites together. In Patricia's classes, for example, she teaches a variety of poses that put your body through its full range of motion. This type of sequencing allows your body to experience flexion and extension, squeezing and soaking, calming and energizing—all opposing actions conjoined to contribute to good, strong circulatory health.

Patricia recommends forward bends to her students suffering from hypertension or high blood pressure, particularly when it's stress-induced. These poses allow you to feel safe, contained, and nurtured, especially if you support yourself in the pose so there is little or no tension in your muscles. Standing or seated forward bends—either a full or modified pose—can help quiet your sympathetic nervous system, relax your body completely, and elongate chronically contracted muscles. In addition, these squeezing postures, according to B. K. S. Iyengar, massage your internal organs and increase circulation to your stomach, liver, intestines, and pancreas.

Each forward bending pose has the important advantage of allowing you to experience what's going on inside of you while you are in the position. Rachel, a friend of mine who has just started taking yoga, told me that she learns a tremendous amount about herself every time she does Seated Forward Bend (Paschimottanasana). Although she strives to stay in the present moment, breathing quietly and fully like her teacher says, sometimes her mind wanders, attaching itself to past or future events. When that happens, she notices how her muscles change (tensing up if a memory is unpleasant, releasing if the memory makes her smile); how her breathing either speeds up or calms down; and how her heart beats more quickly or slowly, depending on what thoughts enter her head. "It helps me in my everyday life," Rachel says. "I try to notice what's going on in my body whenever stressful events happen and now I feel I can do something to calm myself down a lot quicker."

A SEQUENCE FOR HIGH BLOOD PRESSURE

1. Corpse Pose (Savasana)
2. Cross Bolsters Pose
3. Standing Forward Bend (Uttanasana)
4. Downward-Facing Dog Pose (Adho Mukha Svanasana)
5. Child's Pose (Adho Mukha Virasana)
6. Head-on-Knee Pose (Janu Sirsasana)
7. Seated Forward Bend (Paschimottanasana)
8. Reclining Bound Angle Pose (Supta Baddha Konasana)
9. Legs-Up-the-Wall Pose (Viparita Karani)

Generally speaking, the Woman's Restorative Sequence is beneficial to calm your nerves and restore equilibrium. If you choose to do that sequence, omit Headstand (Sirsasana); you should never do unsupported inversions if you have high blood pressure.

1. CORPSE POSE (Savasana) Place a vertical bolster behind you on your mat with a folded blanket at the far end of the bolster for your head. Sit with the end of the bolster touching your buttocks. Lower yourself onto the bolster and rest your head on the blanket. Relax your arms out to the sides, palms up, and let your feet relax away from each other. Focusing on your breathing, completely release your shoulders, neck, and facial muscles. Keep your abdomen soft and relaxed. As you inhale, allow your breath to move into your chest, but keep your throat, neck, and diaphragm free of tension. If you have an eyebag, drape it gently across your eyes to keep out external stimulation and to promote further relaxation. Let your eyes rest and breathe normally for at least 5 to 10 minutes.

To come out, bend your knees and roll slowly to one side. Remain there for a couple of breaths before pushing up to a seated position.

EFFECTS This pose helps lower high blood pressure and soothe your autonomic nervous system.

2. CROSS BOLSTERS POSE Place a bolster on your mat and lay another one across the center of the first to form a cross. Place a folded blanket at one end for your head. Sit on the middle of the top bolster and carefully lie back so your spine is supported on the bolster and the back of your head touches the blanket. Place your arms on either side of your head, palms up, elbows bent, and relax completely. (If you feel any strain in your lower back, raise your feet on a block.)

Relax in this pose for several minutes, breathing deeply. To come out, bend your knees and roll to one side. Help yourself up using your hands.

EFFECTS This posture broadens your chest area, improving circulation and respiration, and helps you open your heart both physically and emotionally.

3. STANDING FORWARD BEND (Uttanasana) Place a padded chair about 2 feet in front of you. Stand facing the chair. Turn your palms outward and lift your arms to the side and over your head, stretching your whole body. As you exhale, extend your spine and bend forward, resting your head on the chair seat and close your eyes. Fold your arms above your head. Relax the base of your skull, your neck, your shoulders, and your abdomen; remain in the pose for 2 minutes, if possible. Come up slowly, using the chair for support.

EFFECTS Because it quiets your whole body and soothes your mind, this pose may help regulate your blood pressure.

4. DOWNWARD-FACING DOG POSE (Adho Mukha Svanasana) Lie facedown and place your palms on the floor by each side of your chest with your fingers well spread and pointing straight ahead. Come up on your hands and knees. That's your position. Now place a bolster or folded blanket or two vertically so your support is in line with your sternum. Your support should be high enough to support your head, but low enough to lengthen your neck. Return to your hands-and-knees position, and turn your toes under.

Exhale, press your hands firmly into the mat and extend up through your inner arms. As you exhale again, raise your buttocks high into the air and move your thighs up and back. Keep stretching through your legs and bring your heels toward the floor. Keep your legs firm and your elbows straight as you lift your buttocks upward and release your head onto your

support. The action of the arms and legs serves to elongate your spine and release your head. Hold this pose for 30 seconds to 1 minute, breathing deeply. To come out, return to your hands and knees, sit back on your heels; go right into the next pose.

EFFECTS With your head supported, this pose helps stabilize your blood pressure, relieve hypertension, and calm your heart physically and emotionally.

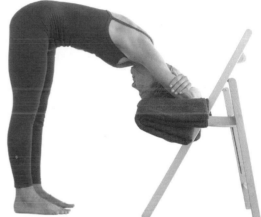

5. CHILD'S POSE (Adho Mukha Virasana) Kneel on the floor with a vertical bolster directly in front of you, the short end between your knees. Spread your knees wide and straddle the bolster, bringing your toes together. Bend forward and stretch your trunk up and over the bolster, pressing it into your abdomen. Fold your arms on the bolster, cradle your head on your arms, and relax completely for 5 to 10 minutes. Use your hands to help you push up to a seated position.

EFFECTS This pose can help counteract breathlessness and reduce hypertension.

6. HEAD-ON-KNEE POSE (Janu Sirsasana) Sit on the floor with your legs stretched out in front of you. Bend your right knee to the side so it is at a 45-degree angle to your left leg and your right heel is near the right side of your groin. Push your right knee as far back as you comfortably can; keep your left leg straight.

Place a bolster or folded blanket on your outstretched leg, and turn your abdomen and chest so your sternum is in line with the center of your left leg. As you inhale, lift your trunk up from the base of your pelvis; as you exhale, lean your trunk forward and rest your arms on the bolster. Cradle your head on your arms. (If that is uncomfortable, add more height to your support.) Your head should rest without straining your neck, and you should feel no pressure or strain in your back or the backs of your legs. Stay in this pose for as long as you are comfortable, preferably 2 to 3 minutes, breathing normally with a slight emphasis on the exhalations. Inhale while coming up, straighten your right leg, and reverse sides by bending your left knee.

EFFECTS This pose may help ease angina pain and normalize blood pressure.

7. SEATED FORWARD BEND (Paschimottanasana) Sit on the floor (or on one or two folded blankets) with your legs stretched out in front of you. Place a bolster or folded blanket across your lower legs. Take a full, deep breath, stretching up through your spine and lifting your sternum and head. Keep your back slightly concave. As you exhale, bend forward and extend your torso over your legs, cradling your head in your arms on your support. (If you feel strain in your back or in your legs, add more height to your support.) Breathe softly, releasing any tension with a little-longer-than-normal exhalation. Stay in this pose as long as you feel comfortable, using your breath to help you release forward without straining. Keep your abdomen soft and relaxed. Rise up on an inhalation.

EFFECTS This pose may help normalize blood pressure, reduce angina pain, and bring deep relaxation to your heart.

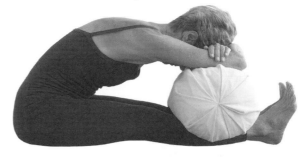

8. RECLINING BOUND ANGLE POSE (Supta Baddha Konasana) Place a bolster vertically on the floor behind you with a blanket on the far end for your head and neck. Sit just in front of the bolster with your knees bent and your sacrum touching the bolster's edge. Place a strap behind your back, at your sacrum; draw it forward over your hips, across your shins, and under your feet (see page xv). Put the soles of your feet together and let your knees and thighs fall to the sides. Cinch the strap securely under your feet. Lie back so your head and torso rest comfortably on the bolster and your buttocks and legs are on the floor. (If you feel any discomfort in your lower back, add some height to your support with a folded blanket or two. If you feel any muscle tension in your legs, roll two blankets vertically and place one under the top of each thigh.) Rest in this pose for at least 3 to 5 minutes, breathing deeply.

To come out, draw your knees together, slip the strap off, and slowly roll to one side. Use your hands to push yourself up to a seated position.

EFFECTS This position gently opens your chest and heart, improves respiration and circulation, helps regulate blood pressure, and brings balance and calm to your entire nervous system.

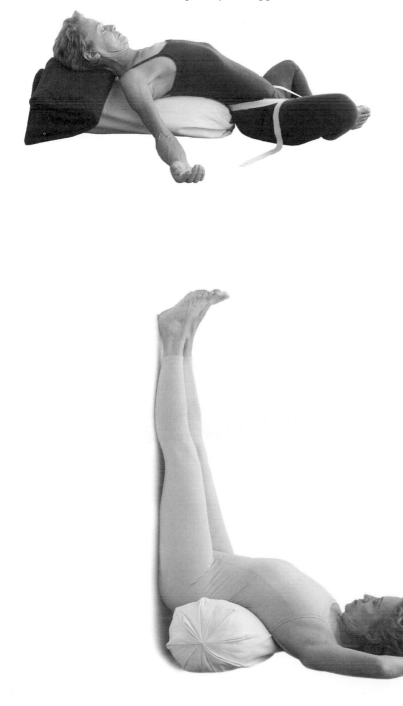

9. LEGS-UP-THE-WALL POSE (Viparita Karani) Place a bolster about 3 inches from the wall. (If you are tall, you may need a higher support, such as a folded blanket on top of the bolster.) Sit on the bolster so your right hip and side are touching the wall. Using your hands to support you, lean back and swivel your body around, taking your right leg and then your left leg up the wall. Keep your buttocks close to or against the wall. (If you feel stiffness or discomfort in your legs, push your buttocks slightly away from the wall.) Lie down so your lower back and ribs are supported by the bolster and your shoulders and head are on the floor. (If your neck is uncomfortable, put a folded towel or blanket under it.) Extend through your legs and place your arms out at your sides in a comfortable position with elbows bent and palms up. Rest in this position, eyes closed, for at least 5 minutes.

To come out, gently push away from the wall until your buttocks are off the bolster and resting on the floor. Roll to one side. Breathe quietly for a few breaths, then use your arms to help you to a seated position.

EFFECTS Practicing this pose may help you relieve heart palpitations, breathlessness, and hypertension.

I have included books, magazines, videos, information sources, and everything else I could think of in this list of resources that might help you on your journey toward wellness.

Resources

READING MATERIAL

This section includes the articles and publications mentioned in the book, as well as some others I think you may find useful.

Books

Balaskas, Janet. *Preparing for Birth with Yoga: Exercises for Pregnancy and Childbirth.* Australia: Element Books, 1994.

Borysenko, Joan. *A Woman's Book of Life: The Biology, Psychology, and Spirituality of the Feminine Life Cycle.* New York: Riverhead Books, 1996.

Cope, Stephen. *Yoga and the Quest for the True Self.* New York: Bantam Books, 1999.

Crawford, Amanda McQuade. *The Herbal Menopause Book.* Freedom, Calif.: Crossing Press, 1996.

Devi, Nischala Joy. *The Healing Path of Yoga: Time-Honored Wisdom and Scientifically Proven Methods That Alleviate Stress, Open Your Heart, and Enrich Your Life.* New York: Three Rivers Press, 2000.

Gladstar, Rosemary. *Herbal Healing for Women: Simple Home Remedies for Women of All Ages.* New York: Simon & Schuster, 1993.

Haas, Elson M., with Eleonora Manzolin. *A Diet for All Seasons.* Berkeley, Calif.: Celestial Arts, 1995.

Iyengar, B. K. S. *Light on Yoga: Yoga Dipika.* New York: Schocken Books, 1979.

———, trans. *Seventy Glorious Years of Yogacharya.* Puna, India: Light on Yoga Trust, 1990.

Iyengar, Geeta. *Yoga: A Gem for Women.* Palo Alto, Calif.: Timeless Books, 1990.

Kornhaber, Arthur, and Kenneth L. Woodward. *Grandparents, Grandchildren: The Vital Connection.* Garden City, N.Y.: Anchor Press/Doubleday, 1981.

Lark, Susan. *Dr. Susan Lark's Menopause Self-Help Book: A Woman's Guide to Feeling Wonderful for the Second Half of Her Life.* Berkeley, Calif.: Celestial Arts, 1990.

———. *The PMS Self Help Book: A Woman's Guide.* Berkeley, Calif.: Celestial Arts, 1984.

Lasater, Judith. *Living Your Yoga: Finding the Spiritual in Everyday Life.* Berkeley, Calif.: Rodmell Press, 2000.

———. *Relax and Renew: Restful Yoga for Stressful Times.* Berkeley, Calif.: Rodmell Press, 1995.

Lee, John R., with Virginia Hopkins. *What Your Doctor May Not Tell You about Menopause: The Breakthrough Book on Natural Progesterone.* New York: Warner Books, 1996.

Lonsdorf, Nancy, Veronica Butler, and Melanie Brown. *A Woman's Best Medicine: Health, Happiness, and Long Life through Ayurveda.* New York: Putnam, 1993.

Love, Susan. *Dr. Susan Love's Hormone Book: Making Informed Choices about Menopause.* New York: Random House, 1997.

Milne, Robert, and Blake More, with Burton Goldberg. *The Definitive Guide to Headaches: An Alternative Medicine.* Tiburon, Calif.: Future Medicine Publishing, 1997.

Monro, Robin, R. Nagarathna, and H. R. Nagendra. *Yoga for Common Ailments.* New York: Simon & Schuster, 1990.

Northrup, Christiane. *The Wisdom of Menopause: Creating Physical and Emotional Health and Healing during the Change.* New York: Bantam Books, 2001.

———. *Women's Bodies, Women's Wisdom: Creating Physical and Emotional Health and Healing.* New York: Bantam Books, 1998.

Ornish, Dean. *Dr. Dean Ornish's Program for Reversing Heart Disease: The Only System Scientifically Proven to Reverse Heart Disease.* New York: Random House, 1990.

Pert, Candace B. *Molecules of Emotion: Why You Feel the Way You Feel.* New York: Scribner, 1997.

Pipher, Mary. *Reviving Ophelia: Saving the Selves of Adolescent Girls.* New York: Putnam, 1994.

Raman, Krishna. *A Matter of Health.* Madras, India: East-West Books, 1998. (Available through Iyengar yoga centers.)

Robertson, Joel C., with Tom Monte. *Natural Prozac: Learning to Release Your Body's Own Antidepressants.* New York: HarperCollins, 1997.

Scaravelli, Vanda. *Awakening the Spine: The Stress-Free New Yoga That Works the Body to Restore Health, Vitality, and Energy.* San Francisco: HarperSanFrancisco, 1991.

Schatz, Mary. *Back Care Basics: A Doctor's Gentle Program for Back and Neck Pain Relief.* Berkeley, Calif.: Rodmell Press, 1992.

Tiwari, Maya. *Ayurveda: A Life of Balance: The Complete Guide to Ayurvedic Nutrition and Body Types with Recipes.* Rochester, Vt.: Healing Arts Press, 1995.

Weed, Susun S. *Menopausal Years: The Wise Woman Way.* Woodstock, N.Y.: Ash Tree, 1992.

Woodman, Marion. *Addiction to Perfection: The Still Unravished Bride. A Psychological Study.* Toronto: Inner City Books, 1982.

———. *The Owl Was a Baker's Daughter: Obesity, Anorexia Nervosa and the Repressed Feminine.* Toronto: Inner City Books, 1980.

Woodman, Marion, with Jill Mellick. *Coming Home to Myself: Daily Reflections for a Woman's Body and Soul.* Berkeley, Calif.: Conari Press, 1998.

Journals, Magazines, and Newsletters

Barensen, Kristen. "The Mind-Bowel Connection." *Yoga Journal.* September/October 1997: 37–38.

Canley, Jane, et al. "Effects of Hormone Replacement Therapy on Clinical Fractures and Height Loss: The Heart and Estrogen/Progestin Replacement Study (HERS)." *American Journal of Medicine* 110, no. 6 (2001): 442–450.

Greenberg, R. P., R. F. Bornstein, M. J. Zborowski, S. Fisher, and M. D. Greenberg. "A Meta-analysis of Fluoxetine Outcome in the Treatment of Depression." *Journal of Nervous and Mental Diseases* 182, no. 10 (1994): 547–51.

Leutwyler, Kristin. "Dying to Be Thin." *Scientific American*. Summer 1998: 17–19.

Schoenen, J., J. Jacquy, and M. Lenaerts. "Effectiveness of High-Dose Riboflavin in Migraine Prophylaxis: A Randomized Controlled Trial." *Neurology* 50, no. 2 (1998): 466–470.

Schatz, Mary. "You Can Have Healthy Bones." *Yoga Journal*. (March/April 1988: 49–50).

Serber, Ellen. "Yoga Care for Headaches." *Yoga Journal*. January/February 1999: 42–43.

Subscription Information

HerbalGram, P.O. Box 144345, Austin, TX 78714. Phone: (512) 926-4900; Web site: herbalgram.org.

The Herb Quarterly, 1041 Shary Circle, Concord, CA 94518. Web site: herbquarterly.com.

The Lark Letter, P.O. Box 60046, Potomac, MD 20897.

Yoga International. Phone: (800) 253-6243; Web site: himalayaninstitute.org.

Yoga Journal, 2054 University Ave., Berkeley, CA 94704. Phone: (800) 600-9642; Web site: yogajournal.com.

ASSOCIATIONS AND WEB SITES

The following organizations provide more detailed information on a variety of health issues and conditions.

American Botanical Council (ABC), P.O. Box 201660, Austin, TX 78720. Phone: (512) 926-4900; Web site: herbalgram.org.

American Heart Association, 7320 Greenville Ave., Dallas, TX 75231. Phone: (214) 373-6300; Web site: americanheart.org.

Bulimia Anorexia Self Help, Inc. (BASH), 6125 Clayton Ave., #215, St. Louis, MO 63139. Phone: (314) 567-4080.

Herb Research Foundation, 1007 Pearl St., #200, Boulder, CO 80302. Phone: (303) 449-2265; Web site: herbs.org.

Largesse: The Network for Size Esteem, P.O. Box 9404, New Haven, CT 06534. Phone: (203) 787-1624; Web site: eskimo.com/~largesse.

National Association of Anorexia Nervosa and Associated Disorders (ANAD), P.O. Box 7, Highland Park, IL 60035. Phone: (708) 831-3438; Web site: anad.org.

National Black Woman's Health Project, 1211 Connecticut Ave. NW, #310, Washington, DC 20036. Phone: (202) 835-0117; Web site: nbwhp.org.

National Headache Foundation, 428 W. St. James Place, 2nd Floor, Chicago, IL 50514. Phone: (888) 643-5552; Web site: headaches.org.

National Institute of Mental Health, NIMH Public Inquiries, 6001 Executive Blvd., Rm. 8184, MSC 9663, Bethesda, MD 20892-966. Phone: (301) 443-4513; Web site: nimh.nih.gov; E-mail: nimhinfo@nih.gov.

National Osteoporosis Foundation, 1232 22nd St. NW, Washington, DC 20037. Phone: (202) 223-2226; Web site: nof.org.

Osteoporosis and Women's Health. Web site: osteoporosis-and-womens-health.com.

Overeaters Anonymous (OA), World Service Office, 6075 Zenith Ct., Rio Rancho, NM 87124. Phone: (505) 891-2664; Web site: oa.org.

Preventive Medicine Research Institute (Dr. Dean Ornish's Opening Your Heart program), 1001 Bridgeway, Box 305, Sausalito, CA 94965. Web site: pmri.org.

Women's Health Initiative (WHI), 1 Rockledge Center, Suite 300, MS 7966, Bethesda, MD 20892. Phone: (301) 402-2900; Web site: hhlbi.nih.gov/whi. (The National Institutes of Health established the WHI in 1991 to study the most common causes of death, disability, and impaired quality of life in postmenopausal women. These studies of 167,000 women will look at the efficacy of hormone replacement therapy, diet, and vitamin supplementation, as well as attempt to identify predictors of disease and understand community approaches to healthful behavior.)

Women's International Pharmacy, 5708 Monona Dr., Madison, WI 54716. Phone: (800) 279-5708; Web site: womensinternational.com; E-mail: info@womensinternational.com.

VIDEOS, AUDIOTAPES, AND OTHER PRODUCTS

Videos

AM and PM Yoga for Beginners with Rodney Yee and Patricia Walden (two-volume set).

Flowing Yoga Postures for Beginners with Lilias Folan.

Prenatal Yoga with Colette Crawford.

Prenatal Yoga with Shiva Rea.

Yoga for Round Bodies (volumes 1 and 2) with Linda DeMarco and Genia Pauli Haddon.

Yoga Journal's Practice Series:

  Yoga Practice: Introduction with Patricia Walden

  Yoga Practice for Beginners with Patricia Walden

  Yoga Practice for Flexibility with Patricia Walden

  Yoga Practice for Strength with Rodney Yee

  Yoga Practice for Relaxation with Patricia Walden and Rodney Yee

  Yoga Practice for Energy with Rodney Yee

  Yoga Practice for Meditation with Rodney Yee

Audiotape

Discover Yoga with Lilias Folan.

Discover Serenity with Lilias Folan.

Yoga for Pregnancy by Janet Balaskas. (Available from Active Birth Centre, 55 Dartmouth Park Rd., London NW5 1SL.)

Products

The following mail-order companies offer a variety of items that may help you with your yoga practice, including yoga mats, blankets, blocks, bolsters, straps, inversion aids, and even clothing. Contact companies directly to find out what they carry.

Body Lift. Phone: (888) 243-3279; Web site: ageeasy.com.
Hugger Mugger Yoga Product. Phone: (800) 473-4888;
    Web site: huggermugger.com.
Lilias products. naturaljourneys.com.
Living Arts catalog. Phone: (800) 254-8464; Web site: gaiam.com.
Tools for Yoga. Phone: (888) 678-9642; Web site: yogapropshop.com.
Yoga Accessories. Phone: (800) 990-9642; Web site: yogaaccessories.com.
Yoga Mats. Phone: (800) 720-9642; Web site: yogamats.com.
YogaPro. Phone: (800) 488-6414; Web site: yogapro.com.
Yoga Props. Phone: (888) 856-9642; Web site: yogaprops.net.
Yoga Shop 4U. Phone: (401) 353-3513; Web site: yogashop4u.com.
Yoga Wear. Phone: (800) 217-0006; Web site: mariewright.net.

Acknowledgments

After writing this book, I feel compelled to acknowledge every conversation I've had, every book I've read, every class I've taken, and every yoga teacher I've practiced with—in short, everyone and everything that has informed my life and my health so far. Since I can't really make the acknowledgments longer than the book itself, I'll have to be content to list the most immediate ones.

First and foremost, I could never have written this book without Patricia Walden. As anyone who has ever taken a class or workshop with her knows, Patricia embodies the yoga teachings with her whole heart and soul. I am, of course, grateful to her for sharing her vast knowledge of yogic principles, asana sequencing, and women's health issues; tirelessly spotting the models on many of the photo shoots; and reviewing the manuscript. But I also feel blessed to have found such a wonderful friend along the way.

Patricia's work and inspiration spring from her long association with B. K. S. Iyengar, her beloved teacher; his daughter Geeta; and his son Prasant. B. K. S. Iyengar, the great modern-day yogi whose yoga asanas and pranayama techniques have been taught throughout the world, is a master at the therapeutic applications of yoga. It is in large part because of his work that yoga is beginning to be taken seriously as a holistic approach to wellness. Geeta Iyengar, a world-renowned teacher in her own right, has tirelessly championed the connection between yoga and women's health. You'll reap the benefits of her pioneering work as you use the sequences Patricia has provided throughout this book.

I want to give special thanks to Chris Saudek, an Iyengar teacher from La Crescent, Minnesota, who not only helped Patricia write the instructions for many of the poses, but generously worked with her on the pregnancy, postpartum, and back care sequences, and spent what little spare time she had helping us in so many ways. I also want to thank Judith Hanson Lasater for writing the foreword. Her knowledge of the human body in general and women's yoga in particular was extremely helpful to me. She even taught me a much better way to do a headstand!

I don't think I've ever met a more generous group of people than those in the yoga community. So many of them offered me their insights, their valuable time, and their unbridled enthusiasm that I'm not sure I'll be able to remember them all. Catherine de los Santos, bless her heart, gave me private lessons to ensure that I stayed healthy through the whole book production process. She modeled, she spotted the other models, and she cheered from the sidelines. Catherine, I salute you. And Eleanor Williams, director of the Harvard Square Yoga Centre in Cambridge, Massachusetts, gave up her studio space and her home for us and traveled all the way to California to model. Very special thanks to Tara Starling, Ilana Rosenberg, Carol Stout, and Mary Quinn, who worked with us early on, and to Amy Stone, Winnie

Chen, Athena Pappas, Ann Austin, Alice Rocky, and Roni Brissette, whose beautiful abilities grace the pages of this book, along with Catherine de los Santos and Eleanor Williams. I'm indebted to Brenda Beebe at Yoga Mats for supplying the props for the photo shoot—at a moment's notice—and to Marie Wright Yoga Wear and Hugger Mugger for generously outfitting the models. Of course, I'll be forever grateful for the opportunity to work with David Martinez and his crew, Kristen Flammer and Frank Gaglione. While David's beautiful photography certainly enlivened the book, his gracious spirit and unflagging sense of humor enriched my life. Also, thanks to stylists Ivan Mendoza and France Dushane for helping the models to look their most beautiful in the photographs.

I'm also grateful to the women whose work has helped inform my own—whose teachings, writings, lectures, and informal conversations with me contributed to these chapters in one way or another: Drs. Christiane Northrup, Susan Love, and Susan Lark, who ceaselessly take on the medical establishment on behalf of us all and whose writings should be required reading for every woman and her physician; Joan Borysenko, whose lectures and books have helped many women discover the power and gifts unfolding at each stage of their lives; Nancy Lonsdorf, M.D., Veronica Butler, M.D., and Melanie Brown, Ph.D., who have published their work on women and ayurveda; psychoneurological immunologist Candace Pert, Ph.D.; my wonderful herbalist friends and colleagues, Rosemary Gladstar, Tierona Low Dog, Amanda McQuade, Susun Weed, Diana de Luca, and Mindy Green, who taught me well; and Dean Ornish, Nischala Devi, Janet Balaskas, Genia Pauli Haddon, Gretchen Newmark, Dr. Mary Schatz, Barbara Kaplan Herring, Judith Hanson Lasater, and others whose therapeutic yoga work has benefited many. I'm so afraid I may have left someone out of this list—if I have, know that I'll wake up one morning with your name in my mind and gratitude in my heart.

Thanks to Bri Maya Tiwari and yoga teachers Jill Edwards Minye, Amy Cooper, Janice Gates, Sarah Powers, Patricia Sullivan, Sharon Gannon, and Angela Farmer, each of whom brings a uniquely feminine touch to this ancient art and contributed in a very special way to my own healing. Thanks also to the teachers and staff at Kripalu Yoga Center, who nurtured me and always made me feel welcome. And a special thank-you to my good friends Mark Dowie and Wendy Schwartz on the West Coast and Richard and Michelle Sterner on the East Coast for offering me a place to write when the distractions in my own world threatened to pull me away from my task.

I'm very thankful to all the people who contributed to the editing process. Kathryn Arnold, editor in chief, and Jennifer Barrett, health editor, of *Yoga Journal*, both read every chapter and gave me important feedback. Baxter Bell, M.D.; Phil Catalfo; Michael Taylor, M.D.; Fran Gendlin; Thomas Alden, D.C.; Amy Cooper; Donna Fone; Genia Pauli Haddon; Gretchen Newmark; and Chris Boskin provided invaluable insights. My agent Joseph Spieler and my "writing buddies" Stephen Cope, Anne Cushman, and the late Rick Fields all helped. I offer my thanks and appreciation to Peter Turner at Shambhala Publications, who believed in this project from the very beginning and encouraged me to forge ahead; to Jennifer Devine for the charming line drawings; to eagle-eyed proofreader DeAnna Satre; to Karen Steib, copyeditor extraordinaire, for keeping all the pieces straight; and most especially to Emily Bower, whose enthusiasm and relentless but loving attention to detail kept me on track and brought the book to completion.

I'm absolutely certain that I could never have finished this book without the love and support I received from my family. Special thanks to my parents for never wavering in their belief that I could do anything I set my mind and heart to; to my daughters, Sarah and Megan, who pitched in wherever they could and distracted me whenever they should to keep me focused and sane while also offering their own particular insights, experiences, and honesty. And of course, to my husband and best friend, Jim Keough, whose lovingly critical eye and amazing ability to synthesize helped more than he knows. I always thought it was a good idea to marry a writer and editor—now I'm certain of it. Especially one who cooks and cleans!

Many thanks to all the women who trusted me with their stories and allowed me to tell those stories here so that other women could benefit from their experiences. And thank you to Marion Woodman, Jungian analyst, who taught me in one evening—with her words, her heart, and her countenance—what it means to be passionately alive, beautifully woman, and truly at home with my body, mind, and spirit.

Linda Sparrowe
December 2001

Index

Alternate nostril breathing, 146

Amenorrhea (Delayed Menses), 91

Angina, 341, 343

Ankylosing spondylitis, 178

Anorexia nervosa, 60, 66–68

Anxiety, 102, 104, 108–109, 140, 209

Arms Overhead (Parvatasana), 154

Arteriosclerosis, 341

Arthritis, 169, 172, 177–179, 181

Back pain, 137, 168, 170, 176

Blood pressure, 341 342, 345

Bound Angle Pose (Baddha
  Konasana), 4, 105, 150, 160,
  242, 247, 292, 312, 316

Bridge Pose (Setu Bandha Sarvangasana), 21, 40, 51, 79, 82, 87,
  95, 104, 107, 112, 120, 152,
  154, 169, 173, 195–196, 200,
  202, 216, 226, 232, 239, 242,
  255, 258, 262, 266, 271, 286,
  294, 309, 314

Bulimia, 61, 66–68

Camel Pose (Ustrasana), 36, 85, 337

Cardiovascular disease, 340–341

Child's Pose (Adho Mukha
  Virasana), 18, 34, 48, 75, 82,
  95, 101, 139, 145, 156, 173,
  197, 202, 215, 230, 239, 285,
  321, 338, 350

Chronic gas, 273

Colitis, 275

Compulsive or binge eating, 61

Constipation, 143, 152, 156, 273,
  275–278

Coronary heart disease, 341

Corpse Pose (Savasana), 23, 41, 66,
  67, 68, 80, 87, 105, 107, 112,
  117, 124, 131, 144, 151–152,
  164, 169, 186, 196–197, 201,
  205, 219, 227, 232, 244, 252,
  255, 259, 262, 266, 272, 287,
  290, 310, 315, 321, 339, 348

Cow-Face (Gomukhasana) Arms,
  154

Cramps, 90, 94, 102, 105, 109

Crohn's disease, 125, 275

Cross Bolsters Pose, 108, 220, 349

Depression, 104, 108–110, 174, 209,
  211–220, 216

Diarrhea, 273

Digestive disorders, 137, 156, 209,
  274–280

Downward-Facing Dog Pose (Adho
  Mukha Svanasana), 15, 32,
  34, 38, 46, 74, 84, 93, 109,
  113, 120, 126, 142, 148, 152,
  166, 177, 188, 221, 224,
  227–228, 239, 242, 248, 255,
  260, 263, 269, 282, 292, 306,
  317–318, 332, 349

Easy Seated Forward Bend (Adho
  Mukha Sukhasana), 153, 196,
  239, 262

Eating disorders, 62–66

Endocrine system, 89, 92, 111, 119,
  129, 137, 146–147

Endometriosis, 93, 106, 176

Expanding Life Force Energy
  Breathing (Ujjayi
  Pranayama), 146, 148, 162,
  215

Extended Side-Angle Pose (Utthita
  Parsvakonasana), 7, 29, 71,
  320

Extended Triangle Pose (Utthita
  Trikonasana), 6, 27, 68, 70,
  142, 159, 173, 177, 183, 245,
  298, 319, 335

Fatigue, 137, 209

Fibroid tumors, 90, 106

Fight-or-flight response, 121, 130,
  146–147, 153, 169

Forward Head Position, 174, 187, 196

Garland Pose (Malasana), 148, 157

Great Seal Pose (Maha Mudra), 152,
  167, 307, 311

Half-Moon Pose (Ardha Chandrasana), 8, 72, 84, 88, 93, 106, 139, 142, 160, 173, 245, 298

Half-Plough Pose (Ardha Halasana), 51, 86, 111, 129, 153, 168, 196–197, 199, 204, 242, 250, 258, 261, 271, 294, 309

Head-on-Knee Pose (Janu Sirsasana), 14, 48, 82, 101, 117, 126, 177, 189, 196, 198, 202, 204, 248, 268, 283–284, 350,

Headaches, 102, 108, 137, 190–203, 205

Headstand (Sirsasana), 16, 33, 47, 76, 85, 93, 97, 110, 114, 120, 127, 143, 196, 222, 239, 249, 256, 261, 264, 270, 284, 293, 327

Headstand with Outstretched Legs (Upavistha Konasana in Sirsasana), 115

Headstand with Soles of Feet Together (Baddha Konasana in Sirsasana), 115

Heart disease, 297, 340–343, 345–347

Heavy bleeding, 105–106

Herbal medicines and headaches, 193

Hero Pose (Virasana), 154

Hero Pose with Cow-Face Arms (Virasana with Gomukhasana Arms), 12, 32, 173, 187

Hot flashes, 209, 234–236, 240, 237–239

Hypertension, 342, 347

Immune system, 118–122, 125, 169

Indigestion, 143, 273

Insomnia, 209

Intense Side Stretch Pose (Parsvottanasana), 10, 31

Interval Breathing (Viloma), 146, 148, 162, 253

Inverted Staff Pose (Viparita Dandasana), 34, 77, 85, 95, 104, 120, 216, 222, 229, 257, 270, 285, 291, 307

Irritability, 104

Irritable bowel syndrome, 273, 276

Kyphosis, 170, 173, 187

Labor and delivery, 146

Legs-Up-the-Wall Pose (Viparita Karani), 22, 40, 52, 67, 80, 87, 93, 120, 130, 152, 146, 163, 169, 196–197, 201, 205, 215, 242, 252, 258, 266, 272, 287, 294, 310, 315, 351

Lordosis, 170, 173

Menopause, 233–237, 241–242, 245–246

Menorrhagia (Heavy Bleeding), 92

Menstrual Back Pain, 175

Menstrual cramps, 90, 94, 102, 107

Menstrual cycle, 112

Menstrual flow, 103

Menstrual problems, 91, 98

Menstruation, 88–91

Migraines, 135, 190–195

Morning sickness, 139, 156, 160

Mountain Pose (Tadasana), 5, 26, 67–69, 142, 159, 298, 305, 326, 331

Mountain Pose with Arms Overhead (Urdhva Hastasana in Tadasana), 5, 26, 70, 318, 331

Myocardial infarction, 341

Nausea, 157, 163

Nursing, 152

Osteoarthritis, 170, 177–178

Osteoporosis, 169–170, 173, 297, 322–324, 328–330

Perimenopause, 209, 233, 239

Plough Pose (Halasana), 20, 39, 79, 93, 97, 116, 216, 230, 242, 265, 314, 330

Postpartum Depression, 153

Pranayama, 65, 89, 124, 146, 151, 162, 197, 219

Pregnancy, 137–147

Premature menopause, 233

Premenstrual syndrome, 90, 95–96

Rebound headaches, 194

Reclining Big Toe Pose (Supta Padangusthasana), 240

Reclining Big Toe Pose I (Supta Padangusthasana I), 45, 179, 185, 317, 338

Reclining Big Toe Pose II (Supta Padangusthasana II), 45, 150, 190

Reclining Bound Angle Pose (Supta Baddha Konasana), 44, 81, 94, 100, 107–108, 124–125, 145, 148, 150, 157, 200, 205, 215, 226, 240, 242, 254, 260, 267, 282, 290, 313, 351

Reclining Easy Seated Pose (Supta Sukhasana), 44, 291

Reclining Hero Pose (Supta Virasana), 145, 151–154, 156, 242, 281, 291

Reclining Knee-to-Chest Pose (Eka Pada Supta Pavanmuktasana), 184

Revolved Triangle Pose (Parivrtta Trikonasana), 9, 173, 187, 336

Rheumatoid arthritis, 125, 177–179

Sacroiliac Pain, 174, 181

Sciatica, 170, 173–174, 181–182, 185

Scoliosis, 176–177, 188

Seated Forward Bend (Paschimottanasana), 15, 49, 83, 102, 151, 196, 198, 203–204, 216, 231, 239, 267, 283, 350

Sequences for
    Anxiety-Driven Depression, 227
    Chronic Depression, 220
    Eating Disorders: Strengthen and Energize, 69
    Eating Disorders: Restore and Renew, 81
    Enhanced Immunity, 125
    Fatigue, 267
    Fuzzy Thinking, 263
    General Back Pain, 181
    Healthy Menstruation, 100
    Heavy or Irregular Periods, 253

Heavy Periods, 105, 253
High Blood Pressure, 348
Hot Flashes, 246
Improving Digestion, 281
Insomnia, 260
Irritable Bowel Syndrome, 290
Joint Stiffness, 316
Migraine Headaches, 202
Postmenstruation, 113
Postpartum Recovery, 165
Pregnancy, 154
Premenstrual Syndrome, 108
Tension Headaches, 197
Urinary Incontinence, 311
Vaginal Health, 304
Shoulderstand (Sarvangasana), 18, 39, 50, 65, 78, 86, 93, 97, 110, 116, 128, 152, 154, 168, 177, 189, 196, 216, 224, 230, 250, 257, 261, 264, 271, 286, 293, 308, 313, 330
Simple Seated Twist Pose (Bharadvajasana), 13, 75, 95, 129, 141–142, 145, 158, 177, 181, 224, 269
Sirsasana (Headstand), 242
Spinal stenosis, 170
Spinal Twist Pose (Marichyasana III), 13, 216, 306
Standing Big Toe Pose I (Utthita Hasta Padangusthasana I), 182

Standing Big Toe Pose II (Utthita Hasta Padangusthasana II), 183
Standing Forward Bend (Uttanasana), 8, 38, 74, 113, 166, 199, 203, 228, 256, 260, 264, 269, 305, 311, 319, 332, 349
Standing Forward Bend with a Twist (Parsva Uttanasana), 38
Standing Spinal Twist Pose (Utthita Marichyasana), 142, 182, 336

Tension headaches, 135, 190–191, 195
Three-Limb Intense Stretch (Triang Mukhaikapada Paschimottanasana), 102
Tree Pose (Vrksasana), 165
Twisted Stomach Pose (Jathara Parivartanasana), 186

Upward-facing bow pose (Urdhva Dhanurasana), 37, 78, 223, 229, 308, 337
Upward-Facing Dog Pose (Urdhva Mukha Svanasana), 36, 152, 173, 184, 318
Upward-Facing Leg Stretch (Urdhva Prasarita Padasana), 168, 185
Urinary incontinence, 302–303

Vaginal dryness, 209, 300 302

Warrior (Virabhadrasana), 68
Warrior I Pose (Virabhadrasana I), 9, 30, 333
Warrior II Pose (Virabhadrasana II), 6, 28, 67, 71, 334
Wide-Angle Seated Pose I (Upavistha Konasana I), 4, 103, 106, 160, 242, 247, 254, 292, 312, 316
Wide-Angle Seated Pose I or II (Upavistha Konasana I or II), 150
Wide-Angle Seated Pose II (Upavistha Konasana II), 103, 111
Wide-Angle Seated Pose with a Twist (Parsva Upavistha Konasana), 103
Wide-Angle Standing Forward Bend (Prasarita Padottanasana), 11, 67, 73, 114, 144, 161, 228, 242, 248, 254, 256, 311, 320
Woman's Energizing Sequence, 25
Woman's Essential Sequence, 3
Woman's Restorative Sequence, 43